KEY TOPICS IN
ANAESTHESIA
THIRD EDITION
CLINICAL ASPECTS

The KEY TOPICS Series

Advisors:

T.M. Craft *Department of Anaesthesia and Intensive Care, Royal United Hospital, Bath, UK*
C.S. Garrard *Intensive Therapy Unit, John Radcliffe Hospital, Oxford, UK*
P.M. Upton *Department of Anaesthesia, Royal Cornwall Hospital, Treliske, Truro, UK*

Anaesthesia, Third Edition, Clinical Aspects
Obstetrics and Gynaecology, Second Edition
Accident and Emergency Medicine
Paediatrics, Second Edition
Orthopaedic Surgery
Otolaryngology, Second Edition
Ophthalmology
Psychiatry
General Surgery
Renal Medicine
Trauma
Chronic Pain
Oral and Maxillofacial Surgery
Oncology
Cardiovascular Medicine
Neurology
Neonatology
Gastroenterology
Thoracic Surgery
Respiratory Medicine
Orthopaedic Trauma Surgery
Critical Care

Forthcoming titles include:

Accident and Emergency Medicine, Second Edition
Acute Poisoning
Ophthalmology, Second Edition
Urology
Evidence Based Medicine

KEY TOPICS IN
ANAESTHESIA
CLINICAL ASPECTS
THIRD EDITION

T.M. CRAFT
FRCA
Consultant in Anaesthesia and Intensive Care,
Royal United Hospital, Bath, UK

P.M. UPTON
MRCP (UK) FRCA
Consultant in Anaesthesia and Intensive Care,
College Tutor, Royal Cornwall Hospital, Treliske, Truro, UK

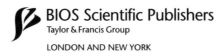

BIOS Scientific Publishers
Taylor & Francis Group

LONDON AND NEW YORK

© 1993, 1995, 2001 BIOS, an imprint of the Taylor & Francis Group

Third edition published in the United Kingdom in 2001
by BIOS, an imprint of the Taylor & Francis Group
11 New Fetter Lane, London EC4P 4EE

Reprinted 2004

Tel.:   +44 (0) 20 7583 9855
Fax.:   +44 (0) 20 7842 2298
E-mail: info@tandf.co.uk
Website: http://www.tandf.co.uk

A CIP record for this book is available from the British Library.

ISBN 1 85996 132 0

Distributed by
Thomson Publishing Services
Cheriton House
North Way
Andover, Hampshire SP10 5BE, UK
Tel.:   +44 (0) 1264 332424
E-mail: salesorder.tandf@thomsonpublishingservices.co.uk

Typeset by Jayvee Computer Services, Trivandrom, India
Printed by The Cromwell Press, Trowbridge, UK

CONTENTS

ABBREVIATIONS

5HT	5-hydroxytryptamine
ACE	angiotensin converting enzyme
ACTH	adrenocorticotrophic hormone
AF	atrial fibrillation
AFE	amniotic fluid embolism
AICD	automatic implantable cardioverter defibrillator
AIDS	acquired immunodeficiency syndrome
AIMS	Australian Incident Monitoring Study
AIP	acute intermittent porphyria
AIS	abbreviated injury scale
ALA	aminoaevulinic acid
ALI	acute lung injury
ALS	advanced life support
APS	acute pain service
APTT	activated partial thromboplastin time
ASA	American Society of Anaesthesiologists
ASD	atrial septal defect
ATLS	advanced trauma life support
BLS	basic life support
BMI	body mass index
BNF	British National Formulary
BP	blood pressure
CABG	coronary artery bypass grafting
CBF	cerebral blood flow
CESDI	The Confidential Enquiry into Stillbirths and Deaths in Infancy
CFM	cerebral function monitor
CHD	congential heart disease
COPD	chronic obstructive pulmonary disease
CPAP	continuous positive airways pressure
CPD	cardiopulmonary bypass
CSE	combined spinal epidural
CTZ	chemoreceptor trigger zone
CVP	central venous pressure
CXR	chest X-ray
DIC	disseminated intravascular coagulopathy
DVT	deep venous thrombosis
ECT	electroconvulsive therapy
EEG	electroencephalogram
ESRD	early stage renal disease
FBC	full blood count
FEV_1	forced expired volume in 1 second
FEP	fresh frozen plasma
FGF	fresh gas flow

F_IO_2	fractional inspired oxygen tension
FRC	functional residual capacity
FVC	forced vital capacity
GA	general anaesthetic
GALT	gut associated lymphoid tissue
GCS	Glasgow Coma Score (Scale)
GDC	General Dental Council
GFR	glomerular filtration rate
GMC	General Medical Council
HBF	hepatic blood flow
HIV	human immunodeficiency virus
HPV	hypoxic pulmonary vasoconstriction
HRT	hormone replacement therapy
ICNARC	The Intensive Care National Audit and Research
ICP	intracranial pressure
ILMA	intubating laryngeal mask airway
IOP	intraocular pressure
IPPV	intermittent positive pressure ventilation
ISS	injury severity score
IVC	inferior vena cava
LFT	liver function tests
LMA	laryngeal mask airways
LSCS	caesarean section
LV	left ventricular
LVEDP	left ventricular end diastolic pressure
MABP	mean arterial blood pressure
MAC	minimum alveolar concentration
MBC	maximum breathing capacity
MEAC	minimum effective analgesic concentration
MG	myasthenia gravis
MH	malignant hyperthermia
MI	myocardial infarction
MIR	minimum infusion rate
MODS	multiple organ dysfunction syndrome
NCEPOD	National Confidential Enquiry into Perioperative Deaths
NICE	National Institute for Clinical Excellence
NMS	neuroleptic malignant syndrome
OLV	one lung ventilation
PAOP	pulmonary artery occlusion pressure
PAP	pulmonary artery pressure
PCA	patient controlled analgesia
PCEA	patient controlled epidural analgesia
PCP	pulmonary capillary pressure
PDT	percutaneous dilatational tracheostomies
PE	pulmonary embolism
PEEP	positive end expiratory pressure

PFC	perfluorocarbons
PIOPED	prospective investigation of pulmonary embolism
PONV	post-operative nausea and vomiting
PTS	paediatric trauma score
RAST	radioallergosorbant tests
REM	rapid eye movement
RF	radio frequency
RFT	respiratory function test
ROSC	return of spontaneous circulation
RTS	revised trauma score
SAPS	simplified acute physiology score
SIRS	systemic inflammatory response syndrome
SMR	standardised mortality rate
SVR	systemic vascular resistance
TENS	transcutaneous electrical nerve stimulator
TIA	transient ischaemic attack
TISS	therapeutic intervention scoring system
TOE	transoesophageal echocardiography
U+E	urea and electrolytes
V/Q	ventilation/perfusion
VAS	visual analogue scale
VC	vomiting centre
VF	ventricular fibrillation
VP	variegate porphyria
VSD	ventral septal defect

PREFACE

The third edition of *Key Topics in Anaesthesia* marks a change in direction. The book has been largely rewritten with a clear focus on the clinical aspects of anaesthesia with particular reference to those working towards the Fellowship of the Royal College of Anaesthetists. New topics included in this edition cover areas such as organ transplantation, TIVA, breast feeding, and drug and tobacco abuse relevant to anaesthesia. In an attempt to provide the reader with as up to date information as possible, many of the references for further reading are to web sites, enabling us all to keep abreast of rapidly evolving advice and guidance from expert organisations.

As always, we are indebted to colleagues who have provided critique and feedback and continue to welcome comment from readers.

T.M. Craft and P.M. Upton, Bath and Truro, 2001

Names of Medical Substances

In accordance with directive 92/27/EEC, this book adheres to the following guidelines on naming of medicinal substances (rINN, Recommended International Non-proprietary Name; BAN, British Approved Name).

List 1 – Both names to appear

UK Name	rINN
[1]adrenaline	epinephrine
amethocaine	tetracaine
bendrofluazide	bendroflumethiazide
benzhexol	trihexyphenidyl
chlorpheniramine	chlorphenamine
dicyclomine	dicycloverine
dothiepin	dosulepin
eformoterol	formoterol
flurandrenolone	fludroxycortide
frusemide	furosemide
hydroxyurea	hydroxycarbamide
lignocaine	lidocaine
methotrimeprazine	levomepromazine
methylene blue	methylthioninium chloride
mitozantrone	mitoxantrone
mustine	chlormethine
nicoumalone	acenocoumarol
[1]noradrenaline	norepinephrine
oxypentifylline	pentoxyifylline
procaine penicillin	procaine benzylpenicillin
salcatonin	calcitonin (salmon)
thymoxamine	moxisylyte
thyroxine sodium	levothyroxine sodium
trimeprazine	alimemazine

List 2 – rINN to appear exclusively

Former BAN	rINN/new BAN
amoxycillin	amoxicillin
amphetamine	amfetamine
amylobarbitone	amobarbital
amylobarbitone sodium	amobarbital sodium
beclomethasone	beclometasone
benorylate	benorilate
busulphan	busulfan
butobarbitone	butobarbital
carticaine	articane
cephalexin	cefalexin
cephamandole nafate	cefamandole nafate
cephazolin	cefazolin
cephradine	cefradine
chloral betaine	cloral betaine
chlorbutol	chlorobutanol
chlormethiazole	clomethiazole
chlorathalidone	chlortalidone
cholecalciferol	colecalciferol
cholestyramine	colestyramine
clomiphene	clomifene
colistin sulphomethate sodium	colistimethate sodium
corticotrophin	corticotropin
cysteamine	mercaptamine
danthron	dantron
desoxymethasone	desoximetasone
dexamphetamine	dexamfetamine
dibromopropamidine	dibrompropamidine
dienoestrol	dienestrol
dimethicone(s)	dimeticone
dimethyl sulphoxide	dimethyl sulfoxide
doxycycline hydrochloride (hemihydrate hemiethanolate)	doxycycline hyclate
ethancrynic acid	etacrynic acid
ethamsylate	etamsylate
ethinyloestradiol	ethinylestradiol
ethynodiol	etynodiol
flumethasone	flumetasone
flupenthixol	flupentixol
gestronol	gestonorone
guaiphenesin	guaifenesin

[1] In common with the BP, precedence will continue to be given to the terms adrenaline and noradrenaline.

hexachlorophane	hexachlorophene
hexamine hippurate	methenamine hippurate
hydroxyprogesterone hexanoate	hydroxyprogesterone caproate
indomethacin	indometacin
lysuride	lisuride
methyl cysteine	mecysteine
methylphenobarbitone	methylphenobarbital
oestradiol	estradiol
oestriol	estriol
oestrone	estrone
oxethazaine	oxetacaine
pentaerythritol tetranitrate	pentaerithrityl tetranitrate
phenobarbitone	phenobarbital
pipothiazine	pipotiazine
polyhexanide	polihexanide
potassium cloazepate	dipotassium clorazepate
pramoxine	pramocaine
prothionamide	protionamide
quinalbarbitone	secobarbital
riboflavine	riboflavin
sodium calciumedetate	sodium calcium edetate
sodium cromoglycate	sodium cromoglicate
sodium ironedetate	sodium feredetate
sodium picosulphate	sodium picosulfate
sorbitan monostearate	sorbitan stearate
stilboestrol	diethylstilbestrol
sulphacetamide	sulfacetamide
sulphadiazine	sulfadiazine
sulphadimidine	sulfadimidine
sulphaguanadine	sulfaguanadine
sulphamethoxazole	sulfamethoxazole
sulphasalazine	sulfasalazine
sulphathiazole	sulfathiazole
sulphinpyrazone	sulfinpyrazone
tetracosactrin	tetracosactide
thiabendazole	tiabendazole
thioguanine	tioguanine
thiopentone	thiopental
urofollitrophin	urofollitropin

CONTRIBUTORS

Peter Berridge
SpR, South Western School of Anaesthesia, UK

Kay Chidley MRCP (UK) FRCA
SpR, South Western School of Anaesthesia, UK

Tim Cook FRCA
Consultant in Anaesthesia, Royal United Hospital, Bath, UK

Claire Gleeson FRCA
SpR, South Western School of Anaesthesia, UK

Steve Hill FRCA
Consultant in Anaesthesia, Royal United Hospital, Bath, UK

Richard Innes FRCA
SpR, South Western School of Anaesthesia, UK

Stephen Laver
Senior House Officer, in Anaesthesia, Royal United Hospital, Bath, UK

Jerry Nolan FRCA
Consultant in Anaesthesia and Intensive Care, Royal United Hospital, Bath, UK

Alison Pickford MRCP (UK) FRCA
Consultant in Anaesthesia and Intensive Care, Royal Cornwall Hospital, Treliske, Truro, UK

Dave Pogson FRCA
SpR, South Western School of Anaesthesia, UK

Ruth Spencer FRCA
SpR, South Western School of Anaesthesia, UK

Richard Struthers FRCA
SpR, South Western School of Anaesthesia, UK

Jenny Tuckey FRCA
Consultant in Obstetric Anaesthesia, Royal United Hospital, Bath, UK

Adrian Walker FRCA
Consultant in Anaesthesia and Intensive Care, Royal Cornwall Hospital, Treliske, Truro, UK

ADRENOCORTICAL DISEASE

The adrenal cortex produces glucocorticoid, mineralocorticoid and sex hormones (mainly testosterone). Cortisol, the principal glucocorticoid, modulates stress and inflammatory responses. It is a potent stimulator of gluconeogenesis and antagonizes insulin. Aldosterone is the principal mineralocorticoid. It causes increased sodium reabsorption, and potassium and hydrogen ion loss at the distal renal tubule. Adrenal androgen production increases markedly at puberty, declining with age thereafter. Androstenedione is converted by the liver to testosterone in the male and oestrogen in the female. Cortisol and androgen production are under diurnal pituitary control (adrenocorticotrophic hormone – ACTH). Aldosterone is released in response to angiotensin II, produced following renal renin release and subsequent pulmonary angiotensin I conversion.

Clinical diseases result from relative excess or lack of hormones.

Adrenocortical excess

1. Cushing's syndrome. This may result from steroid therapy, adrenal hyperplasia, adrenal carcinoma or ectopic ACTH.

2. Cushing's disease. This is due to an ACTH secreting pituitary tumour.

Clinical features of adrenocortical excess include; moon face, thin skin, easy bruising, hypertension (60%), hirsutism, obesity with a centripetal distribution, buffalo hump, muscle weakness, diabetes (10%), osteoporosis (50%), aseptic necrosis of the hip and pancreatitis (especially with iatrogenic Cushing's syndrome).

3. Problems
- Control of blood sugar (insulin may be required).
- Hypokalaemia resulting in arrhythmias, muscle weakness and postoperative respiratory embarrassment.
- Hypertension, polycythaemia, congestive heart failure. The patient may require central venous and/or pulmonary artery occlusion pressure monitoring.
- Atrophic skin and osteoporosis demand care when positioning the patient during anaesthesia and with vessel cannulation.

Adrenocortical deficiency

1. Acute. This may follow sepsis, pharmacological adrenal suppression or adrenal haemorrhage associated with anti-coagulant therapy. Critically ill patients normally have raised mineralocorticoid levels, but if their adrenal glands are involved in the septic process or they usually receive supplementary steroids, an acute deficiency may occur.

Clinical features include; apathy, hypotension, coma, and hypoglycaemia.

2. Chronic. Chronic deficiency may follow surgical adrenalectomy, auto-immune adrenalitis (Addison's disease), adrenal infiltration with tumour, leukaemia, infection (TB, histoplasmosis), amyloidosis, or may be secondary to pituitary dysfunction.

Clinical features include; fatigue, weakness, weight loss, nausea and hyper-pigmentation. Hypotension, hyponatraemia, hyperkalaemia, eosinophilia and occasionally hypoglycaemia may also be found on further investigation.

A short synacthen test, giving 250 µg of synthetic ACTH, is used to assess the adrenal gland's ability to produce cortisol at 0, 30 and 60 minutes.

3. Problems
- Hypotension, a low intravascular volume and a small heart may precipitate circulatory collapse with minor fluid overload.
- Hypoglycaemia.
- Hyperkalaemia – potential risk with suxamethonium.
- Steroid replacement therapy.

Hyperaldosteronism

1. Primary (Conn's syndrome).
This is caused by an adenoma in the zona glomerulosa secreting aldosterone.

Clinical features include, hypokalaemia, muscle weakness and hypertension.

2. Problems
- Hypokalaemia may result in cardiac arrhythmias, postoperative muscle weakness and respiratory embarrassment.
- Hypertension.
- Hormone replacement following adrenalectomy.

Anaesthetic management

1. Assessment and premedication.
The state of the disease must be assessed preoperatively and electrolyte and glucose disorders corrected.

Steroid supplementation will be required for patients with Addison's disease, or if pituitary ablation or adrenalectomy is to be performed. If a patient stopped taking supplementary steroids more than 3 months ago, or is on less than 10 mg/day of prednisolone, no perioperative supplements are required.

If a patient is on more than 10 mg/day of prednisolone then 25 mg of hydrocortisone is given at induction. If the patient is having minor surgery then no further supplements are required. If a patient is having moderate surgery then 100 mg hydrocortisone is given over the next 24 hours. If major surgery is performed this is continued for 2–3 days. Patients who are taking high dose steroids to produce immunosuppression should remain on the same doses perioperatively.

Excess supplementation can cause immunosuppression, glucose intolerance and delayed wound healing.

2. Conduct of anaesthesia.
A single dose of etomidate may interfere with corti-sol synthesis for at least 24 hours in the critically ill patient, but the clinical signifi-cance of these findings is not clear. Epidural anaesthesia may reduce the stress response, providing the level of block is adequate and it is continued into the post-operative period. Blood volume, glucose and potassium should be monitored.

3. Postoperatively.
The problems described continue into the postoperative period and demand continual reassessment. Steroid replacement will be required

following bilateral adrenalectomy and those on regular steroid therapy (>10 mg prednisolone daily – see above). Pneumothorax may occur following adrenalectomy.

Further reading

Masterson GR, Mostafa SM. Adrenocortical function in critical illness. *British Journal of Anaesthesia*, 1998; **81**: 308–310.

Nicholson G, Burrin JM, Hall GM. Peri-operative steroid supplementation. *Anaesthesia*, 1998; **53**: 1091–1104.

Related topics of interest

Phaeochromocytoma (p. 203); Preoperative preparation (p. 209); Stress response to surgery (p. 248)

ADVERSE DRUG REACTIONS

Adverse drug reactions may be classified as either predictable or unpredictable.

Predictable reactions
- They are dose dependent.
- They are related to the known pharmacological actions of the drug.
- They occur in otherwise healthy individuals.
- They account for approximately 80% of adverse drug reactions and are usually toxic in nature.
- They are due either to an excessive amount of drug in the body (overdosage), unintentional route of administration (e.g. intravascular local anaesthetic), or impaired metabolism or excretion.

Unpredictable reactions
- Unrelated to dose.
- Not related to the drug's known pharmacological effects.
- Related to an immune response on behalf of the patient. They are occasionally related to a genetic idiosyncrasy (e.g. suxamethonium apnoea).

Life-threatening reactions
Immunological responses to drugs may be anaphylactic (IgE mediated) or anaphylactoid (non-IgE mediated and often following first exposure to the drug). Such reactions are an adverse response of lymphocytes and are detrimental to the host. Reactions may be as a consequence of direct activation of mast cells by the drug (pharmacological histamine release) and do not involve complement activation (e.g. after certain muscle relaxants including curare).

They may also occur following 'classical' pathway complement activation. Previous exposure to the antigen with antibody formation is required.

'Alternative' pathway activation occurs when the drug directly triggers the cascade; previous exposure to the antigen is not necessary (e.g. dextrans or contrast media).

Immediate hypersensitivity is an IgE (reaginin) mediated type 1 reaction.

Anaesthetic management
1. *Assessment.* Atopic patients are more at risk. A high IgE level may also positively correlate with a risk of reaction. Preoperative prophylaxis with H_1 and H_2 antihistaminergic agents has been recommended.

2. *Conduct of anaesthesia.* Intravenous agents should be injected slowly into a fast-flowing crystalloid infusion sited in a large vein. Drugs which have a low incidence of adverse reactions should be used. The diagnosis of an acute adverse reaction under general anaesthesia may be difficult. It is strongly suggested by cardiovascular collapse with hypotension, tachycardia, vasodilatation and arryhthmias. Once suspected the following immediate management should be instituted.

3. Management of a drug reaction
- Stop administration of the suspected antigen.
- Maintain the airway and give 100% O_2.
- Commence external cardiac compressions if there is no palpable pulse regardless of the cardiac rhythm.
- Give intravenous epinephrine (adrenaline). Adult dose = 50–100 µg (0.5–1.0 ml of 1:10000 solution). Repeat as indicated especially if bronchospasm or hypotension persist.
- Commence intravascular volume expansion.
- Discontinue surgery and anaesthesia if feasible.
- Secondary management includes hydrocortisone, antihistamines, salbutamol or aminophylline and bicarbonate in the presence of continued acidosis. Arterial blood gases should be measured before considering extubation.

4. Follow up.
Resuscitation and recovery from the initial event should be followed by investigation to establish a cause.

Non-specific tests

An elevated blood C3 and C4 complement level suggests an immune mediated response. Elevation of C3 alone suggests alternative pathway activation. Total IgE antibody levels may also be measured. Blood histamine levels may be elevated for a short time only, but its metabolite methylhistamine has a longer half-life and is measurable in urine up to 2–3 hours following a reaction. Tryptase, a mast cell specific protease released during degranulation, may also remain in the blood for about 3 hours.

Specific tests

Drug specific antibodies may be quantified using labelled anti-human IgE antibody by radioallergosorbant tests (RAST).

Skin tests

These tests should only be performed where full resuscitation facilities are immediately available. The optimum time for testing is six weeks following a reaction. The patient should not be taking drugs which may interfere with the response (e.g. corticosteroids, antihistamines).

Intradermal testing utilizes dilute solutions of potential antigens. Solutions of the test agents are diluted to 1:1000 and 1:100 and a control solution (e.g. saline) prepared. A 1 mm weal of each solution is then raised on the forearm of the patient. A positive result occurs when a weal >10 mm persists for more than 30 min.

Skin prick testing is safer, quicker and easier to perform (the test agent does not require dilution). A drop of solution is placed on the skin and a puncture made through it (<1 mm). A weal >3 mm after 15 minutes is considered a positive result.

Further reading

Association of Anaesthetists of Great Britain and Ireland and Clinical Immunology. *Suspected anaphylactic reactions associated with anaesthesia.* Revised edn., 1995.

McKinnon RP, Wildsmith JAW. Histaminoid reactions in anaesthesia. *British Journal of Anaesthesia,* 1995; **74:** 217–28.

Related topics of interest

CPR (p. 75); Preoperative preparation (p. 209); Sequelae of anaesthesia (p. 232)

AIDS AND HEPATITIS

Acquired immunodeficiency syndrome (AIDS) was first reported in 1981. An exponential increase in the numbers of seropositive people infected with human immunodeficiency virus (HIV) has been seen world-wide with 30 million thought to be infected by 1998. The virus, a retrovirus, is transmitted through sexual contact, perinatally, and via blood and blood products. It is becoming more common in the heterosexual population and in children. Infection preferentially affects T helper lymphocytes resulting in immunosuppression and the eventual development of 'AIDS' in most people infected with the virus. The appearance of symptomatic immunosuppression takes a variable length of time. Opportunistic infections, malignancies (Kaposi's sarcoma, non-Hodgkin's lymphoma) and neurological manifestations occur.

Problems

1. **Patients.** HIV positive patients may require surgery for tumour excision, diagnostic biopsy, drainage of foci of infection or for non-related disease, for example trauma. Preoperative assessment should seek respiratory, neurological, gastrointestinal and haematological complications as well as secondary infections. Drug therapy such as protease inhibitors, nucleoside and non-nucleoside reverse transcriptase inhibitors are often used in combination. Side effects such as neutropenia, anaemia, diarrhoea, and abnormal hepatic, glucose and lipid metabolism are common. Aseptic techniques are vital, and the risks of sepsis from invasive monitoring should be balanced against the potential benefits. The psychological implications of HIV infection must not be forgotten.

2. **Staff.** High risk body fluids are blood, amniotic fluid, vaginal secretions, semen, breast milk, CSF, peritoneal, pleural, pericardial and synovial fluid. Saliva in association with dentistry, and unfixed organs and tissues also are classified as high risk and may transmit the virus. It is presently considered unethical to test all patients for evidence of HIV infection prior to surgery. 'Universal precautions' which assume that all patients may be infected are recommended. Identical precautions are taken with other bloodborne infective agents, e.g. hepatitis B, and their success suggests that they are likely to be equally effective against the less infective HIV virus. Other precautions include the use of gloves when there is any risk of contact with infective body fluids, the wearing of masks and protective glasses when infective fluids may become airborne and gowns if there is any chance of being splashed. If contact with body fluids occurs the affected part should be washed immediately. Open or exudative wounds should be covered and contact with potentially infective fluids avoided. To reduce the risk of needle stick injuries, needles are immediately disposed of in a suitable container. They are not resheathed, or passed from one person to another. The risk of seroconversion following a needle stick injury is 0.3%. Postexposure prophylaxis with zidovudine, lamivudine and indinavir is given as soon as possible (within 1–2 hours) after exposure and continued for 4 weeks.

3. **Protection for uninfected patients.** Where possible single use items should be used, and if not high level disinfection or sterilization should be employed.

All blood and blood products are screened for antibodies to HIV. Transmission can occur in the 3 month 'window' between infection and seroconversion, or due to clerical errors in reporting results or labelling blood. This transmission risk is less than one in a million per transfused unit of blood. The isolation of seropositive patients is not appropriate unless the patient is bleeding or requires isolation due to immuno- suppression or a contagious secondary infection. Cases of drug resistant TB should be managed in a specialized unit.

4. *Infected staff.* All health care workers should be immunized against hepatitis B, and carry out universal precautions. An individual who thinks they may be infected should seek confidential expert advice. HIV or hepatitis B-infected individuals should not carry out exposure-prone procedures where the hands are not completely visible. They are therefore likely to be allowed to continue their clinical practice in anaesthesia.

Further reading

Association of Anaesthetists of Great Britain and Ireland. HIV and other bloodborne viruses – guidance for anaesthetists. 1996.   http://www.aagbi.org

Avidan MS, Jones N, Pozniak AL. The implications of HIV for the anaesthetist and the intensivist. *Anaesthesia* 2000; **55:** 344–354.

Related topics of interest

Blood (p. 32); Blood salvage (p. 34)

AIR EMBOLISM

Air embolism is a potential complication of many operations. An open vein, gravity, a low CVP and poor surgical technique predispose to its development. The outcome depends on the volume and rate of air entrainment, the cardio-respiratory health of the patient, the use of N_2O, and the presence of a patent foramen ovale thus permitting systemic embolization (up to 27% of adults have a potentially patent foramen ovale). A right to left shunt may be precipitated by the use of PEEP as this increases right atrial pressure. Children are more likely to develop air embolism, and to suffer more profound hypotension.

Predisposing factors

1. **Neurosurgical.** Incidence of up to 76%, detected by transoesophageal echo for sitting procedures. Operating on the skull and dura (the beginning and end of the operation) place the patient at most risk, as this is when small veins are open.

2. **Orthopaedic.** Especially hip and knee replacement and arthrograms.

3. **Pregnancy related.** Termination of pregnancy, manual removal of placenta and while the uterus is open during Caesarean section.

4. **Abdominal.** Especially with laparoscopy or uterine insufflation.

5. **Thyroid and head and neck surgery.**

6. **Others.** For example endoscopic surgery, epidurals, bronchoscopy, jet ventilation and central line insertion.

Diagnosis

In the conscious patient coughing, dyspnoea, chest pain and dizziness progressing to loss of consciousness may occur. In the unconscious patient diagnosis is based on the signs of developing hypotension, tachycardia, jugular venous distension and decreased pulmonary compliance during an 'at risk operation'. It may also be made using the specific monitoring aids listed below.

Monitoring

1. **Basic senses.** Hissing may be heard or bubbles seen being sucked into open veins.

2. **Heart sounds.** The classical 'millwheel' murmur may be heard using an oesophageal or precordial stethoscope. It is insensitive (1.5–4.0 ml of air/kg) and may be preceded by cardiovascular collapse.

3. **ECG.** May show development of right ventricular strain and arrhythmias, and ST segment depression.

4. **CVP.** Obstruction of right heart filling by the embolism will cause a rise in central venous pressure.

5. Capnography. As emboli are trapped in the lung, perfusion falls causing an increase in physiological dead space. This results in a sudden fall in the peak end expired CO_2 concentration. Capnography allows the detection of an air embolism before cardiovascular compromise occurs (1.5 ml air/kg).

6. Expired gas analysis. Once alveolar denitrogenation has been completed, the detection of further nitrogen in expired gas signifies the occurrence of an air embolism.

7. Pulmonary artery pressure (PAP). Raised PAP occurs with air embolism. Return to 'pre-embolism' levels can be used as an indication of successful treatment and the timing of the recommencement of surgery.

8. Doppler. Ultrasonic detection of air embolism is very accurate, permitting the detection of 0.5 ml of air. A change from the usual swishing noise to a roaring sound is heard. Accurate placement (4th right intercostal space or in the oesophagus) and testing of its ability to detect 0.5 ml of injected air is confirmed preoperatively. The problems are diathermy interference, maintenance of good patient contact, and the recognition of a changing noise pattern and potential oversensitivity (it is able to detect inconsequential air embolism).

9. Transoesophageal echocardiography. This is even more sensitive than Doppler, but is not specific, being unable to differentiate between air, fat and blood micro-emboli. It is able to localize intracardiac air to a specific chamber, therefore detecting paradoxical air embolism.

Treatment

1. Surgical. Once air embolism is detected the surgeon is informed and the wound flooded with saline. A careful search for open veins is then made.

2. Nitrous oxide. This is discontinued and 100% O_2 given. Being 35 times more soluble than nitrogen, N_2O is rapidly transported to intravascular air and increases the bubble size.

3. Neck compression. This obstructs the venous drainage preventing further air entering during head and neck and neurosurgery. It also increases local venous pressure, filling potentially open veins with blood.

4. CVP. A multi-orifice catheter with the tip at the caval–atrial junction is optimal for aspiration of the air embolus. Accurate positioning can be confirmed by X-ray, pressure changes (enter right ventricle and then withdraw the catheter), or by intravascular ECG (risk of cardiac microshocks).

5. Drugs are given as indicated to support the cardiovascular system.

6. Position. The left lateral head down position may prevent a large air embolus from entering the pulmonary artery by 'trapping' it in the right ventricle.

7. CPR may become necessary.

Further reading

Ho AM, Ling E. Systemic air embolism after lung trauma. *Anesthesiology* 1999; **90:** 564–575.

Porter JM, Pidgeon C, Cunningham AJ. The sitting position in neurosurgery: a critical appraisal. *British Journal of Anaesthesia* 1999; **82:** 117–128.

Related topics of interest

Neuroanaesthesia (p. 167); Positioning (p. 207)

AIRWAY SURGERY

Surgery to the upper airway presents a special challenge to the anaesthetist.

Problems
- Shared airway between anaesthetist and surgeon.
- Prevention of tracheal and bronchial soiling with blood and debris.
- Upper airway disease is associated with other pulmonary disease.

Anaesthetic management

1. Assessment and premedication. The likely ease of intubation should be assessed, with reference to CT or MRI scans and previous ENT assessment. Evidence of obstructive pulmonary symptoms should be sought together with their timing and frequency. Pulmonary function tests are then required. Upper airway obstruction is usually worse at night when supine and asleep, with decreased tone in the oropharyngeal musculature. A history of sleep disturbance or sleep apnoea should be sought especially in children for tonsillectomy. They may develop airway obstruction with opioids and require post-operative ventilation. Sedative premedication is avoided. The ECG may show right ventricular strain and hypertrophy.

Patients with nasal polyps are more likely to be atopic and allergic to anti-prostenoids, in particular aspirin. Those with airway malignancies are almost always smokers and may have other smoking-related diseases.

Premedication should allay anxiety and prevent pre-operative hypertension. It should not depress airway reflexes. Antisialagogues dry the airway making anaesthesia and surgery easier.

2. Conduct of anaesthesia. A smooth induction without coughing maintains haemodynamic stability and reduces operative haemorrhage. Oxygen saturation and end tidal CO_2 should be maintained in the patient's normal range. A pharyngeal pack soaks up blood and secretions and is used where surgical access will not be impeded. Care must be taken to ensure the tracheal tube does not become dislodged or obstructed. A pre-formed or reinforced tube may be helpful. Eye and teeth protection should be considered, although some surgeons prefer to see the eyes during nasal operations. The use of 10–15° of head-up tilt (reverse Trendelenburg) will increase venous drainage and decrease haemorrhage.

At the end of surgery the larynx is inspected and the airway suctioned under direct vision. Extubation is performed in the left lateral position with the head positioned to drain blood and secretions away from the larynx.

3. Postoperatively. Supplemental O_2 is given in a quiet recovery area monitored by experienced staff. When conscious and in control of their airway, patients are sat up to reduce haemorrhage. Blood in the pharynx should be suctioned or spat out as swallowed blood is strongly emetic. Postoperative airway oedema may occur and may be treated with dexamethasone 0.25 mg/kg initially, repeated if necessary. Nebulized epinephrine (adrenaline) may also be of benefit.

Special considerations

1. *Oral surgery*. Nasal intubation offers the best surgical access but an oral tracheal tube does not preclude most procedures. Nasal intubation requires antibiotic prophylaxis if a cardiac lesion is present. A pharyngeal pack is positioned prior to commencing surgery. Tracheal tubes with pre-formed angles (e.g. RAE tube) permit optimal positioning of the breathing system. For some oral surgery, a flexible LMA can be used after discussion with the surgeon.

2. *Nasal surgery*. Vasoconstriction of the nasal mucosae will reduce intraoperative bleeding. This may be achieved by regional or topical techniques. A regional block to the sphenopalatine ganglion will include the vasodilator fibres of the nasal blood vessels. Topical vasoconstrictors include 25% cocaine paste or 10% cocaine with an equal volume of 1:1000 epinephrine (adrenaline).

Moffett's solution consists of 2 ml 8% cocaine hydrochloride, 2 ml 1% sodium bicarbonate and 1 ml 1:1000 epinephrine (adrenaline). While awake, the patient lies supine with their head over the end of the trolley, neck fully extended and head supported by an assistant. An angled needle is used to direct the solution towards the roof of the nose and the patient kept in that position for 10 minutes. They then sit up and spit out any remaining solution. Moffett's solution may also be administered during anaesthesia with the patient placed in a steep head-down tilt. Any remaining solution is suctioned from the pharynx before the patient is returned to a head-up position. Although very effective Moffett's solution is now rarely used due to the complexity of mixing the solution and time required to prepare it.

Local anaesthetic agents combined with adrenaline may be injected into the submucosa. The strength of epinephrine (adrenaline) solution varies from 1:200 000 to 1:80 000. Epinephrine (adrenaline) contraindicates the use of halothane due to the likelihood of cardiac arrhythmias. Phenylephrine may be used as an alternative vasoconstrictor.

Most nasal surgery is now performed with anaesthesia administered via a reinforced laryngeal mask airway and a pharyngeal pack.

3. *Airway endoscopy*. Fibreoptic instruments may be passed under local or topical anaesthesia. Rigid instruments require relaxation of the jaw and are usually passed under general anaesthesia. Instrumentation of the larynx commonly causes a rise in blood pressure and manipulation may precipitate cardiac arrhythmias.

Endoscopy under general anaesthesia may be performed with the patient breathing spontaneously and unintubated. This may be particularly important for removal of a foreign body from the airway, especially in children. Positive pressure ventilation in such circumstances may result in the foreign body being forced further into the airway. The patient will 'lighten' during the endoscopy and from time to time the surgeon will be asked to stand back whilst anaesthesia is deepened and the patient's inspired O_2 increased. TIVA may also be used. Rigid laryngoscopy may be performed with a microlaryngeal tracheal tube in situ. As the internal resistance of these tubes is high, and therefore also the work of breathing, IPPV is required.

Apnoeic oxygenation may be employed to permit endoscopic procedures. Following preoxygenation an 8 French gauge catheter is passed through the vocal cords and O_2 supplied to the lungs at a flow rate of 6 l/min. This technique is only useful for short operations as there is no facility for removal of CO_2. Arterial CO_2 will rise by 0.26–0.66 kPa (2–5 mmHg) per minute of apnoea.

Intermittent jet ventilation using a hand-held injector will entrain room air via the Venturi principle and can be used with either a catheter through the cords or attached to the side of a ventilating rigid bronchoscope. Transtracheal jet ventilation, either with a hand held injector or a high frequency jet ventilator, may be used via a crico-thyroid cannula to maintain oxygenation where the anatomy of the larynx is severely abnormal. With jet ventilation a clear expiratory pathway must be present to avoid barotrauma. Apnoeic oxygenation and methods of jet ventilation require incremental doses or infusions of intravenous anaesthetic agents to prevent awareness.

4. *Post-tonsillectomy haemorrhage.* Reactionary haemorrhage occurs within 24 hours of surgery and may be fatal. Delayed haemorrhage suggests infection and may be a less serious anaesthetic problem. The role of antiprostenoid analgesics (NSAIDs) in the aetiology of post-tonsillectomy haemorrhage remains controversial.

Blood loss is difficult to assess as much of it is swallowed, and hypovolaemia may develop. With blood in the stomach, the patient is not 'starved'. A difficult intubation can occur due to clot or active bleeding in the pharynx. The residual effects of recent anaesthetic agents may reduce airway reflexes. Children with post-tonsillectomy haemorrhage will be frightened and the parents anxious.

Ensure adequate resuscitation and blood volume replacement before re-anaesthetizing, with further cross-matched blood available. A nasogastric tube may be passed (although this may cause further distress and exacerbate bleeding).

Establish whether the child suffers from sleep apnoea. This will not have been cured by the tonsillectomy. Consider the use of atropine and an antiemetic. Intravenous access prior to induction is essential. The nasogastric tube is aspirated and removed. There are two choices of induction technique.

- Inhalational with halothane or sevoflurane and O_2 in the lateral position with head down tilt and wide bore suction. Intubation is performed when sufficient depth of anaesthesia is achieved. However, deep volatile anaesthesia causes hypotension. Attempts to intubate the trachea too soon will cause coughing and laryngospasm.
- Conventional rapid sequence induction, although the dose of induction agent required is likely to be reduced.

The size of tracheal tube required may be reduced as a consequence of glottic oedema from the previous intubation. Once intubated, a large bore orogastric tube should be passed and the stomach emptied. Extubate awake in the lateral head down position.

Further reading

Fagan JJ, James MFM. A prospective study of anaesthesia for quinsy tonsillectomy. *Anaesthesia* 1995; **50:** 783–785.

Plummer S, Hartley M, Vaughan RS. Anaesthesia for telescopic procedures in the thorax. *British Journal of Anaesthesia* 1998; **80:** 223–234.

Related topics of interest

Asthma (p. 27); Depth of anaesthesia (p. 86); Emergency anaesthesia (p. 109); Epiglottitis and croup (p. 111); Intubation – awake (p. 138); Intubation – difficult (p. 141); Laryngectomy (p. 144); Laser surgery (p. 146); Sleep apnoea (p. 237); TIVA (p. 264); Tracheostomy (p. 266)

ALCOHOL

Dave Pogson

Acute and chronic alcohol abuse is extremely common in the UK. The incidence is increasing. All groups of adult patients may be affected. Many definitions of alcoholism exist. The anaesthetist must obtain a drinking history from the patient and identify any deleterious effects.

Chronic alcohol abuse can lead to social deterioration and malnutrition. Coexisting conditions include obesity and smoking-related lung disease. Alcohol abuse is especially common among victims of trauma. Five ml of blood in a glucose sampling tube is required to measure blood alcohol. Alcohol skin swabs must not be used. Eighty mg/dL is the UK limit for driving.

Alcohol (ethanol) is metabolized at a rate of 0.1 mg/kg/h by zero order kinetics. It depresses the activity of excitable membranes, initially causing euphoria followed by somnolence and diminished laryngeal reflexes. Alcohol tolerance is largely behavioural. There is increased cellular resistance to toxic effects but the rate of metabolism is increased only in chronic alcoholism. There is no increase in the lethal dose. Alcohol increases hepatic microsomal enzyme activity, resulting in cross-tolerance to benzodiazepines. When intoxicated the effects of other sedative drugs are additive. Prolonged alcoholism will eventually precipitate hepatic failure and coagulopathy.

Alcohol has a direct diuretic effect while the blood level is rising, increasing free water clearance. There may be a fall in serum potassium and magnesium. Gluconeogenesis is inhibited and glycogenesis enhanced. This may result in hypoglycaemia up to 30 hours after alcohol consumption in the fasted patient.

Chronic alcoholism leads to leucopenia and thrombocytopenia. Megaloblastic anaemia occurs due to folate antagonism, but reverses rapidly with supplementation. The incidence of lung pathology, especially aspiration pneumonia, is increased. Alcoholism accounts for up to 80% of cardiomyopathies. The adrenocortical response to surgery is diminished in chronic alcohol abusers. Intravenous alcohol infusion was found to suppress some withdrawal symptoms but did not alter the stress response.

Problems

- Gastric residual volume and acidity are increased.
- Coexisting morbidity.
- Potential hypoglycaemia and electrolyte disturbance.
- Cross-tolerance to anaesthetic drugs.

Anaesthetic management

1. *Assessment and premedication.* Assessment of the usual drinking habit is required, with the amount and timing of the most recent episode. Intoxicated patients should not be anaesthetized except in true emergencies. The state of hydration should be assessed and any hypoglycaemia treated with a glucose infusion. Anaemia, low potassium and magnesium should be sought and corrected. Coagulopathy is rare except in severe chronic abuse. Cardiomyopathy may manifest with ECG changes such as extrasystoles or abnormal QRS morphology.

2. *Conduct of anaesthesia.* A rapid sequence induction is performed. Regional anaesthesia may not be feasible because of lack of co-operation. Peripheral neuropathy must also be considered. The sedative effects of alcohol are additive with barbiturates. In chronic abuse, no effect on the pharmacodynamics or pharmacokinetics of thiopental was observed. MAC of volatile anaesthetics is reduced in the intoxicated patient. An increased volume of distribution may increase requirements of muscle relaxants, but not if there is profound muscle atrophy. Diminished pseudocholinesterase is not a clinical problem, however electrolyte disturbance can potentiate non-depolarizing blockade. Thermoregulation is impaired and warmed fluids and a forced warm air blanket should be considered.

3. *Postoperatively.* The recovery of the intoxicated patient may be prolonged. Alcohol may contribute to postoperative nausea and vomiting. Body temperature should be maintained.

Alcohol withdrawal

Minor withdrawal phenomena occur 6–8 h after alcohol with tremor, anorexia, nausea and sleep disturbance. Major withdrawal phenomena occur in 5% of hospitalized alcoholics after 3–4 days. Onset is slow with severe hallucinations, confabulation, agitation, pyrexia and sympathetic activity. Seizures may occur.

Treatment involves correction of electrolytes, magnesium replacement and use of sedatives such as chlordiazepoxide. Intravenous clomethiazole therapy is associated with a poorer outcome in ventilated patients due to fluid overload.

Further reading

Bruce D. Alcoholism and anaesthesia. *Anesthesia and Analgesia* 1983; **62:** 84–96.
Edwards R, Mosher V. Alcohol abuse, anaesthesia and intensive care. *Anaesthesia* 1980; **35:** 474–489.

Related topics of interest

Drugs of abuse (p. 97); Liver disease and anaesthesia (p. 151)

ANAEMIA

Anaemia is defined as a haemoglobin (Hb) concentration below the normal limit. Normal Hb levels vary with age, sex, and in pregnancy.

Age vs Hb

Age	Hb (g/dl)
Birth	16–18
3 months	9–12
1 year	11–13
12 years	12–15
16 years	13–17 (male) 11–16 (female)

Anaemia may be acute or chronic and may be caused by:

- Acute or chronic blood loss.
- Lack of factors, e.g. iron, vitamin B_{12}, folate, vitamin C, protein, thyroxine.
- Marrow failure (hypoplastic anaemia) due to haemopoietin deficiency, drugs, irradiation, or idiopathic.
- Marrow infiltration by carcinoma, leukaemia, myeloma, or myelofibrosis.
- Increased haemolysis due to red cell anomalies (spherocytosis, sickle cell disease, glucose-6-phosphate dehydrogenase deficiency), mechanical trauma (burns, prosthetic heart valves), chemicals (lead, venoms), sepsis, antibodies, uraemia and hypersplenism.

Oxygen transport is dependent on haemoglobin, yet when the haematocrit (Hct) falls to 0.2 (normal 0.37–0.52) and the blood volume remains constant, tissue O_2 delivery may remain unchanged or even be increased. This may be due to:

- Increased capillary blood flow as viscosity decreases.
- Increased O_2 extraction.
- Right shift of the oxygen–haemoglobin (oxy–Hb) dissociation curve.

Anaemia and anaesthesia

It is frequently stated that anaesthesia may safely be undertaken with Hct levels above 0.3 (equivalent to Hb ~10 g/dl). Proponents of normovolaemic haemo-dilution, however, claim far lower Hct levels as safe (e.g. 0.21–0.24). The difficulty is that the critical level of Hb or Hct at which to trigger transfusion is an individual and not a generally valid figure. The most important organ when considering the safety of anaesthesia and anaemia is the heart. Cardiac arteriovenous oxygen extraction is nearly maximal even at rest. Any perioperative increase in myocardial oxygen demand must be met with an increase in myocardial blood flow. About 1 in 25 asymptomatic middle-aged men suffer silent myocardial ischaemia and represent a high risk group when considering the consequences of reduced myocardial oxygen delivery secondary to anaemia. For this group a Hct level only as low as 0.3 in the perioperative period may be associated with fatal complications. There is thus no absolutely safe Hct when considering anaesthesia for populations, it can only be addressed on an individual patient basis.

Problems

- Maintenance of O_2 delivery in anaemia depends on increasing the cardiac output and/or Hb saturation. (NB 10% of a smoker's Hb may be HbCO.)
- Hb is an important buffer for CO_2-induced pH change, acidosis is thus more likely in anaemia.
- The oxy-Hb dissociation curve will be adversely affected by hypocapnia.
- Transfused Hb has 70% of the normal 2,3-DPG level and therefore 'unloads' O_2 poorly. Twenty-four hours is required to restore 2,3-DPG to normal levels.

Anaesthetic management

Cardiac output falls during surgery and blood loss is common. Oxygen carriage should be optimized preoperatively (Hct >0.3, Hb >10 g/dl). Non-urgent surgery should be postponed pending investigation and/or transfusion.

Initial resuscitation following acute blood loss should be with colloid and crystalloid rather than blood. Blood should be given to keep the Hct above 0.25. Surgery may commence once the patient is haemodynamically stable. Avoid respiratory depressant and anticholinergic premedicants to prevent hypoventilation and thus haemoglobin desaturation.

Monitoring with oximetry indicates haemoglobin saturation and not oxygen delivery. CVP and urine output should be monitored in acute blood loss. Critically ill patients require intra-arterial blood pressure and Hct monitoring. Consider a pulmonary artery catheter and inotropic agents to maintain a high cardiac index.

Select a technique to preserve cardiac output and O_2 delivery. This may necessitate a high inspired O_2 concentration. Hyperventilation should be avoided.

Postoperatively

- Continue O_2 therapy until stable.
- Consider ITU/HDU for continued resuscitation or observation.

Useful formulae

- Oxygen content (CaO_2) is the volume of O_2 present in a known volume of blood (100 ml). Units = ml/dl.
- $CaO_2 = Hb \times 1.34 \times \%$ saturation $+ 0.0225(PaO_2 \text{ [kPa]})$
- Available O_2 (O_2 flux) is the O_2 delivered to the tissues per minute.
- Available $O_2 = CaO_2 \times$ cardiac output.

Further reading

Lunsgaard-Hansen P. Safe haemoglobin or haematocrit levels in surgical patients. *World Journal of Surgery*, 1996; **20**: 1182–1188.

Soni N, Fawcett WS, Halliday FC. Beyond the lung: oxygen delivery and tissue oxygenation. *Anaesthesia*, 1993; **48**: 704–711.

Related topics of interest

Blood salvage (p. 34); Cardiac surgery (p. 65); Hypotensive anaesthesia (p. 133); Sequelae of anaesthesia (p. 232)

ANAESTHETIC RECORDS

Alison Pickford

A permanent record of an anaesthetic must be made and filed in the notes. This may be hand written or printed and should contain details of the pre-operative assessment and anaesthetic plan, the anaesthetic episode and the postoperative recovery period.

In addition to giving warning of previous difficulties and hazards, the anaesthetic record is also a medicolegal document. The standard of documentation is clearly important, what is not recorded will not be recalled accurately in the future. In the past the courts have interpreted the standard of documentation as reflecting the overall standard of anaesthetic care provided; scanty documentation being viewed as an indication of inadequate care, resulting in the plaintiff being awarded damages.

There is no standard data set which should be recorded and the appropriate level of documentation will increase with the complexity of the case. The content appropriate for a minor procedure in a fit patient will differ from that for a major procedure in a compromised patient. The following is based on current guidelines produced by The Royal College of Anaesthetists.

Anaesthetic record set

Pre-operative information

1. Patient details. Name, hospital number (national health service number) and date of birth. Weight.

2. Assessment and risk factors. Past anaesthetic, medical and family history. Drug history, allergies and addictions (alcohol, tobacco and other drugs). An assessment of the patient's cardiorespiratory fitness and potential airway problems, including prostheses, crowns and teeth. Investigations and their results. Assessment of the patient's ASA.

3. Consent to anaesthesia. The anaesthetic technique proposed and agreed with the patient (general, regional or local anaesthesia, administration of suppositories, etc.) should be documented, together with a list of the risks discussed. Current guidelines suggest that verbal consent to anaesthesia is adequate.

Per-operative information

1. Pre-operative checks. Nil by mouth, consent. Check of anaesthetic equipment in anaesthetic room and theatre.

2. Operation details. Proposed and actual operation performed. Urgency of procedure (scheduled – listed on a routine list, urgent – resuscitated, not on a routine list, emergency – not fully resuscitated). Personnel – all anaesthetists involved (including consultant staff informed of the case), anaesthetic assistants, and surgeons. Place of operation, date, start and end times.

3. Anaesthesia. Airway: airway type, size, cuff and shape used. Breathing system used. Ventilation – type and mode. Use of humidifier, filter, throat pack. Difficulties encountered. Intravenous cannula used – type, size and site. Drugs and fluids used together with doses, route of administration and time given.

4. *Regional anaesthesia.* The block performed, type and size of needle, aids to location (peripheral nerve stimulator, loss of resistance, etc.) together with whether the patient was awake, sedated or under general anaesthesia. Problems encountered should be documented (paraesthesia, location of blood vessel, inadvertent dural tap, etc.) Assessment of block prior to surgery (modality tested and extent of block).

5. *Monitoring.* The anaesthetist should detail which monitors were in use during the case, and keep an accurate record of the information that those monitors provided. In emergency situations it is clearly difficult to keep contemporaneous records, although a printed record obtained from the monitor goes some way to alleviating this problem. If a printed record is used it must be annotated to indicate anomalous readings and attached to the hand-written record. The anaesthetist should specify what monitoring is required during the postoperative period.

6. *Patient position and attachments.* The position of the patient should be noted together with any measures taken to protect eyes, nerves and pressure points. Prophylaxis against thrombosis and method of temperature control should be recorded.

Postoperative instructions

Special airway instructions, including oxygen, and suggested monitoring for the postoperative period should be documented together with prescriptions for analgesic drugs and fluids.

Critical incidents and hazard flags

These form an important part of risk management. A record of any difficulties or untoward events which could have or did lead to a negative outcome for the patient must be made. This includes any event occurring in the pre-, per- and post-operative period. Some attempt should be made to put the event in context and define contributing and causative factors, as well as document the response of the anaesthetist and the eventual outcome.

Anaesthetic hazards such as adverse drug reactions, difficult airway or intubation, malignant hyperpyrexia susceptibility, etc. should be recorded clearly in both the anaesthetic record and again in the patient notes.

Patient transfers

Many sedated or anaesthetized patients are transferred either within a hospital or between hospitals. Appropriate documentation is essentially the same as for an anaesthetic, with particular attention to the following:

- Patient name, age, weight and condition.
- Transferring and receiving hospitals.
- Method of transportation.
- Times – departure and arrival.
- Personnel responsible – doctor and nursing staff.

- Care of the airway and breathing, including method of ventilation.
- Intravenous access available.
- Drugs given during transfer.
- Monitoring used and a record of these parameters.
- Emergency equipment checked and available – airway equipment (i.v. equipment, drugs, suction, defibrillator).
- Problems encountered.

References

Anaesthetic Reference Set. *The Royal College of Anaesthetists.* April 1996. http://www.rcoa.ac.uk/training/goodpract.html

Guidelines for the Provision of Anaesthetic Services. *The Royal College of Anaesthetists.* July 1999. http://www.rcoa.ac.uk

Information and Consent for Anaesthesia. *The Association of Anaesthetists of Great Britain and Ireland.* 1999. http://www.aagbi.org

Related topics of interest

Critical incidents (p. 78); Preoperative preparation (p. 209); Transfer of the critically ill (p. 268)

ARDS and ALI

Tim Cook

Acute respiratory distress syndrome (ARDS) is a syndrome of respiratory failure associated with severe hypoxia and low respiratory compliance. The characteristic radiological changes are of widespread pulmonary infiltrates. Pulmonary artery occlusion pressure (PAOP) measurements may be low or normal. The plasma oncotic pressure is usually normal. The reported annual incidence of ARDS is variable, 5:100000 being quoted in the UK, but 75:100000 in the USA. This reflects differing thresholds for diagnosis.

ARDS is usually the pulmonary manifestation of the systemic inflammatory response syndrome (SIRS). Sepsis and trauma are the commonest causes. Other causes include haemorrhage with hypotension, transfusion, obstetric emergencies, cardiopulmonary bypass, pancreatitis, DIC, fat embolus and following cardiac arrest or head injury. Local insults such as aspiration or smoke inhalation may also result in ARDS. Onset of the disease is rapid; most cases develop within 24 hours of the initial insult. The clinical presentation is one of tachypnoea, laboured breathing and cyanosis.

The pathophysiological features of ARDS are initially due to epithelial injury and include a severe protein-rich alveolar oedema with inflammatory infiltrates (principally neutrophils), although ARDS may occur in the neutropenic patient. Surfactant denaturation by protein leaking into the alveolus leads to atelectasis, a reduced FRC and hypoxia. Type I alveolar cells are damaged and type II cells proliferate. Later, fibroblast infiltration and collagen proliferation lead, in some cases, to an accelerated fibrosing alveolitis and microvascular obliteration. This disease process does not affect the lung in a uniform fashion; there may be considerable functional variation between different lung regions.

Diagnosis

There are strict definitions for the diagnosis of acute lung injury (ALI) and ARDS. The triad of hypoxia, low lung compliance and widespread infiltrates on CXR should be accompanied by a known precipitant of the syndrome and a normal left atrial pressure (PAOP). A $PaO_2/FiO_2 \leq 40$ kPa defines ALI and a $PaO_2/FiO_2 \leq 27$ kPa defines ARDS.

Prognosis

The reported mortality for ARDS is variable. This in part is related to lack of consistency in diagnosis. Sepsis is associated with the greatest mortality at any stage of the disease whilst fat embolism alone is associated with a low mortality (90% survival). ARDS associated with bone marrow transplant or liver failure has negligible survival. Over 80% of deaths in ARDS are not as a result of respiratory failure. The presence of other organ failure thus has great bearing on the prognosis. Recent studies suggest that the mortality rate has fallen in the past decade from ~60% to 40%.

Management

Inspired O_2 concentrations greater than 0.5, high tidal volumes (>10 ml/kg) and high plateau airway pressures (>35 cmH$_2$O), may cause lung damage. Avoiding these risk factors may improve outcome.

Treatment is supportive, but control of infection is vital. Bacteriological specimens should be cultured and every effort made to prevent nosocomial infection. Prevention of gastric colonization by avoiding the use of H_2 receptor antagonists may reduce the incidence of nosocomial pneumonia. Nursing and medical hygiene must be scrupulous. Positive blood cultures should be followed by an extensive search for the site of infection.

Ventilation

The principles of mechanical ventilation are to provide adequate oxygenation and CO_2 removal while minimizing the risk of barotrauma and volutrauma. Dependent, collapsed alveoli should be recruited using positive end expiratory pressure (PEEP) of 5–18 cmH$_2$O. The use of prolonged inspiratory times (i.e., inverse ratio ventilation) will increase intrinsic PEEP (PEEPi) and may be beneficial. Relatively small tidal volumes (< 7 ml kg^{-1}) will minimize peak inspiratory pressures and reduce the potentially damaging shear forces in the alveoli. Inspired O_2 concentrations should be reduced to 0.5 as soon as possible by setting targets for acceptable hypoxaemia (e.g. SaO$_2 > 0.88$).

Arterial pCO$_2$ may therefore be allowed to rise to 10 kPa or higher providing renal compensation minimizes the accompanying acidosis (permissive hypercarbia). With one exception, prospective controlled studies of protective ventilation strategies and permissive hypercarbia have not, however, shown an improvement in outcome. Refractory hypoxia is often improved by the use of reversed I:E ratios and/or nursing the patient prone. Although extracorporeal membrane oxygenation with CO_2 removal (ECMO) is of benefit in infantile ARDS, its use in adults remains controversial.

Pulmonary artery catheterization may be valuable initially to exclude cardiogenic pulmonary oedema, in assessing optimum preload, and to guide inotrope, vasodilator and vasopressor therapy. Measurement of cardiac output, mixed venous saturation, and lactate or base deficit help to assess oxygen consumption. Extravascular lung water may be controlled by judicious administration of fluids to prevent high left atrial pressures. Controversy still surrounds the choice between colloid and crystalloid.

Specific treatment

The exact role of prostaglandin inhibitors, anti-TNF antibodies, surfactant therapy, and oxypentifylline is uncertain in this condition. Steroid therapy may be beneficial during the fibrosing stage of ARDS (late steroid rescue). This benefit appears to be limited to a narrow therapeutic window of between 7 and 15 days after the onset of ARDS.

Nitric oxide

Nitric oxide is a potent vasodilator. When it is inhaled it enters only ventilated areas of the lung and causes appropriate vasodilatation so improving ventilation:perfusion matching and oxygenation. This is in contrast to intravenous vasodilators that tend to do the converse and so increase shunt. It has a great affinity for haemoglobin (15 000 times that of carbon monoxide) and combines rapidly with it on entering the bloodstream. As a result it does not cause systemic vasodilatation. It is given directly into the ventilated gas mixture at a concentration of 5–20 ppm. The use of nitric oxide has not been shown to improve outcome from ARDS.

Survivors

The outlook for survivors is good. At 1 year 50% of survivors have abnormal lung function but few have functional respiratory disability. Late deaths in ARDS are secondary to pulmonary fibrosis (55%) and sepsis/multiple organ failure (69%).

Further reading

Bernard GR, Artigas A, Brigham KL, *et al.* Report of the American–European Consensus Conference on ARDS: definitions, mechanisms, relevant outcomes and clinical trial coordination. *Intensive Care Medicine*, 1994; **20**: 225–32.
Sair M, Evans T. ARDS: are we winning at last? *Anaesthesia*, 1998; **53**: 831–2.

Related topics of interest

Burns (p. 44); Sepsis and SIRS (p. 229); Ventilation (p. 276)

ASTHMA

Asthma is a chronic disease characterized by increased responsiveness of the tracheobronchial tree to various stimuli (e.g. inhaled allergens, infection, exercise, anxiety, cold or drugs). It manifests as widespread airway narrowing with mucosal oedema and a cellular infiltrate. Reversibility of airway obstruction is characteristic and distinguishes asthma from the fixed obstruction of chronic bronchitis and emphysema. The severity of airflow obstruction varies widely over short periods of time but airway resistance may be normal for long periods. The prevalence of asthma is 3–6%.

Problems

- Anxiety, anaesthetic drugs and airway manoeuvres may precipitate bronchoconstriction.
- Mucous trapping.
- Adrenal suppression from chronic steroid therapy.

Preoperative assessment

The goal of preoperative assessment is to determine the severity of the disease, the effectiveness of its management, and to formulate a plan for perioperative care. Episodic wheezing, dyspnoea and cough are the most common symptoms. The signs of an acute exacerbation include sweating, anxiety, the use of accessory muscles of respiration, pulsus paradoxus, cyanosis, and insufficient breath to speak. Disease severity is best determined by lung spirometry (FEV_1, FEV_1/FVC, PEFR) and its response to bronchodilator therapy. A normal PEFR in adults is ~600 ml. Rises in $PaCO_2$ occur only in severe cases ($FEV_1 < 25\%$ normal). ECG changes (sinus tachycardia, right ventricular strain, right axis deviation) are non-specific and only present in severe cases. The CXR is of little use in the diagnosis or assessment of the severity of asthma but may indicate atelectasis due to mucous trapping, pneumonia, pneumothorax, heart failure, or a foreign body in children. The commonest abnormality on CXR is overinflation of the lungs.

Physiotherapy, antibiotics and hydration may be required preoperatively to optimize the patient's condition. Bronchodilator therapy by aerosol should be administered prior to anaesthesia and be available for nebulization into the breathing system intraoperatively. H_2 receptor antagonists are best avoided as they may unmask H_1 receptor mediated bronchoconstriction. There is no evidence that opioids produce direct or reflex bronchoconstriction of clinical importance, but the respiratory depressant effect should be considered. Agents that cause the release of histamine (e.g. morphine) should be avoided. Anticholinergics may increase viscosity of airway secretions. Steroid supplementation may be required. Hypokalaemia may occur due to the actions of β-adrenoceptor agonists, steroids and hyperventilation.

Anaesthetic management

Regional anaesthesia is the technique of choice dependent on the surgical site. A high subarachnoid or epidural block that affects chest wall muscle function should, however, be avoided. Regional anaesthesia in an otherwise awake asthmatic may still be associated with intraoperative bronchospasm, possibly precipitated by anxiety.

Thiopental induction has been controversial because bronchospasm has been reported following its use. Too little thiopental (i.e. light anaesthesia) rather than the drug itself is the more likely factor producing bronchospasm. Methohexitone is more conventionally used barbiturate. Propofol appears not to precipitate bronchoconstriction. Lidocaine (lignocaine), 1–2 mg/kg i.v., or as a topical spray, or a volatile agent may be used following induction to prevent airway reflexes at intubation. Ketamine is least likely to cause bronchoconstriction, although this protective effect is abolished by β-blockade. Ketamine increases airway secretions. Gaseous induction may increase anxiety.

Halothane, enflurane, isoflurane and sevoflurane all exert beneficial effects on bronchoconstriction, probably to a similar extent. Halothane should be used with caution in patients receiving theophylline as cardiac arrhythmias and cardiac arrest have been reported. The volatile agents are of benefit in asthma because of their anticholinergic effects. Theophylline may lead to increased renal potassium excretion.

Muscle relaxation and mechanical ventilation provide the best arterial oxygenation and a volume-controlled ventilator should be available. Non-depolarizing relaxants that do not result in histamine release should be chosen. Care should be taken to ensure the tracheal tube lies in the upper trachea and does not stimulate the carina. Consideration of a spontaneously breathing technique without the use of tracheal intubation should be made, thus avoiding the stimulating effect of airway instrumentation. Ventilation should be at a slow rate to aid gas distribution and with a long expiratory time to allow full expiration. PEEP and intrinsic PEEP should be avoided. All gases should be warmed and humidified. Airway pressure, arterial O_2 saturation, expired CO_2, and arterial blood gas tensions should be closely monitored.

Intraoperative bronchospasm may manifest as increased inflation pressures or wheeze. Adequacy of oxygenation is the first priority. Other causes of intraoperative wheezing should be excluded (e.g. endobronchial intubation, pulmonary oedema, pneumothorax, anaphylaxis). Bronchodilatation may be achieved by increasing the concentration of volatile agent, or administering a non-anaesthetic bronchodilator. β-adrenergic agonists are the drugs of choice, stimulation of the $β_2$ receptors on bronchial smooth muscle causing muscle relaxation. Administering the agents via inhalation produces less systemic toxicity. Salbutamol and epinephrine (adrenaline) remain the agents of choice with newer, longer-acting agonists being too slow in onset to be of use in the acute attack.

Extubation should be performed at a plane of anaesthesia sufficient to prevent airway response.

Analgesia using local anaesthesia has the advantage of a lack of respiratory depression. Opioids should be titrated with care and may be delivered best by infusion systems.

Hydration should be maintained with crystalloid infusions. Consider elective ITU admission and ventilation for severe asthmatics requiring postoperative care.

Aminophylline: loading dose 5 mg/kg;
maintenance 0.5–0.9 mg/kg/hour;
therapeutic level 10–20 µg/ml.

Further reading

Short JA, Barr CA, Palmer CD, Goddard JM, Stack CG, Primhak RA. Use of diclofenac in children with asthma. *Anaesthesia*, 2000; **55**(4): 334–7.

Smyth RJ. Ventilatory care in status asthmaticus. *Can Respir J*, 1998; **5**(6): 485–90.

Related topics of interest

Adrenocortical disease (p. 1); Emergency anaesthesia (p. 109); Preoperative preparation (p. 209); Ventilation (p. 276)

AUDIT – National

Clinical audit is defined as systematically looking at the procedures used for diagnosis, care and treatment, examining how associated resources are used and investigating the effect care has on the outcome and quality of life for the patient. Audit is conducted in each hospital, and the discussion will be limited to national audit projects.

Confidential enquiry into maternal deaths

Confidential enquiries were started in 1952 and a maternal mortality report is produced every 3 years. It covers the entire United Kingdom and receives support from all relevant Royal Colleges. Death rates have fallen dramatically as a result of improved obstetric and anaesthetic care. In the 1952–4 report anaesthesia caused 49 deaths. In the 1994–6 report only one death was attributed to anaesthesia. The leading causes of direct maternal deaths in the 1994–6 report were thrombosis and thromboembolism (48), hypertensive disease of pregnancy (20), amniotic fluid embolism (17), early pregnancy deaths (15), sepsis (14) and haemorrhage (12). These deaths occurred from an estimated 2.9 million pregnancies.

Although only one death was attributed to anaesthesia, anaesthetists are involved in the multidisciplinary care of the critically ill pregnant woman.

CESDI

The Confidential Enquiry into Stillbirths and Deaths in Infancy was established in 1992. It collects information on late fetal losses, stillbirths and deaths in infancy. The aim is to identify ways in which these deaths may be prevented. Regional panels and focus groups analyse data in order to investigate particular problems.

ICNARC

The Intensive Care National Audit and Research Centre reports annually on outcomes and activity of participating intensive care and high dependency units in England, Wales and Northern Ireland. Data are collected according to the ICNARC Case Mix Programme Database, which includes PRISM, APACHE II and III, and SAPS II (Simplified Acute Physiology Score) data. This data is valid-ated, and by 1999, the report contained validated data on 22000 admissions to 62 units. Ongoing validation of data from 134 units of 60000 admissions would be considered in future reports.

A national report is produced, with a report for each unit on its performance. Age distribution, past medical history, illness severity scores, outcome, length of stay, and treatments given are analysed. The database can be further investigated for specific conditions, patient ages, type of hospital etc.

NCEPOD

The National Confidential Enquiry into Perioperative Deaths is overseen by a steering group of representatives from a wide range of professional bodies including the Association and the Royal College of Anaesthetists. It is based on case collection and peer review. The first 12-month study commenced in November 1985 (CEPOD) and was made of all patients who died within 30 days of an operative procedure carried out by an anaesthetist and/or a surgeon in three Health Regions. Since then the study has been conducted on a national basis and is now funded by the National Institute for Clinical Excellence (NICE). Each year the study is given a different emphasis by enquiring about deaths in different groups of patients. 'Extremes of age' were examined in 1997/8, and a 10% sample of reported deaths in 1998/9 and 1999/2000 to enable comparison with the 1990 data.

General recommendations from previous reports

1. Consultant involvement in complex cases.
2. Consultant supervision of trainees, with advice being sought.
3. Appropriately specialized and trained surgical and anaesthetic teams for the patient's condition.
4. Preoperative visiting and appropriate preoperative preparation, which may include intensive care.
5. Locum appointments.
6. Competent non-medical assistance for anaesthetists should be invariable.
7. Specific medical issues e.g. DVT/PE prophylaxis, NSAIDs, fluid management, monitoring before and during the induction of anaesthesia, fibreoptic intubating laryngoscopes, laparoscopic surgery and postoperative pain relief.
8. Inappropriate operations are sometimes done when there is no realistic hope of survival.
9. Shortages of resources, on a single site, of operating theatres dedicated to emergencies, ITU facilities, 24 hour recovery, and general staffing deficiencies.
10. Regular audits of operative results, with joint meetings with surgeons, with morbidity and mortality discussed. Good clinical records.
11. Increase is needed in the hospital postmortem rate of 8% in 1996. Approximately 50% of postmortems find new and unexpected findings which are relevant.

Further reading

The National Confidential Enquiry into Perioperative Deaths, annual reports from 1989. 35–43 Lincoln's Inn Fields, London.   http://www.ncepod.org.uk

Department of Health. *Why Mothers Die. Report on Confidential Enquires into Maternal Deaths in the United Kingdom*, 1994–1996, HMSO.

Related topics of interest

Ethics and duty of care (p. 115); Governance (p. 121); Scoring systems (p. 223)

BLOOD
Claire Gleeson

Enhanced screening of blood donors and testing procedures on donated blood have resulted in substantial improvements in the safety of blood supply. Nonetheless, human donor blood is expensive, in short supply, antigenic, requires crossmatching, has a limited shelf life, requires a storage facility and carries a risk of disease transmission. Homologous blood transfusion is immunosuppressive and may independently increase the risk of infection after trauma.

Screening

- Potential donors are screened with a health questionnaire.
- Donated blood is screened for HIV 1 and 2 antibodies, Hepatitis B surface antigen, Hepatitis C antibody, syphilis serology, CMV and HTLV1.

Collection and storage

One unit of blood (approximately 430 ml) is collected into a closed triple bag system containing CPD-A (citrate, phosphate, dextrose-adenine). From this first collection bag plasma and red cells can be separated by centrifugation if required (the closed system prevents exposure to infection and air). The red cells are then resuspended in SAG-M (sodium chloride, adenine, glucose and mannitol). Mannitol prevents haemolysis. The shelf life in this suspension is 42 days and the haematocrit is 0.6–0.7. The temperature at which blood should be stored is 2–6°C. The addition of glycerol allows blood to be frozen and stored for many years. This is expensive and although not appropriate for routine use has a place for use by the armed forces.

Effects of storage

After collection continued metabolic activity results in the following:

- Reduced pH.
- Reduced levels of 2,3-DPG and ATP.
- Increased potassium ion concentration (due to increased osmotic fragility resulting in cell rupture).
- Reduced viability of blood constituents, e.g. platelets and coagulation factors (factor XI is reduced, IX and X are reduced after one week, V and VIII are almost completely destroyed).
- Formation of microaggregates.

Blood products

Whole blood can be separated into its various constituents thus allowing appropriate products to be given to individual patients according to their needs. Following centrifugation, whole blood can be separated into packed red cells and platelet-rich plasma. The platelet-rich plasma can then be separated into platelets and plasma. Platelets have a shelf life of up to 7 days; one unit of platelets will increase the platelet count by approximately 7×10^9/l.

Fresh frozen plasma (FFP) lasts for a year, it contains all the clotting factors. To produce a clinically significant increase in serum levels of clotting factors 4–8 units of FFP are required.

FFP can further be separated into cryoprecipitate and supernatant. Cryoprecipitate is rich in factor VIII and fibrinogen. Supernatant contains albumin, factor IX and immunoglobulins. Human albumin solution has a shelf life of about 2 years and is available as 4.5% and 20% solutions.

Red cell substitutes

Red cell substitutes (oxygen-carrying volume replacement solutions) are being developed. Potential advantages include:

- Sterilization of bacterial and viral contaminants.
- Long shelf life.
- Room temperature storage.
- Universal biocompatibility.

Red cell substitutes under investigation include soluble haemoglobin solutions and emulsions of perflurocarbons.

1. Haemoglobin solutions. There are three principal sources of haemoglobin; human (out-of-date blood), bovine, and genetically engineered haemoglobin. Potential problems with these solutions include short half life, increased affinity for oxygen due to lack of 2,3-DPG, and vasoactive properties resulting in hypertension.

2. Perflurocarbons. Perflurocarbons (PFCs) are chemically inert, water insoluble hydrocarbons with fluoride ions substituted for all the hydrogen ions. They have a low viscosity which can improve oxygenation of ischaemic tissues. Fluosol DA 20% has been approved for coronary angioplasty. Side effects of its use include anaphylaxis. PFCs accumulate in the reticuloendothelial system with poorly understood long term effects.

Further reading

Goodenough LT, Brecher ME, Kanter MH, AuBuchon JP. Transfusion medicine. Blood transfusion. *New England Journal of Medicine*, 1999; **340**: 438–47.
Waschke KF, Frietsch T. Modified haemoglobins and perflurocarbons. *Current Opinion in Anaesthesiology*, 1999; **12**: 195–202.

Related topics of interest

AIDS and hepatitis (p. 7); Anaemia (p. 18); Blood salvage (p. 34)

BLOOD SALVAGE
Claire Gleeson

Perioperative anaemia may result in morbidity, mortality and functional impairment due to inadequate oxygen delivery to tissues. Preoperative autologous blood donation, intraoperative and postoperative blood salvage, acute normovolaemic haemodilution and recombinant human erythropoietin can be used to reduce the need for allogenic blood transfusion.

Predonation

The volume of blood that a patient can donate preoperatively is a function of the total circulating red cell mass and the rate of recovery of the packed cell volume after collection. A mean decrease of 1g/dl of haemoglobin occurs with each unit of autologous blood collected (350–450 ml). The number of units of autologous blood obtained preoperatively is based on the number of units that would be crossmatched before surgery if allogenic blood were being used. Preoperative autologous donation is inherently wasteful as not all donated blood is reinfused at the time of surgery. A British consensus conference concluded that autologous blood donation should only be considered if the likelihood of transfusion exceeds 50%. The time between the last donation and the date of surgery should be maximized to reduce the risk of anaemia. Iron must be administered during the time of blood donation. Exclusion criteria include systemic infection, unstable angina and a packed cell volume < 34%.

1. Advantages of autologous blood donation:
- Prevents transfusion-transmitted disease.
- Avoids red cell alloimmunization.
- Provides compatible blood for patients with alloantibodies.

2. Disadvantages:
- Does not eliminate the risk of bacterial contamination.
- Does not eliminate the risk of clerical error resulting in ABO incompatibility.
- Causes perioperative anaemia increasing the likelihood of transfusion.
- Expensive.

Intraoperative blood salvage

Blood is collected into a reservoir using an aspirator and a collection bag attached to the inferior edge of the wound. The blood is anticoagulated with heparin as it is retrieved. The red cells are then washed and packed by centrifugation, removing cellular debris and heparin. The packed red cells can then be reinfused into the patient, during surgery or postoperatively. Relative contraindications include infection, contaminants (e.g. ascitic or amniotic fluid), and malignancy.

Postoperative blood salvage

Postoperative blood salvage may be used if there is significant blood loss postoperatively, in particular with certain orthopaedic and thoracic procedures. Blood is collected from surgical drains. The survival and quality of autotransfused red cells has been shown to be equal to autologous banked red cells. Hyperthermic or hypotensive reactions can occur during reinfusion.

Acute normovolaemic haemodilution

Whole blood is collected immediately prior to surgery and simultaneously replaced with crystalloid or colloid, to maintain normovolaemia. The blood is collected in standard bags containing anticoagulant and is infused after any major blood loss has ceased. It should be considered when the potential blood loss is likely to exceed 20% of the blood volume and only in patients with a preoperative haemoglobin >10 g/dl and who do not have severe myocardial disease. In theory there should be less red cell loss because the blood lost intraoperatively has a lower Hct as a result of haemodilution, however, in practice savings are small unless profound haemodilution is accompanied by large blood loss (> 2 l). Advantages over autologous predonation include lower cost (no testing required) and negligible chance of administrative error.

Erythropoietin

Recombinant human erythropoietin accelerates erythropoiesis resulting in an increased red blood cell production, haematocrit level and haemoglobin concentration. The efficacy of recombinant erythropoietin is undeniable but its cost-effectiveness is debatable.

Blood transfusion

Direct antiglobulin testing is used to determine the ABO group and rhesus status of a patient. To confirm ABO compatibility between recipient and donor, recipient serum and donor cells are mixed together, an immediate spin cross-match is performed and agglutination observed. This takes approximately 5 minutes to perform. A full cross-match takes approximately 45 minutes and involves incubation of donor cells and recipient sera for at least 15 minutes (observing for agglutination) followed by a Coombs' test to detect antibody on donor red cells. In an emergency group-specific blood or failing that Group O blood can be administered to a patient. For premenopausal females Group O negative must be used to avoid sensitization to Rh D antigen.

Hazards of allogenic blood transfusion

1. *Acute haemolytic transfusion reaction.*   Due to ABO, Lewis, Kell or Duffy incompatible transfusion. Symptoms include bronchospasm, chest pain, urticaria, fevers, rigors, back pain, cardiovascular collapse, pulmonary oedema and cyanosis. If a clinically important reaction occurs the transfusion must be stopped and the unused blood returned to the laboratory with a 10 ml sample of the patient's blood for investigation.

Half of all deaths caused by ABO incompatibility are as a result of administrative errors.

2. *Non-haemolytic transfusion reaction*   is due to recipient antibody to donor white cell antigens. It occurs in 1–5% of all transfusions and results in fever, chills and urticaria.

3. **Delayed immune reactions.** Due to undetected antibody. Symptoms can be similar to acute reactions but are generally more benign.

4. **Infection – viral.** The current estimated infection risks are: HIV 1 in 1 000 000, Hepatitis B 1 in 100 000, Hepatitis C 1 in 100 000. HTLV types 1 and 2, non-A, non-B, non-C hepatitis, parvovirus B19, CMV and Epstein Barr virus can also be transmitted. Risks of transfusion transmitted disease are expected to fall even further when donors are screened using polymerase chain reaction assay, thus shortening the window period.

5. **Infection – Bacterial.** *Yersinia enterocolitica* is the organism most commonly implicated in the contamination of red cells. Contamination is directly related to length of storage.

6. **Immunosuppression.** Allogenic transfusion results in the suppression of cell mediated immunity resulting in an increased risk of postoperative infection.

7. **Acute lung injury.** Non cardiogenic pulmonary oedema caused by recipient antibody to donor leucocyte HLA antigens.

Massive transfusion

The following complications are more commonly associated with massive transfusion (>10 U or a transfusion of more than the patient's blood volume):

- Coagulopathy – massive transfusion results in dilutional effects on platelets and clotting factors (V and VIII). DIC may also occur. FFP and platelets may need to be administered.
- Biochemical abnormalities – hyperkalaemia, metabolic acidosis, metabolic alkalosis (as citrate is converted to bicarbonate), hypocalcaemia secondary to citrate toxicity and hypoalbuminia.
- Hypothermia – results in a shift of the oxygen dissociation curve to the left.
- Volume overload.
- Iron overload occurs following multiple transfusions over a long period of time. It causes myocardial and hepatic damage as a result of haemosiderin deposition.

The Serious Hazards of Transfusion initiative (SHOT) concluded that transfusion is extremely safe and resources should be directed to evaluation of methods for identification of blood and patient. The chance of a severe adverse reaction remains less than 1 in 10 000.

Further reading

Chen AY, Carson JL. Perioperative management of anaemia. *British Journal of Anaesthesia*, 1998; **81** (suppl 1): 20–4.
Goodenough LT, Becher ME, Kanter MH, AuBuchon JP. *Transfusion medicine*, 1999; **340**: 438–47.

Related topics of interest

BRAIN DEATH AND ORGAN DONATION

Brain stem death is defined as the irreversible cessation of brain stem function, but not necessarily the physical destruction of the brain. In the UK, it has been agreed that brain stem death = death (i.e. despite the presence of a beating heart). Prior to the diagnosis of brain stem death it is necessary to consider certain preconditions and exclusions. Head injury and intracranial haemorrhage account for approximately 80% of cases.

Preconditions
- Apnoeic coma requiring ventilation.
- Irreversible brain damage of known cause.

Exclusions
- Hypothermia (temperature > 35°C).
- Drugs (no depressant or muscle relaxant drugs present).
- Acid–base abnormality.
- Metabolic/endocrine disease, e.g. uncontrolled diabetes mellitus, uraemia, hyponatraemia, Addison's disease, hepatic encephalopathy, thyrotoxicosis.
- Markedly elevated $PaCO_2$.
- Severe hypotension.

The brain stem death tests
These should be performed by two doctors but not necessarily at the same time. Neither should belong to the transplant team and both should have been registered for 5 years or more. One must be a consultant. More than 6 hours should have elapsed since the event that caused the suspected brain stem death. Two sets of tests must be performed. They may be carried out by the doctors separately or together. Careful records should be kept.

1. **Pupillary responses.** There are no direct or consensual reactions to light. This tests the 2nd cranial nerve and the parasympathetic outflow.

2. **Corneal reflex.** No response to lightly touching the cornea. This tests the 5th and 7th cranial nerves.

3. **Painful stimulus to the face.** A motor response in the cranial nerve distribution of the stimulus is looked for. Tests the 5th and 7th cranial nerves.

4. **Caloric tests.** After visualizing both ear drums (wax may need to be removed first), 30 ml of ice cold water is injected into each external auditory canal. No response is seen if the 8th nerve and brain stem are dead. Nystagmus occurs if the vestibular reflexes are intact. (Tests 8th, 3rd and 6th cranial nerves.)

5. **Gag reflex.** Tests the 9th and 10th cranial nerves.

6. **Apnoea test.** The patient is ventilated with 100% O_2 and then disconnected

from the ventilator, while observing for respiratory effort. A tracheal catheter may be used to supply oxygen. The patient is left disconnected for 10 minutes or until the $PaCO_2$ is >6.65 kPa. If marked bradycardia or haemodynamic instability occur the test is discontinued. The SaO_2 should not fall below 90%. It may help the patient's relatives come to terms with the concept of brain death if they witness the apnoea test.

Other tests

Doll's eyes movement. The head is moved rapidly from side to side. If the brain stem is dead the eyes remain in a fixed position within the orbit. This is the oculocephalic reflex and tests the 8th cranial nerve. If the cortex is dead but the brain stem is intact the eyes appear to move to the opposite side and then realign with the head. It does not form part of the legally required brain stem death tests.

Some countries require other tests for the diagnosis of brain death. These include EEG, 'four vessel' cerebral angiography, radioisotope scanning and transcranial Doppler ultrasound. There is no evidence that these tests increase the accuracy of diagnosis. Their use may be limited but they may be helpful in situations where the clinical testing described above cannot be undertaken (e.g. local cranial nerve injuries, an inability to perform the apnoea test because of severe hypoxia).

Problems

- Spinal reflexes may be present. However, decerebrate posturing means some brain stem activity exists.
- The presence of drugs or other unresponsive states may lead to a false diagnosis of brain death.
- Communication with relatives. The discussion of a 'hopeless prognosis' being misinterpreted as brain stem death. A subsequent survival may then be ascribed to an incorrect diagnosis of brain stem death.
- Death of the cortex leading to a vegetative state is not brain death.
- Elective ventilation. A patient who is dying should not commence assisted ventilation simply to allow organ donation where this ventilation is of no therapeutic benefit to the dying patient. This practice is considered unacceptable in the UK.

Anaesthetic management of organ donation

Organ retrieval takes place in the operating theatre. Organ perfusion is maintained, with fluids and inotropes if necessary. High-dose inotropes are, however, detrimental to subsequent organ function. During surgery the MAP, SVR and PAOP increase initially and then fall below preoperative levels. A pulmonary artery catheter should be considered for multi-organ donors. Ventilation to keep the PaO_2 > 10 kPa is continued.

Spinal reflexes and autonomic haemodynamic responses require the use of neuromuscular blockers and opioids for control.

Potential complications in brain stem dead organ donors that may require intra-operative correction include:

- Cardiovascular instability.
- Hypoxaemia.
- Diabetes insipidus.
- Endocrine abnormalities (e.g. thyroid, adrenal or pancreatic function).
- Electrolyte imbalances.
- Acid–base disorders.
- Hypothermia.
- Hyperglycaemia.
- Coagulopathy.

Once the organs have been removed ventilation is stopped. The emotional needs of the staff and relatives involved in organ harvesting should not be overlooked especially if the donor is a child.

Further reading

Working Party for the Department of Health. A code of practice for the diagnosis of brain stem death. *Department of Health*, March 1998.

Young PJ, Matta BF. Anaesthesia for organ donation in the brainstem – why bother? *Anaesthesia*, 2000; **55:** 105–106.

Related topics of interest

Head injury (p. 124); Neuroanaesthesia (p. 167); Organ transplantation (p. 187)

BREAST FEEDING

A growing appreciation of the benefits of breast feeding coupled with incentives and encouragement from the government for women to breast feed babies means that anaesthetists are frequently asked to anaesthetize nursing mothers.

Problems

- Derangement of an established feeding schedule.
- Passage of drugs into milk and subsequent risks to the infant.

Unbound drug in the maternal circulation is free to cross into milk. Changes in maternal protein levels in late pregnancy and the early postpartum phase may alter drug binding. Having entered human milk drugs may then bind to protein in milk, partition into milk lipid, or remain free in the aqueous component of milk. Plasma concentration of the total dose of a drug ingested by the infant will be influenced by the oral bioavailability and clearance of the drug.

Anaesthetic management

1. Preoperative assessment. Breast feeding mothers should be told that all drugs given to them, by whatever route, might pass into breast milk. They should be reassured, however, that they do so in only small amounts and that those drugs used in anaesthesia carry very minor risks to the infant. The operation should be timed to allow the mother to feed her child just prior to surgery. It may be possible to express milk preoperatively to be stored for administration to the infant whilst the mother is unable to breast feed.

2. Perioperative care. Premedicants should be avoided if possible. Benzodiazepines may safely be given to an anxious breast feeding patient but there is a risk of postoperative drowsiness interfering with the smooth recommencement of a feeding regimen. Anti-emetics should be avoided. Metoclopramide is concentrated in milk by comparison with plasma. There is a theoretical risk of anti-dopaminergic reactions in the infant following ingestion of milk containing such agents.

Induction with thiopental and propofol is safe. All volatile agents and muscle relaxants are thought to be safe. Analgesia is best achieved with combination therapy, thus limiting the use of opioids. Non-steroidal anti-inflammatory drugs (anti-prostenoids) are not contraindicated with the exception of aspirin. There is a theoretical risk of Reye's syndrome with the latter.

A low threshold for the administration of intravenous fluids should be adopted as dehydration will reduce milk production.

The normal feeding regimen should be established as soon as is practicable in the immediate postoperative period.

Further reading

Gin T. Anaesthesia and breast feeding. *Anaesth Intensive Care*, 1993; **21(2):** 256–257.
Lee JJ, Rubin AP. Breast feeding and anaesthesia. *Anaesthesia*, 1993; **48:** 616–625.

Related topics of interest

Day surgery (p. 80); Preoperative preparation (p. 209)

BREATHING SYSTEMS

The ideal breathing system would maintain oxygen delivery, remove carbon dioxide, and deliver anaesthetic gases with no resistance to spontaneous respiration or increase in internal resistance in those ventilated. It would limit the wastage of volatile agents and be lightweight and easy to handle.

Classification of breathing systems has been based on the restriction of fresh gas flow (FGF) and expired gases. Systems are said to be:

- Open – no restriction to FGF.
- Semi-open – some restriction to FGF.
- Closed – a fully bounded system with no provision for gas overflow (whether expired or excess FGF).
- Semi-closed – fully bounded system with provision for venting gas.

Closed and semi-closed systems may be further classified as rebreathing or absorption systems. Non-absorber systems may also have the Mapleson classification applied to them.

Circle systems

Circle systems are closed or semi-closed breathing systems with or without absorbers. In some countries it is common practice to switch the absorber out of the circle towards the end of an anaesthetic to allow the carbon dioxide concentration to increase within the system. They permit the administration of low flow anaesthesia. Low-flow anaesthesia is defined as a FGF of less than half the minute volume and is usually less than 3 l/min. Circle systems and low-flow anaesthesia reduce the cost of gaseous anaesthesia, increase humidification of the FGF, reduce patient heat loss via the lungs, and can reduce potential environmental damage from anaesthetic agents. Concerns about the use of low-flow anaesthesia include the risks of a gradually falling FiO_2 in the breathing system both as a result of oxygen consumption and dilution by nitrogen from the patient. There is also the risk of production of toxic by-products from the breakdown of anaesthetic vapours in the absorber.

Carbon dioxide absorption

Soda lime is the commonest absorption agent in use. It is a mixture of calcium hydroxide (94%), sodium hydroxide (5%), and potassium hydroxide (1%). Silica may be added to increase the overall hardness of the soda lime and thus reduce dust formation. Indicators that change colour as the soda lime expires and produces acids are also often added. Carbon dioxide is absorbed by the chemical reactions:

$$CO_2 + 2NaOH \rightarrow H_2O + Na_2CO_3 + heat$$
$$Na_2CO_3 + Ca(OH)_2 \rightarrow 2NaOH + CaCO_3$$

To a lesser extent carbon dioxide reacts with calcium hydroxide directly:

$$CO_2 + Ca(OH)_2 \rightarrow H_2O + CaCO_3 + heat$$

The byproducts of water and heat aid in humidifying and warming the inspired gases. Soda lime may react with volatile agents to form carbon monoxide. This may be a particular risk with sevoflurane. An alternative absorption material is baralyme which uses barium hydroxide in place of sodium hydroxide. It is less efficient as an absorber of carbon dioxide and more expensive than soda lime.

Circle systems in use

The safety of a circle system at low flow depends on the correct functioning of the unidirectional valves in the inspiratory and expiratory limbs as well as the ability to accurately monitor the FiO_2, $PE'CO_2$, and the inspired and expired volatile agent concentrations.

At the extreme of its design a circle system can be used as a fully closed system in which there is no overspill of gas. Since carbon dioxide is absorbed, the FGF can be reduced to the basal metabolic oxygen requirement ($\sim$250 ml/min). In reality circle systems leak and most users run FGF slightly higher than basal oxygen requirements.

Vaporizers and circle systems

Vaporizers may be either outside the circle (VOC) or in the circle (VIC). Plenum vaporizers have a high internal resistance and are not suitable for use in the circle. The FGF is split as it enters a plenum vaporizer, with only part passing into the vaporizer chamber, and thus mixing with fully saturated vapour. The split parts are recombined before entering the circle system. When a vaporizer is used outside the circle its setting must compensate for the FGF. The lower the FGF, the greater the dilution of the fresh gas vapour concentration by the gas in the breathing system. This is because at low flows the patient has largely extracted the vapour in the breathing system.

Drawover vaporizers have low resistance to gas flow and can be used inside the circle. All the fresh gas flows through the vaporizer. The output of a drawover vaporizer is variable depending in part on the volume of vapour in the vaporizer as well as the fresh gas flowing through it.

Further reading

Anaesthesia Under Examination: The Efficiency and Effectiveness of Anaesthetic and Pain Relief Services in England and Wales. Audit Commission, July 1998.
http://www.audit-commission.gov.uk/ac/NR/Health/clinic2.

Related topic of interest

TIVA (p. 264)

BURNS
Stephen Laver

Without skin the body is open to infection, and to a breakdown of important physiological functions. The skin forms a protective barrier against physical, chemical and bacterial agents that may harm deeper structures. It maintains body temperature, prevents water loss, acts as a sensory organ providing information about the environment and plays a role in activating vitamin D.

In the United Kingdom, there are 200 000 people burnt per year, with 8000 patients presenting to Accident and Emergency departments, of whom 300 die. Most fatalities still occur in house fires from smoke inhalation. Mortality has dramatically reduced since the introduction of smoke detectors. Deaths are more likely to occur in patients from lower socio-economic groups. Once successfully resuscitated, patients most commonly die of infection, usually burn-wound sepsis or pneumonia.

Definition of a burn

- A first-degree burn affects only the epidermal layer and is red, painful, dry and is absent of blisters.
- A second-degree burn involves the epidermal and dermal layers, and can be classified as superficial or deep depending on the extent of damage to the dermis. The skin is red, blistered and painful and oedema is present.
- A third-degree (full thickness) burn destroys all layers of the skin and also some of the underlying tissues. The burn appears white and is painless. Pricking the skin with a needle causes no bleeding.

Assessment of a burn

1. History. There are several key aspects to the history. Firstly the mechanism of injury is important (i.e. flame, chemical, etc.). This will make the medical team aware of any potential hazards to themselves. Secondly, the location of injury. If the burn occurred in an enclosed area, there is more likely to be an inhalation injury or blast injury if there was an explosion. Thirdly, in the case of a paediatric burn, detailed questioning may elicit evidence of abuse (10% of abuse cases involve burns and severe scalds). The time of injury is also important, as it will inform the time from which fluid resuscitation should have commenced.

2. Total body surface area (TBSA) burnt. The 'rule of nines' is used to approximate the TBSA burnt. Head 9%, arms 9% each, legs 18% each, trunk 18% front and 18% back, and perineum 1%.

3. Major burn. Defined as:

- Full thickness burn involving >10% TBSA.
- Partial thickness burn involving >25% TBSA in adults or >20% TBSA at the extremes of age.
- Burns to the face, hands, perineum or feet.

- Burns affecting a major joint.
- Inhalation, chemical or electrical burns.

Initial management of a major burn

1. Airway and breathing. Assessment of the airway should include looking for direct burns to the face, singeing of eyebrows, eyelashes and nasal hair, swelling of the face, lips, tongue or oropharynx, a cough, wheeze or stridor, or soot in the nose, mouth or sputum. The patient may be drooling or dribbling saliva. Carbon monoxide has an affinity for haemoglobin 250 times that of oxygen. Thus, the oxygen carrying capacity will be reduced dramatically. Tissue hypoxia occurs by displacement of oxygen from haemoglobin, and the inhibition of complex IV in the respiratory chain in mitochondria. A pulse oximeter is unable to detect different haemoglobin moieties and will give inappropriately high saturations in the event of severe hypoxia. A co-oximeter is the only way to get an accurate measure of oxygen content as it uses spectroscopy at various wavelengths and can differentiate carboxyhaemoglobin from oxyhaemoglobin.

If any of the above are found, the minimum treatment is humidified high-concentration oxygen (the half life of carboxyhaemoglobin falls from 4 hours to 30 minutes if the FiO_2 is 1.0), but early intubation may be considered before gross swelling of the upper airway occurs.

Smoke inhalation with toxic substances such as cyanide, ammonia, hydrochloric acid and phosgene may also occur. They may cause marked inflammatory change or be specific poisons (e.g. cyanide blocks mitochondrial aerobic reactions and produces histotoxic hypoxia and acidosis). Antidotes to cyanide include amyl nitrate (forms methaemoglobin to reduce cyanide binding), thiosulphate (provides substrate for cyanide metabolism) and dicobalt edetate (binds to from an inert complex).

If the airway is very swollen, and if intubation is required, an awake fibreoptic intubation or inhalational induction should be considered.

A perforated tympanic membrane suggests a blast injury, and the likelihood of a chest injury and increased fluid requirements. A blast rapidly expands air-filled structures such as the middle ear, airways and abdominal organs which can cause rupture.

2. Circulation. A burn is associated with large fluid flux, and prompt fluid resuscitation of a major burn reduces potential organ failure and maintains cardiac output. Failure of fluid resuscitation may convert a second-degree burn into a third-degree burn. Oedema results from loss of plasma fluid into the interstitium. There are a number of regimens for fluid resuscitation. The Parkland regimen specifies the use of 4 ml/kg% burn^{-1} per day of crystalloid, giving 50% in the first eight hours, continued for 48 hours. This is only a guide, and much more may be needed, especially if there are other injuries or a blast injury. The use of colloids is controversial and may increase mortality in the burns patient. In addition, regimens that use hypertonic solutions may be used and have the advantage of producing less oedema in non-burnt tissue, but have no effect on burn oedema. During episodes of sepsis, vasoconstrictors or vasodilators may be needed to stabilize the cardiovascular system.

3. Renal. The maintenance of renal output is imperative. Mannitol may be needed if there is myoglobinaemia. Renal failure in the burns patient requiring renal replacement therapy is a poor prognostic indicator.

4. Metabolic changes. The euthermic temperature is rapidly reset to approximately 38.5°C after a major burn due to changes in the hypothalamic–adrenal axis. Oxygen consumption and carbon dioxide production increases as a marker of increased basal metabolic rate. Enteral nutrition will reduce bacterial translocation and infection by maintenance of the gut mucosal barrier. Feeding during grafting may also be beneficial.

5. Infection. Burns are initially virtually free from bacteria, which have been killed by the heat, but the dead tissue soon becomes heavily colonized by bacteria. This is not significant in superficial burns, but is the major cause of death in more major burns. The usual organisms are *Streptococcus pyogenes, Pseudomonas aeruginosa* and *Staphylococcus aureus.*

The first line of defence against infection involves protecting the patient against microbial contaminants. This is either through primary excision and skin grafting, antisepsis with antibacterial substances such as 1% silver sulphadiazine and asepsis with regular dressings changes, isolation of patients and good ward hygiene. The second line of defence is to prevent invasion of the tissues and bloodstream by bacteria growing on the burn with antibiotic therapy and active or passive immunization.

Secondary management

A first-degree burn heals within a week. A superficial second-degree burn heals in 14 days with no scarring in the superficial burn and in 4 weeks with scarring if it is deep. Excision and grafting may be required for the latter. A deep second-degree burn is in danger of being converted to a third-degree burn with inadequate resuscitation. Skin grafting is required to treat a third degree burn.

1. Surgical management. The only definitive management of major burns is excision and skin grafting to prevent infection. The graft may be harvested from the patient or be from a human donor or porcine in origin. Artificial 'skins' also can be placed over the burn after excision. Circumferential contraction of burns can be life-threatening, especially on the neck, chest, abdomen or the limbs, and requires immediate escharotomies.

Anaesthetic management

It may be difficult to apply monitoring to a burns patient. The burnt skin may necessitate the use of transcutaneous electrodes and difficult placement of venous and arterial lines to avoid burnt skin. Central venous monitoring may only be possible by long line placement or femoral lines.

Induction with propofol and ketamine is common. The use of ketamine is especially good in repeated anaesthetics and dressing changes by injection or nasal spray, as it gives long-lasting analgesia and does not compromise the airway.

Suxamethonium is contraindicated following a burn from six hours to two years after the insult. There is an increase in the requirements for muscle relaxants due to an up-regulation of α_1-glycoprotein.

An awake fibreoptic intubation may be needed as the airway swells quickly after fluid resuscitation has commenced even without an airway burn. The ambient temperature in the theatre should be at least 30°C and greater than 80% humidity to minimize heat loss mainly through evaporation.

Debridement and grafting will result in large blood losses and hypothermia, and the operation should stop to allow compensation of blood losses, and be terminated when the patient gets cold (it is not possible to cover the patient up for surgery, as the good skin may be harvested to make grafts).

Opioids will be needed for analgesia. Third-degree burns do not cause pain, but there will be areas that still have an active nerve supply, and hence require analgesia. Ketamine may be used to reduce morphine requirements.

Further reading

Judkins K. Burns treatment in the 21st century: a challenge for British anaesthesia. *Anaesthesia*, 1999; **54:** 1131–5.

Related topics of interest

Intubation – difficult (p. 141); Pain relief – acute(p. 199); Sepsis and SIRS (p. 229); Temperature – hypothermia (p. 255)

CARCINOID SYNDROME

Carcinoid tumours may secrete 5 hydroxytryptamine (5HT), bradykinin, histamine, substance P or prostaglandins. Various clinical manifestations may therefore be seen. Tumours arise in enterochromaffin (argentiffan) cells and produce symptoms when peripheral levels of 5HT, etc. are high. In 36% the tumour is of the small bowel (metastasizing to the liver before causing the carcinoid syndrome), but other sites such as the lung, pancreas, large bowel and stomach are described. They are frequently multiple in number and generally slow growing, utilizing dietary tryptophan (causing nicotinamide deficiency manifesting as pellagra). The classic syndrome is of diarrhoea, flushing with hypotension, telangectasia and bronchospasm. Less commonly, hypertension and right-sided valvular lesions (endocardial fibrosis) occur. The $5HT_2$ receptor mediates vasoconstriction. Attacks may be precipitated by exercise, anxiety and alcohol. Diagnosis is confirmed by a raised urinary 5-hydroxyindole acetic acid on a low serotonin diet. The incidence is 8:100 000.

Problems
- Electrolyte imbalance and malnutrition (diarrhoea).
- Haemodynamic effects of tumour products.
- Cardiac lesions especially pulmonary stenosis and tricuspid regurgitation.
- Bronchospasm.
- Of the primary tumour, e.g. bleeding, gastro-intestinal obstruction.

Anaesthetic management

Assessment and premedication
It is important to determine what substance the tumour is predominantly secreting as this will allow prediction of the likely effects. The preoperative assessment should include a search for all the features of the syndrome. Treatment is aimed at blocking the release or effects of vasoactive substances. Somatostatin analogues, such as octreotide, block gastroenteropancreatic peptide release. Octreotide is a tetra-decapeptide and is commonly used. It may cause hypoglycaemia. Patients may be treated with methysergide, ketanserin or cyproheptadine as 5HT antagonists. Ketanserin is also an alpha-1 antagonist. Aprotinin, a kallikrein trypsin inhibitor, has been used to prevent the conversion of kininogens to bradykinin. Investigations should include FBC, U+E, blood sugar, LFT, clotting, ECG and CXR, with more specific tests as indicated by the symptoms and signs. Premedication may be with an oral benzodiazepine, H_1 and H_2 antagonists, together with continuation of specific treatments. Octreotide is given subcutaneously, one hour preoperatively if patients are not regularly receiving it. Patients who have received steroids will require further supplementation.

Conduct of anaesthesia

1. *Regional anaesthesia.* Hypotension may cause release of bradykinin and is thus not recommended, although the cautious use of an epidural has been described.

2. *General anaesthesia.* Monitoring should include invasive CVS monitoring for fluid balance, arterial blood pressure and gases. Smooth, unstimulating anaesthesia and surgery is required. Avoid histamine-releasing and cardiovascularly unstable drugs. Consider fentanyl plus etomidate or a benzodiazepine, with vecuronium as the muscle relaxant of choice. Isoflurane is the recommended volatile agent. Infusions of octreotide and aprotinin may be given during the procedure. Hypertension should be treated with ketanserin or labetolol while hypotension is managed with fluid replacement, octreotide or angiotensin. Sympathomimetics are conventionally avoided as they may precipitate release of peptides by alpha adrenergic stimulation. However, the cautious use of methoxamine and adrenaline has been described if other measures are unsuccessful.

Postoperatively

ITU/HDU care should be available for the immediate postoperative period as CVS instability is likely. Octreotide is continued and good analgesia ensured.

Further reading

Veall G et al. Review of the anaesthetic management of 21 patients undergoing laparotomy for carcinoid syndrome. *British Journal of Anaesthesia* 1994; **72:** 335–341.

Kam PCA, Chang GWM. Selective serotonin reuptake inhibitors. Pharmacology and clinical implications in anaesthesia and critical care medicine. *Anaesthesia* 1997; **52:** 982–988.

Related topic of interest

Asthma (p. 27)

CARDIAC ARRHYTHMIAS

Although most arrhythmias occurring during anaesthesia require little intervention, serious arrhythmias can occur and need urgent treatment. Certain stimuli tend to cause specific arrhythmias and a combination of precipitants can occur.

Types of arrhythmia

1. Supraventricular. Sinus bradycardia, sinus tachycardia, ectopic beats, atrial flutter, atrial fibrillation, junctional tachycardia.

2. Ventricular. Ventricular ectopics, idioventricular rhythm, ventricular tachycardia, ventricular fibrillation.

3. Conduction problems. Sick sinus syndrome, sinus arrest, 1st degree block, 2nd degree block (Wenckebach; progressively longer PR intervals followed by a P wave that is not conducted [Mobitz type I] or regular failure of A-V conduction e.g. 2:1 or 3:1), 3rd degree block (complete heart block), bundle branch blocks.

4. Asystole.

5. Electromechanical dissociation (pulseless electrical activity).

Preoperative causes

- Pre-existing cardiac lesions, e.g. IHD, valvular heart disease or cardio-myopathy.
- Endocrine disorders, e.g. hyperthyroidism, phaeochromocytoma.
- Drugs, e.g. β-blockers, digoxin, tricyclics.
- Acid–base disorders and electrolyte disturbances, e.g. hypokalaemia causing ectopic beats.
- Anxiety with high levels of endogenous catecholamines.
- Raised ICP.

Peroperative causes

Any preoperative cause may extend into the peroperative period. Others include:

1. Anaesthetic causes.
- Depth of anaesthesia, i.e. too light or too deep.
- Hypoxia or hypercarbia.
- Hypo and hyperthermia.
- Hypo and hypertension.
- Stimulation of the larynx.
- Hypo and hyperthermia.
- Drugs, e.g. volatile agents (especially halothane) suxamethonium, local anaesthetics with epinephrine (adrenaline), inotropes.

2. Surgical causes.
- Stimulation, especially of the eye, carotid body, throat, peritoneum, anus and cervix. CVP line insertion.

(b) Diathermy and pacemakers.

(c) Manipulation of endocrine tumours.

*3. **Intraoperative crises.*** e.g. air emboli, pulmonary emboli, myocardial infarction, intracranial bleeding, pneumothorax.

Postoperative causes

Any of the pre- or peroperative causes may extend into the postoperative period. Others include:

- Hypoxia.
- Pain.
- Drugs used intraoperatively.

Perioperative management

Stabilization or correction of the arrhythmia should be undertaken and any precipitating factors corrected prior to elective surgery. Anti-arrhythmic therapy is continued until surgery. Potassium and digoxin levels should be optimized. Beta blockers and calcium channel antagonists can interact with volatile agents causing a decreased cardiac output and hypotension. Cardiological advice should be sought for complex arrhythmias, e.g. Wolf-Parkinson-White syndrome with atrial fibrillation. A sedative premedicant may prevent excessive tachycardia.

Careful CVS monitoring is needed for patients with arrhythmias. Precipitating anaesthetic or surgical causes are sought and corrected. Treatment is needed if the arrhythmia causes circulatory compromise, could precipitate a more serious rhythm disturbance, or if myocardial perfusion may become critical in patients with IHD.

Postoperative care

The development of a new, serious rhythm disturbance may necessitate admission to a critical care bed and further investigation, e.g. electrolytes, cardiac enzymes, ECG and CXR.

Peri-arrest arrhythmias

The development of certain arrhythmias at any time in the perioperative phase warrants urgent treatment. For the management of arrhythmias associated with cardiac arrest.

Further reading

Bossaert L (ed). Peri-arrest arrhythmias: management of arrhythmias associated with cardiac arrest. In: *European Resuscitation Council Guidelines for Resuscitation.* Amsterdam, Elsevier, 1998, pp. 159–168.

Related topics of interest

Cardiac assessment (p. 55); Cardiac pacemakers (p. 62); Cardiac surgery (p. 65); CPR (p. 75); Minimally invasive surgery (p. 154)

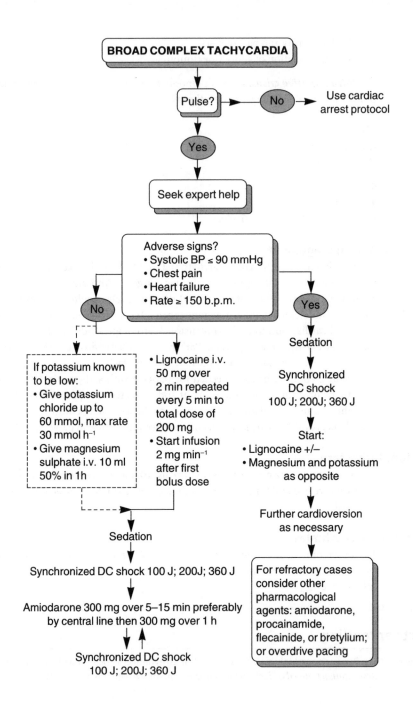

Reprinted from *Resuscitation*, Volume 37, 1998 with permission from Elsevier Science.

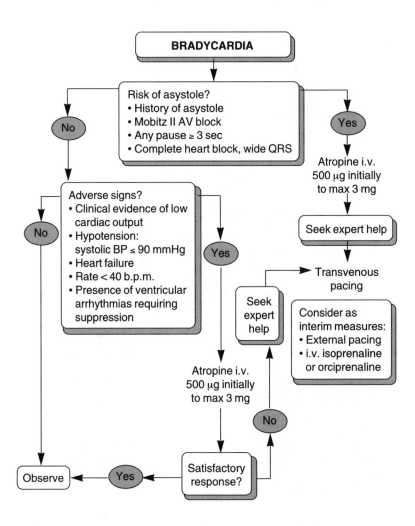

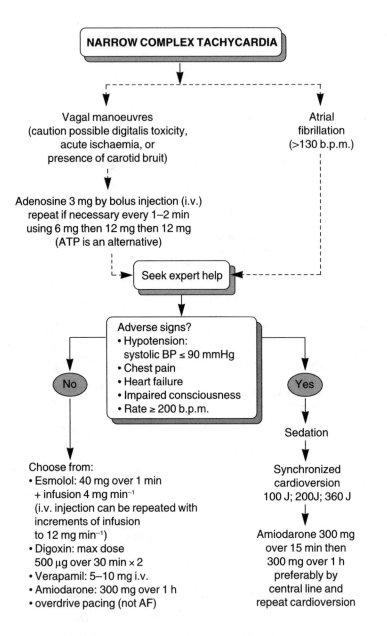

NARROW COMPLEX TACHYCARDIA

Vagal manoeuvres
(caution possible digitalis toxicity,
acute ischaemia, or
presence of carotid bruit)

Atrial
fibrillation
(>130 b.p.m.)

Adenosine 3 mg by bolus injection (i.v.)
repeat if necessary every 1–2 min
using 6 mg then 12 mg then 12 mg
(ATP is an alternative)

Seek expert help

Adverse signs?
• Hypotension:
  systolic BP ≤ 90 mmHg
• Chest pain
• Heart failure
• Impaired consciousness
• Rate ≥ 200 b.p.m.

No

Yes

Sedation

Choose from:
• Esmolol: 40 mg over 1 min
  + infusion 4 mg min⁻¹
  (i.v. injection can be repeated with
  increments of infusion
  to 12 mg min⁻¹)
• Digoxin: max dose
  500 µg over 30 min × 2
• Verapamil: 5–10 mg i.v.
• Amiodarone: 300 mg over 1 h
• overdrive pacing (not AF)

Synchronized
cardioversion
100 J; 200J; 360 J

Amiodarone 300 mg
over 15 min then
300 mg over 1 h
preferably by
central line and
repeat cardioversion

Notes: *Vagal manoeuvres include the Valsalva manoeuvre, and carotid sinus massage (performed unilaterally and only after a carotid bruit has been excluded).*
β-blockade after verapamil may result in AV node standstill.

Reprinted from *Resuscitation*, Volume 37, 1998 with permission from Elsevier Science.

CARDIAC ASSESSMENT
Ruth Spencer

The high prevalence of cardiac disease in the general population makes peri-operative cardiac morbidity the leading cause of death following anaesthesia and surgery. Accurate assessment allows the identification of high-risk patients who will need further investigations and optimization of their treatment prior to surgery. Assessment will also allow planning for appropriate monitoring, senior surgical and anaesthetic personnel and the provision of high dependency or intensive care postoperatively. In addition to ischaemic heart disease and valvular problems, an increasing number of patients with corrected congenital heart defects now survive into adult life and present for surgery. Preoperative investigations should be limited to those that will alter case management.

History

Hypertension is common and usually without symptoms. A record of the blood pressure (BP) over a few months is more reliable than a single admission level. Angina which is unstable and limits functional activity is more significant than stable angina. Twenty-five per cent of myocardial infarctions may be silent, a feature especially common in diabetes. Symptoms of arrhythmias, left or right cardiac failure, cerebrovascular and peripheral vascular disease should be sought. Drug history and current treatment may indicate the severity of the disease especially if there has been a recent escalation in therapy.

Previous cardiac investigations should be noted and the need for antibiotic prophylaxis considered.

Examination

Signs of persistent hypertension, right or left heart failure, valvular lesions and peripheral vascular disease should be sought. Even in the hands of experienced physicians, clinical findings do not correlate well with measured haemodynamic parameters.

Investigations

The medical history and examination alone may underestimate the severity of coronary artery disease and left ventricular function. Further evaluation is needed to determine cardiac reserve prior to the haemodynamic stresses imposed by surgery.

1. ECG. A 12 lead ECG should be recorded routinely in those over a given age (e.g. 60 years, according to local protocols) and in younger patients with known cardiac disease, diabetes, hyperlipidaemia, heavy smokers or a strong family history. Twenty-four hour ambulatory ECG monitoring demonstrates that the majority of ischaemic ST depression is silent and its presence correlates with the likelihood of developing peri-operative ischaemia. It also allows detection of arrhythmias such as premature ventricular beats, which are predictive of serious pathology if frequent, multi-focal or 'R on T'. Temporary pacing may be required. Episodes of VT or VF indicate severe myocardial pathology. ECG stress testing assesses functional capacity and may be done by exercise or by dobutamine. Positive test results include ST depression of greater than 0.2 mV, little increase in BP or heart rate or the development of hypotension and may be an indication for further investigation.

2. CXR.   70% of patients with radiological evidence of cardiomegaly have an ejection fraction of less than 50%. Other abnormalities to be excluded are pulmonary oedema, thoracic or ventricular aneurysms and valvular calcification.

3. *Echocardiography.*   Two-dimensional ECHO allows dynamic assessment of the heart including left ventricular function, abnormal wall motion and direction of blood flow via colour flow doppler. It provides estimates of ventricular volumes, ejection fraction (EF) and the gradient across stenotic valves. Stress echocardiography using dobutamine can be used to demonstrate cardiac reserve pre-operatively. Transoesophageal ECHO provides superior images with reduced image degradation and less interference from bone, fat and lung. It can provide a continuous view of heart function during anaesthesia and surgery.

4. *Nuclear imaging.*   A MUGA scan (multi-gated acquisition) obtained by IV injection of technetium[99] demonstrates volumes and dimensions of the ventricles, the amplitude and synchronicity of contractions and areas of regional dysfunction. Technetium[99] is also taken up by acutely infarcted tissue and then appears as 'hot spots'.

Dipyridamole/thallium scanning relies on thallium being taken up by myocardial tissue in proportion to the degree of perfusion. Underperfused areas appear as 'cold spots'. Dipyridamole induces coronary artery vasodilatation, dilating normal coronary arteries more than atherosclerotic vessels, creating a steal syndrome. Two thallium scans are taken at 0 and 2 hours. Redistributed thallium (a defect on the first image which fills on the second) indicates hypoperfused myocardium whereas a fixed defect indicates nonviable myocardium. Such areas of hypoperfusion strongly correlate with a high risk of myocardial ischaemia peri-operatively.

5. *MRI scanning.*   The development of ultra fast imaging sequences has made MRI an accurate, non-invasive test providing high-resolution, three-dimensional images that can also be combined with dobutamine stress testing. Its real strength is the potential to encompass cardiac anatomy, function, perfusion, metabolism and coronary angiography in a single test that may make it cost-effective.

6. *Angiography.*   This remains the 'gold standard' despite the associated morbidity and mortality. It allows insertion of stents and balloon angioplasty as well as defining coronary anatomy and pressures prior to bypass grafting.

Risk factors

In 1996 the American College of Cardiology developed guidelines for the perioperative cardiovascular evaluation of non cardiac surgery. A set of clinical indicators for increased perioperative risk and stratified risk for non cardiac surgery was established. This index may supersede that of Goldman (1977, modified by Detsky in 1986).

1. *Major risk factors*
- The presence of cardiac failure.
- Recent myocardial infarction (within six months).
- Significant arryhthmias.
- Severe valvular heart disease.
- Unstable or severe angina.

2. *Intermediate risk factors*
- Mild angina.
- Previous myocardial infarction (greater than six months previously).
- Diabetes.
- Previous coronary surgery.

3. *Minor risk factors*
- Advanced age.
- Abnormal ECG (e.g. rhythm other than sinus).
- History of stroke.
- Uncontrolled hypertension.

The major surgical contributions to potential cardiac complications are: duration of surgery, blood loss, volume shifts, violation of visceral cavities, loss of thermo-regulation and the type of surgery involved (vascular surgery being high risk).

Further reading

Belzberg H, Rivkind AI. Preoperative cardiac preparation. *Chest*, 1999; **115:** 82s–95s.
Juste RN, Lawson AD, Soni N. Minimising cardiac risk. *Anaesthesia*, 1996; **51:** 255–62.

Related topics of interest

Cardiac arrhythmias (p. 50); Cardiac ischaemia (p. 58); Cardiac pacemakers (p. 62); Cardiac surgery (p. 65); Cardiac valvular disease (p. 67); Cardioversion (p. 70); Preoperative preparation (p. 209); Vascular surgery (p. 273)

CARDIAC ISCHAEMIA
Kay Chidley

Coronary artery disease is the most common cause of premature death in the UK. Its cause is unknown but a number of reversible risk factors including smoking, hypertension and hyper-cholesterolaemia, have been identified. Coronary artery disease is common in the surgical population with up to 30% of perioperative complications and 50% of postoperative deaths being due to a primary cardiac event. Overall about 4% of patients suffer serious perioperative cardiac morbidity following non-cardiac surgery.

Reducing the incidence of perioperative myocardial ischaemia is associated with a significant reduction in adverse cardiac outcome during the hospital admission and for up to 2 years afterwards.

Pathology

An atheromatous plaque causes stenosis of a coronary artery lumen sufficient to reduce blood flow to the heart resulting in myocardial ischaemia. Plaque rupture results in a focus for platelet aggregation and the formation of a thrombus. Complete occlusion of the lumen will result in irreversible muscle damage and the patient will sustain a myocardial infarction due to lack of muscle perfusion. When myocardial oxygen demand exceeds supply the imbalance will result in myocardial ischaemia.

Myocardial oxygen supply is determined by arterial oxygen saturation, coronary blood flow and myocardial oxygen extraction. Coronary blood flow depends on the difference between diastolic blood pressure and left ventricular end diastolic pressure (LVEDP). Oxygen demand is determined by heart rate, wall tension (dependent on LVEDP and systolic BP), muscle mass and contractility.

Coronary blood flow at 250 ml/min occurs mainly in diastole. Myocardial oxygen consumption (on a tissue weight basis) is high even at rest (10 ml/100 mg/min) and, despite an oxygen extraction ratio of 75%, any increased demand can only be met by an increase in flow.

Problems

1. Coexisting morbidities such as diabetes mellitus and peripheral vascular disease.
2. Other factors that may influence myocardial oxygen supply such as haematocrit, blood flow, coronary collateral blood flow and lung disease.
3. Anaesthesia and surgery may alter the myocardial supply:demand ratio with an increase in sympathetic nervous system output especially when in pain and/or cold, precipitating arrhythmias.
4. The patient may already be taking a number of drugs setting the scene for drug interactions.

Anaesthetic management

1. Preoperative risk stratification. A patient's cardiac risk should be defined before deciding when and how to proceed with surgery as identification of risk factors may then enable perioperative interventions which improve outcome.

The degree of haemodynamic change is a major determinant of surgery-specific stress and outcome i.e. major vascular operations are associated with an increased cardiac morbidity and mortality due to the significant haemodynamic stresses accompanying these operations.

2. *Preoperative therapy.* Evidence for the prophylactic use of β-blockers to reduce myocardial ischaemia is compelling.

Perioperative β-blockers are the only drugs found to reduce myocardial ischaemia, non-fatal cardiac events and mortality, reducing short- and long-term cardiac complications. They reduce the amount of silent ischaemia as well as producing favourable intraoperative haemodynamic effects. The anti-ischaemic mechanism of β-blockers is related to a reduction in heart rate and myocardial contractility, reducing myocardial oxygen consumption. They also have anti-arrhythmic properties. β-blockers should be considered in all high-risk patients undergoing non-cardiac surgery. They should be started 2 weeks before surgery and continued in the postoperative period.

α-blockers may also limit perioperative ischaemia. They act by reducing sympathetic output causing mild sedation as well as a reduction in heart rate and blood pressure.

Control of arrhythmias, which usually occur secondary to electrolyte disturbances, should be achieved prior to surgery.

Appropriate metabolic control is also important in reducing the incidence of perioperative ischaemia. Perioperative normoglycaemia in diabetics and maintenance of normothermia during and after surgery in all patients improve cardiac outcome.

3. *Anaesthetic technique.* Aims include:
- The maintenance or improvement of the oxygen supply:demand ratio.
- Avoiding extremes of blood pressure (hypertension increases oxygen demand and hypotension reduces coronary flow).
- Avoidance of tachycardia (increases oxygen demand and reduces myocardial perfusion time).
- Avoidance of a high preload which increases LVEDP and also oxygen demand.

Routine monitoring is instituted and invasive monitoring, ST segment trend analysis and transoesophageal echocardiography considered. Evidence does not support the use of pulmonary artery flotation catheters and invasive haemodynamic monitoring to reduce perioperative morbidity and mortality in non-cardiac surgery, although this is controversial. Those patients achieving a high cardiac output and oxygen delivery have an improved outcome, often obtained by administration of fluids and maintaining a normal haemoglobin alone. The benefit of using inotropic support to reach these end-points is less clear.

Debate exists regarding the choice of regional or general anaesthesia for high-risk patients. Advocates of regional anaesthesia propose a greater reduction in the stress response to surgery, but general anaesthesia using volatile agents may be equally efficacious. Animal experiments suggest that volatile anaesthetic agents have cardio-protective effects that may aid the recovery of ischaemic myocardium. Ischaemia may follow regional anaesthesia with hypotension and excess use of vasoactive drugs or an inadequate block permitting pain postoperatively. However, effective regional anaesthesia will reduce preload, improve peripheral circulation and decrease sympathetic stimulation in the postoperative period.

For general anaesthesia, pre-oxygenation is followed by the slow administration of a titrated dose of induction agent as the arm–brain circulation time may be prolonged. Increases in sympathetic stimulation at induction, tracheal intubation, skin incision, and extubation may produce unacceptable cardiovascular instability. Administration of high-inspired concentrations of volatile agents may also increase sympathetic activity. The pressor response to intubation should be controlled. Isoflurane is probably the best volatile agent to use in these patients as it causes minimal myocardial depression, increases coronary flow, decreases afterload by systemic vasodilatation, with little effect on baroreceptors and almost no sensitization to catecholamines. Despite the theoretical risk of coronary steal, isoflurane does not appear to cause any more ischaemic episodes than other agents. Intraoperative infusions of ultra-short acting opioids offer an alternative means of controlling sympathetic stimulation during general anaesthesia.

Intraoperative ischaemia should be promptly treated with 100% oxygen and normalization of cardiovascular parameters using GTN, β-blockers and fluids. Provision for HDU/ITU care should be considered.

4. Postoperative care. Postoperative ischaemia and myocardial infarction have a peak incidence at 48 hours. This ischaemia is silent in 90% of cases, occurs in the early hours of the morning, is not associated with a tachycardia and does not appear to be a simple supply and demand phenomenon.

Inflammatory responses occurring during surgery continue into the postoperative period. There may be an increase in sympathetic nervous system activation following extubation or as a result of inadequate postoperative analgesia. There may be a role for α_2-agonists in the postoperative period.

5. Treatment of myocardial ischaemia. Suspicion should be high in the postoperative period. Oxygen administration for five days and nights postoperatively decreases the frequency of ischaemic episodes in high-risk groups. The diagnosis of an acute MI in the postoperative period is made on the history, ECG changes, a rise in the creatinine kinase (MB fraction) or troponin I. Measurement of troponin I is likely to be a more accurate indicator than creatinine kinase following surgery as it is not influenced by muscle damage.

Short-term therapy should be the same as standard medical practice with the exception of thrombolytic therapy which may be contraindicated depending on the nature of the surgery. Cautious heparinization is usually acceptable. Intravenous GTN, beta- and calcium channel blockers should be used to control abnormal haemodynamics. Abnormal cardiac rhythms should be managed with antiarrhythmic agents such as amiodarone. ACE inhibitors are of clear benefit if left ventricular function is impaired.

Antiplatelet agents such as inhibitors of the glycoprotein IIb–IIIa receptor are an effective strategy in the treatment of unstable angina or non-Q wave MI. These agents inhibit platelet function by occupying the fibrinogen binding site, promoting stabilization of ruptured plaque and stopping further platelet activity thus preventing further cardiovascular events. There does not appear to be an increase in major bleeding, stroke or thrombocytopenia, so there may be a role for such agents in the postoperative period.

6.   The future.   Traditional approaches to the problem of myocardial ischaemia address the problem of myocardial oxygen balance. New cardioprotective therapies may instead reduce the metabolic, mechanical and electrophysical consequences of ischaemia. Drugs shifting the oxyhaemoglobin dissociation curve, antiplatelet drugs, inhibitors of the glycoprotein IIb–IIIa receptor, K_{ATP} channel agonists, certain volatile agents and δ_1-opioid receptor agonists may all have a future role in the prevention of perioperative ischaemia.

Further reading

Potyk DK. Perioperative assessment and management of patients with coronary artery disease. *Texas Medicine*, 2000; **96**(3): 58–66.

Warltier DC *et al.* Approaches to the prevention of perioperative myocardial ischemia. *Anesthesiology*, 2000; **92**: 253–9.

Related topics of interest

Cardiac arrhythmias (p. 50); Cardiac assessment (p. 55); Cardiac pacemakers (p. 62); Cardiac surgery (p. 65); Cardiac valvular disease (p. 67); Cardioversion (p. 70); Congenital heart disease (p. 72); Sequelae of anaesthesia (p. 232); Stress response to surgery (p. 248); Vascular surgery (p. 273)

CARDIAC PACEMAKERS

Information regarding the pacemaker must be available preoperatively and elective surgery should be deferred until it is. Pacemakers are classified using a four or five letter code. The first letter refers to the paced chamber and the second to the sensed chamber. The chamber codes are A (atrium), V (ventricle), D (dual), or O (none). The third letter signifies the pacemaker's response to sensing and may be T (triggered), I (inhibited), D (dual), or O (none). The fourth letter refers to pacemaker programmability and the fifth to anti-tachyarrhythmia functions such as cardioversion. The most common mode in use is VVI.

Problems

- Induction of anaesthesia may alter pacemaker function.
- Surgical diathermy may alter pacemaker function (e.g. by mimicking arrhythmias).
- Diathermy currents may be conducted down the pacemaker lead(s) and result in destruction of the control unit, myocardial burns with a subsequent increase is threshold potential, or may even be fatal.

Assessment

The indication for cardiac pacing should be sought together with the classification of the unit implanted. An ECG with a rhythm strip should be examined to determine whether there is an intrinsic cardiac rhythm or if the patient is pacemaker dependent. A CXR will reveal the position of the pacemaker and its lead(s). An over-penetrated radiograph may also reveal the make and type of unit implanted.

Conversion of VVI pacemakers to a fixed rate (VOO) may be achieved by placing a magnet over the control box (usually found subcutaneously in the axilla or infra-clavicular region). This will render it less susceptible to electrical interference per-operatively. Such a manoeuvre will, however, place a growing number of pro-grammable pacemakers in to a mode that permits reprogramming of the unit, thus making them more susceptible to external stimuli.

Peroperative management

Peroperative cardiac monitoring is essential. A modern ECG monitor will filter diathermy noise and permit continuous monitoring of pacemaker function. Patients with pacemakers in situ are likely to have abnormal cardiac haemodynamic function as well as conduction deficiencies. The use of a pulmonary artery catheter should be dictated by the patient's cardiac function but the benefits must be weighed against the risk of inducing ventricular tachyarrhythmias in a susceptible heart. The pacemaker lead system may be dislodged during insertion of the catheter. Strict maintenance of the intravascular volume will optimize cardiac function and a lower threshold for CVP monitoring may be adopted. Antibiotic prophylaxis against endocarditis should be considered.

Induction of anaesthesia may depress cardiac conduction and result in the triggering of a previously inhibited pacemaker. Muscular contractions at induction may be sensed by a pacemaker and cause inappropriate inhibition resulting in asystolic episodes in a patient without intrinsic rhythm.

Volatile agents raise the stimulation threshold and may do so to a level resulting in loss of capture. Hypercarbia, hypoxaemia, and high concentrations of volatile agents all predispose to ventricular extrasystoles or tachyarrhythmias which may result in competition between the intrinsic rhythm and the pacemaker. A ventilated, low dose volatile anaesthetic technique is thus recommended.

Surgical diathermy may produce continuous interference of sufficient intensity during the pacemaker's sampling (refractory) phase as to reset its refractory period continuously resulting in asynchronous pacing. The use of bipolar diathermy should be encouraged whenever possible. If unipolar diathermy must be used, the indifferent electrode should be placed as far from the heart as possible in a position that will ensure current flow is not across the chest. Some software-driven pacemakers may completely dump their programmes after sensing diathermy interference. Under these circumstances surgery with the use of diathermy should take place with an external pacer attached to the patient or a pacemaker technician in attendance that is capable of reprogramming the pacemaker very quickly.

Atrial systole occurring during ventricular systole results in cannon waves, poor ventricular filling and hypotension. This is known as the pacemaker syndrome. In the event of pacemaker failure in a patient without intrinsic rhythm, atropine has no effect and isoprenaline is the drug of choice in resuscitation. If direct current cardioversion is required shocks should be given at 90° to the pacing wire.

Transcutaneous electrical nerve stimulator (TENS) devices should not be used for analgesia.

The patient's pacemaker clinic should be informed that they have undergone a procedure involving the use of diathermy and pacemaker function should be checked.

Indications for temporary peroperative pacing

The indications for this are broader than those for permanent pacing. They include:

- Sinus node disease.
- Mobitz type II second degree heart block.
- Third degree heart block.
- Unexplained recurrent syncope.
- Trifasicular heart block.
- Bifasicular heart block associated with symptoms.

Asymptomatic first-degree heart block and Mobitz type I (Wenckebach) second-degree block do not require pacing. The latter is usually only seen in healthy people below the age of 30 years.

Automatic implantable cardioverter defibrillators (AICDs)

Survivors of cardiac arrest due to ventricular tachyarrhythmias (the most common rhythm for adults to arrest in) have a 40% chance of re-arresting within 2 years.

AICDs are more efficacious than best pharmacological antiarrhythmic therapy at preventing death from secondary arrests. With advancing technological developments that mean thoracotomy is no longer required for their insertion, increasing numbers of patients will present for non-cardiac surgery with an AICD in situ. As with pacemakers, an assessment of the patient's cardiac function is essential. In general, AICDs should be deactivated prior to surgery as they can discharge inappropriately following the detection of extraneous signals such as myopotentials (shivering), fasiculations (suxamethonium) or surgical diathermy. AICDs being implanted currently may have the facility to selectively deactivate the antitachy-cardia mode, leaving the pacing/antibradycardia function intact. No adjustments in the performance of cardiopulmonary resuscitation are necessary in patients with an AICD in situ. Personnel administering chest compressions may experience a mild electric shock if the arrest is due to VT or VF as the unit discharges but this poses no risk. Internal defibrillation may damage the AICD.

The use of TENS machines is contraindicated in these patients as they may lead to the inappropriate delivery of shocks.

Further reading

Anderson C, Madsen GM. Rate-responsive pacemakers and anaesthesia. *Anaesthesia*, 1990; **45**: 472–476.
Kam PCA. Anaesthetic management of a patient with an automatic implantable cardioverter defibrillator *in situ*. *British Journal of Anaesthesia*, 1997; **78**: 102–106.

Related topics of interest

Cardiac arrhythmias (p. 50); Cardiac assessment (p. 55); Diathermy (p. 92)

CARDIAC SURGERY
Peter Berridge

Successful cardiac surgery depends on good communication between cardiologists, surgeons, anaesthetists, perfusionists and ITU staff. Approximately 40 000 cardiac procedures were carried out in the NHS in 1997/98, with a mortality rate of 4%. Patients presenting for cardiac surgery are increasingly older, with multi-organ disease and may be undergoing revision surgery. Smoking, obesity, diabetes, hypertension, cerebrovascular, renal and lung disease are common.

Problems

1. *Cardiac.* Ventricular dysfunction, secondary to ischaemic or mechanical disease, leading to perioperative haemodynamic instability should be anticipated. Optimal preload, afterload, contractility, rhythm and rate vary according to the disease process(es) involved.

2. *Cerebral.* Neurological complications increase with age and may be related to the degree of hypotension (not pump flow rate) or rate of rewarming. Minor neuro-behavioural changes are common. Major cerebrovascular events may occur due to emboli (air, clots, aortic plaques), poor O_2 delivery or hypocarbia. Transoesophageal echocardiography (TOE) or epiaortic scanning to detect aortic plaques prior to instrumentation and alpha-stat pH strategy for the management of blood gas results may reduce complication rates.

3. *Renal.* Pre-operative dysfunction is the biggest risk factor for postoperative renal impairment. Haemodynamic disturbance, embolization, nephrotoxins and a direct effect of extra-corporeal circulation may contribute. Fluid load from the bypass pump prime and potassium load from cardioplegia make the maintenance of renal output imperative.

4. *Pulmonary.* Sternotomy, surgical manipulation, potential pneumothorax, fluid loads/shifts and bypass may adversely affect pulmonary function.

5. *Cardiopulmonary bypass (CPB).* Cannulae are inserted at various sites (central or femoral). The circuit consists of venous drainage, a pump, an oxygenator, a heat exchanger and arterial return. It is primed with about 2 l of fluid causing haemodilution to haematocrits of 0.2–0.25. Priming the lines with blood may be undertaken for paediatric surgery. Volatile anaesthetics may be added to the circuit to maintain unconsciousness. CPB alters the pharmacokinetics of drugs, causes trauma to blood components and initiates a systemic inflammatory response. It may be pulsatile or non-pulsatile.

6. *Temperature.* Body cooling reduces cellular oxygen requirements (50% normal at 28°C), protecting organs from hypoperfusion damage. Cold cardioplegia (using potassium-rich solutions) protects the myocardium and arrests the heart in diastole. Rewarming is associated with a risk of awareness, increased blood coagulability, electrolyte instability and haemodynamic lability.

7. *'Fast-tracking'.* The pressure on and cost of intensive care resources has prompted the drive towards 'fast-tracking'. Minimally invasive procedures and surgery without CPB using modified anaesthetic techniques in selected patients may allow early extubation and the avoidance of post-operative ITU admission.

Anaesthetic management

1. Assessment and premedication. The symptoms and signs of cardiovascular and related disease are sought. Investigations include angiography, echocardiography, radioisotope imaging, MRI, arterial blood gases and respiratory function tests. Pre-operative drug therapy is continued (except aspirin and anti-coagulants). An anxiolytic may be prescribed.

2. Conduct of anaesthesia. The aim is to minimize perioperative myocardial ischaemia by maintaining oxygen supply–demand balance in the face of intense surgical stimulation. The patient is transferred to the operating theatre breathing supplementary oxygen. Intravenous access and direct arterial pressure monitoring are established (a radial artery may be needed as a graft). Following pre-oxygenation, anaesthesia is induced. The choice of anaesthetic drugs is less important than the manner of use. A CVP line, urinary catheter, temperature probes and occasionally a pulmonary artery catheter or transoesophageal echocardiography probe are inserted. The use of a thoracic epidural is controversial but may provide stress response attenuation, cardiac sympathetic blockade and intense post-operative analgesia. Concern arises over epidural haematoma formation. After anticoagulation with heparin (3 mg/kg), CPB is usually established and the patient may be cooled. Activated clotting time is measured to ensure adequate anticoagulation throughout. Ventilation is then stopped. Drugs may be used to manipulate heart rate, contractility and vascular tone pharmacologically. At the end of the procedure the patient is weaned from CPB. This may necessitate inotropic support or intra-aortic balloon pump counterpulsation. Anticoagulation is reversed with protamine. Epicardial pacing wires and a left atrial pressure line may be left in situ.

3. Postoperatively. The timing of extubation varies between units and patients. Criteria include stable cardiovascular system (rhythm, cardiac output), core temperature >36°C, adequate gas exchange, minimal bleeding and a neurologically appropriate patient.

Further reading

Lampa M, Ramsay J. Anaesthetic implications of new surgical approaches to myocardial revascularization. In: Biebuyck JF, Van Aken H, eds. *Current Opinion in Anaesthesiology*, 1999; **12:** 3–8.

Ross S, Foex P. Protective effects of anaesthetics in reversible and irreversible ischaemia-reperfusion injury. *British Journal of Anaesthesia*, 1999; **82:** 622–632.

Related topics of interest

Cardiac assessment (p. 55); Cardiac pacemakers (p. 62); CPR (p. 75); Stress response to surgery (p. 248); Temperature – hypothermia (p. 255)

CARDIAC VALVULAR DISEASE

Patients presenting for non-cardiac surgery may have valvular heart disease. Valvular lesions alter cardiac haemodynamics resulting in symptoms and signs. Longstanding valvular heart disease of any severity results in morphological and functional changes in the heart. The heart requires an adequate returning supply of blood (preload) and a 'normal' resistance to pump against (afterload) to pump efficiently. In addition, heart rate affects the adequacy of diastolic filling. An abnormal valve may result in hypertrophy, dilation or alteration in contractility of related chambers. Myocardial tissue oxygenation depends on the balance between the supply and the utilization of O_2 (see cardiac surgery). Valvular heart disease may alter this balance. The aim of anaesthetic management of patients with valvular heart disease is firstly to ensure that heart rate and haemodynamic parameters are optimized preoperatively and secondly to select an anaesthetic technique that will result in the least disturbance of this optimized state.

Prior to elective surgery severely diseased valves may need replacement. Valvular disease carries an increased risk of infective endocarditis and prophylaxis should always be given. Invasive monitoring including direct arterial blood pressure, a CVP and pulmonary artery catheter may be required regardless of the nature of the proposed surgery.

Aortic stenosis

The commonest aetiology is degenerative (calcification and fibrosis), others include congenital, rheumatic, or bicuspid valve calcification. The onset of dyspnoea, angina and syncopal attacks imply advanced disease with a risk of sudden death. The risk of death is greatest in those with associated heart failure. A slow rising pulse of low pressure is found with concentric left ventricular hypertrophy and a systolic ejection murmur, maximal in the 2nd right intercostal space and radiating to the neck. The ECG and CXR confirm cardiac hypertrophy. Echocardiography may demonstrate the abnormal valve, estimate the pressure gradient across it, the ventricular ejection fraction and the impaired compliance. The cardiac output is 'fixed' with the blood pressure being proportional to the SVR. Perioperatively, preload is maintained to ensure adequate atrial and ventricular filling while the SVR must not be allowed to fall or severe hypotension may occur. Sinus rhythm, with atrial systole assisting in filling the poorly compliant ventricle, must be maintained. Bradycardia and tachycardia are avoided to optimize myocardial oxygenation and ventricular filling. Regional techniques that decrease afterload are relatively contraindicated.

Aortic regurgitation

This can occur with rheumatic heart disease, infective endocarditis, syphilis, seronegative arthropathies, Marfan's syndrome and trauma. The regurgitant valve leads to ventricular overload and symptoms develop when the myocardium is damaged. Dyspnoea, a wide pulse pressure with a collapsing pulse, left ventricular hypertrophy, an early diastolic murmur and a quiet second heart sound are found. A systolic flow murmur and a diastolic Austin Flint murmur may also occur. ECG, echocardiography and CXR reflect hypertrophic dilation of the left ventricle. The percentage of blood that regurgitates into the ventricle depends on the pressure across the valve, the size of the defect in the valve and the diastolic time. Bradycardia allows more time for blood to regurgitate. Preload must be maintained while an increase in afterload, myocardial depression and bradycardia are avoided. Vasodilators, inotropes and chronotropic agents may be needed. If cardiomegaly and failure are present, invasive monitoring, including a pulmonary artery catheter, is recommended.

Mitral stenosis

This almost exclusively follows rheumatic heart disease although the typical history may not be found in 30%. The effects of the stenotic valve may remain static or may progress. Blood flow from the left atrium to the left ventricle is obstructed leading to an increase in left atrial pressure and size, and this may lead to pulmonary hypertension and RVH. Dyspnoea and pulmonary oedema develop. Haemoptysis, fatigue, palpitations and recurrent bronchitis are common. Atrial systole is important for left ventricular filling and 'decompensation' may occur if sinus rhythm is acutely lost (atrial fibrillation occurs in 40%). Anticoagulation is often used as there is a high risk of systemic emboli. Evidence of a low systemic cardiac output (due to chronic underfilling of the left ventricle) with right ventricular failure may be found. An opening snap is followed by a diastolic murmur (the length is proportional to the severity) and there is a loud first heart sound. Presystolic accentuation may occur when in sinus rhythm. The ECG may show atrial fibrillation, p-mitrale and right ventricular hypertrophy. The CXR may demonstrate a calcified valve, left atrial enlargement and signs of pulmonary volume overload. Preload should be maintained to maximize ventricular filling, although diuretic therapy may result in pre-operative hypovolaemia. As cardiac output is 'fixed', the systemic blood pressure becomes proportional to the SVR. Tachycardia must be prevented (digoxin and β-blockade) to allow adequate diastolic time for ventricular filling. Although LV function is normal, RV function may not be and this may necessitate invasive monitoring. Inotropes and pulmonary vasodilators may be required to assist RV function. Hypoxia causing pulmonary vasoconstriction must be avoided.

Mitral regurgitation

Rheumatic heart disease, mitral valve prolapse and dilation of the mitral ring with LVH may all result in chronic mitral regurgitation. Papillary muscle damage following an infarct or bacterial endocarditis may cause acute mitral regurgitation. It may be associated with mitral stenosis in the chronic state. Regurgitation results in left atrial enlargement which may progress to pulmonary congestion, hypertension and right ventricular failure with the anticipated symptoms and signs. Volume overload of the left ventricle results in dilation and hypertrophy. The soft first heart sound is followed by a pansystolic murmur which radiates to the axilla. A third heart sound may be present due to the large volume of blood entering the left ventricle.

The ECG may show LVH and p-mitrale. Large V waves may be seen on the pulmonary catheter trace. The percentage of blood regurgitated depends on the pressure gradient across the valve, the size of the defect, the heart rate and the SVR. Bradycardia and a raised SVR will increase the regurgitation. Anaesthesia is well tolerated unless pulmonary hypertension has developed. A mild tachycardia, systemic and pulmonary vaso-dilatation and inotropic support may be needed.

Infective endocarditis

This may be acute or subacute. Abnormal valves (congenital or acquired) predispose to infection with *Streptococcus viridans* or more rarely with *Haemophilus influenzae, Staphylococcus aureus, Streptococcus faecalis,* Coxiellae or fungi. Infection often follows surgical procedures, particularly dental. Lethargy and a low-grade fever are associated with the symptoms and signs of mitral or aortic incompetence. Infective emboli or immune complex emboli may cause cerebral abscesses, splinter haemorrhages, or renal impairment. Diagnosis is clinical and is confirmed with blood cultures and echocardiography. High-dose antibiotics are given for six weeks after sensitivities are known (if possible). Surgical replacement of a damaged valve may be needed. This may have to occur during the acute illness due to severe valve destruction resulting in cardiac failure, but carries a high mortality.

Prophylaxis for those at risk undergoing surgical procedures under general anaesthesia should be amoxicillin 1 g i.v. at induction with 500 mg oral given six hours later. Alternatively 3 g may be given orally both before and after the procedure. For patients at special risk (prosthetic valve or previous endocarditis) gentamicin 120 mg i.v. at induction is added to the above regimen. If patients are penicillin-allergic or have received more than one dose of penicillin in the previous month then vancomycin, teicoplanin or clindamycin may be given.

The British National Formulary gives regimens and should be consulted.

Further reading

British National Formulary 40. BMJ Publishing, September 2000.
Hwang NC, Sinclair M. *Cardiac anaesthesia.* Oxford University Press, Oxford, 1997.

Related topics of interest

Cardiac arrhythmias (p. 50); Cardiac assessment (p. 55); Cardiac ischaemia (p. 58); Cardiac pacemakers (p. 62); Cardiac surgery (p. 65); Congenital heart disease (p. 72); Hypertension (p. 131); Vascular surgery (p. 273)

CARDIOVERSION

Dave Pogson

Cardioversion is a common minor procedure performed electively or as an emergency. It is most often performed to convert atrial fibrillation (AF), which affects 1 in 40 patients in the general population. The risk of stroke in patients with AF is increased fivefold. Warfarin reduces this risk by two-thirds, but significantly increases the risk of intracranial haemorrhage. If AF is present for a year or more the chance of successful cardioversion is much less.

Cardiac arrhythmias are converted to sinus rhythm by DC countershock. The current causes a proportion of myocardial cells to depolarize. These cells then enter the recovery phase of the cardiac cycle and the sinoatrial node is then able to regain control as the pacemaker. Cardioversion results in improved LV ejection fraction and exercise capacity and greatly reduces the risk of stroke. Sedation and analgesia are required for the procedure, which can be painful.

The patient may present electively or *in extremis* with a full stomach. A short period of anaesthesia is required with rapid emergence, avoiding myocardial depression. Successful cardioversion is more likely if acidaemia and hypokalaemia are corrected and the transthoracic impedance, caused by the chest wall and lungs, is minimized. Transthoracic impedance varies from 10 to 150 ohms and as little as 4% of the charge energy may traverse the heart. Less energy is required to cardiovert atrial arrhythmias than those affecting the ventricles but 200 J increases success to 80% from 50% at 50 J.

Indications for cardioversion

1. Ventricular tachycardia.
2. Atrial flutter.
3. Wolf–Parkinson–White arrhythmias.
4. Supraventricular tachycardia with failed therapy.
5. Atrial fibrillation. (a) Onset less than 1 year.
   (b) With systemic emboli.
   (c) After failed drug therapy.
   (d) After treated thyrotoxicosis or cardiac surgery.

Beta blockade, hypokalaemia, digoxin toxicity or inadequate anticoagulation are relative contraindications.

1. Problems
- The patient may have a history of cardiac disease including recent myocardial infarction, ventricular failure and angina.
- The patient may present in incipient cardiovascular collapse, with a full stomach.
- The procedure is often performed in a remote site.

Anaesthetic management

1. Assessment and premedication.
A history of cardiovascular disease should be elicited. Clinical examination may reveal cardiac failure. ECG and CXR may help to assess ventricular enlargement and pulmonary oedema. Serum potassium should be within normal limits. Elective cases should be adequately anticoagulated (INR 1.6–2.5) for three weeks before and four weeks after cardioversion. The presence of

antiarrhythmic therapy such as lidocaine may increase the energy required. Monitoring should include ECG, oximetry and blood pressure. A tipping trolley and checked equipment are required. The defibrillator should be checked and staff appropriately trained. It is not usually necessary to premedicate the patient. Vagolytics have been used. Nitrate patches must be removed from the patient as they can ignite.

2.   Conduct of anaesthesia.   Preoxygenation will provide a margin of safety and maximize oxygen delivery to the heart. Rapid sequence induction and intubation will be required if the patient is not fasted. Careful titration of the induction agent is more important than the choice of agent itself. Midazolam in low dosage will not reduce cardiac output in a very sick patient, but may cause prolonged sedation. Ketamine should be avoided. Repeated boluses of barbiturate may accumulate. Etomidate is stable but may cause nausea and vomiting and adrenocortical suppression. Propofol titrated carefully combines cardiovascular stability and rapid emergence. Infusion may be more stable than repeated boluses.

The countershock should be administered once the eyelash reflex is lost, with the oxygen source removed from the patient. Transthoracic impedance is lowest at the end of expiration. The countershock should be synchronized with the R wave, but in fact the incidence of VF/VT is less than 5% when unsynchronized. Repeated shocks can be given on the same dose of induction agent. In AF the procedure should be abandoned if two 360 J shocks fail. The therapy itself does not cause persistent pain and short-acting opiates may not be needed as they may prolong recovery. Post countershock myocardial depression can occur, but is usually short-lived as restoration of sinus rhythm improves cardiac output.

3.   Postoperatively.   A rapid return of consciousness with airway reflexes is desirable. Oxygen should be administered and analgesia is occasionally necessary. Respiratory acidosis should be avoided as it may provoke arrhythmias. A trained nurse should stay with the patient until they are fully recovered.

Further reading

Bourke ME. The patient with a pacemaker or related device. *Canadian Journal of Anaesthesia* 1996; **43:** R24–41.
Stoneham M. Anaesthesia for cardioversion. *Anaesthesia* 1996; **51:** 565–570.

Related topics of interest

Cardiac arrhythmias (p. 50); Cardiac assessment (p. 55); CPR (p. 75); ECT (p. 105)

CONGENITAL HEART DISEASE

Eight per 1000 live births have a congenital heart defect (CHD). The most common being VSD (35%), ASD (9%), patent ductus arteriosus (8%), coarctation of the aorta (6%), pulmonary stenosis (8%), aortic stenosis (6%), Tetralogy of Fallot (5%), transposition of the great arteries (4%) and others (19%). Patients with CHD may present for non-cardiac procedures prior to their corrective surgery with arrhythmias, failure to thrive, heart failure or cyanosis. They may also be encountered after their cardiac surgery which may leave residual defects. The latter are most commonly encountered in obstetrics and gynaecology, dental and orthopaedic surgery.

General considerations

1. Age. Neonates or young children for initial surgery, with increasing numbers surviving into adult life.

2. Infective endocarditis. Antibiotic prophylaxis is required.

3. Balance between systemic and pulmonary vascular resistance. This may be critically altered by anaesthetic manoeuvres e.g. the cyanotic child will benefit from a decreased pulmonary vascular resistance but not a decreased SVR (e.g. regional anaesthesia). Nitric oxide may have a role as selective pulmonary vasodilator.

4. Air emboli. Increased risk of cerebral air emboli, especially if a right to left shunt is present.

5. Fluid balance. Cyanotic children and those with heart failure need careful fluid balance.

6. Speed of induction of anaesthesia. Patients with right to left shunts have a faster induction time than normal with intravenous agents and slower than normal with inhalational agents.

7. Duct patency. Lesions requiring ductus arteriosus patency may need PGE1 infusions (e.g. pulmonary outflow tract obstruction, severe coarctation and hypoplastic left heart syndrome).

8. Arrhythmias. These are common following corrective surgery.

Special considerations

1. Ventricular septal defect (VSD). Usually a perimembranous lesion causing left-to-right shunting. A small VSD presents asymptomatically as a loud pan-systolic murmur, loudest at the left sternal edge. Moderate VSDs will, in addition, cause dyspnoea and fatigue. Large VSDs lead to pulmonary hypertension causing cardiomegaly with large 'pruned' pulmonary arteries on CXR. Shunts >3:1 may lead to pulmonary pressures exceeding systemic pressures. The murmur may disappear as the right and left pressures equate. If the shunt reverses becoming right-to-left, cyanotic Eisenmenger's syndrome will develop. Full assessment of the lesion by cardiac catheterization is followed by Dacron patching via the right ventricle using cardiopulmonary bypass. In 50% the lesion is small and will close spontaneously.

2.   *Atrial septal defect (ASD).*   Ostium primum ASD is associated with atrio-ventricular canal defects. Ostium secundum ASD is far more common, usually has a sole defect due to failure of closure of the foramen ovale. It has a higher incidence in females, is often asymptomatic but may cause dyspnoea, fatigue, atrial arrhythmias and an increase in pulmonary infections. The second heart sound has fixed splitting, with loud systolic pulmonary and diastolic tricuspid flow murmurs. The murmurs may decrease if pulmonary hypertension develops. The ECG shows right bundle branch block and right axis deviation (with ostium secundum) or left axis deviation (with ostium primum). Except for small lesions surgical correction is needed using either a primary repair or Dacron grafting via the right atrium with cardio-pulmonary bypass.

3.   *Coarctation of the aorta.*   This is more common in males, but has an association with Turner's syndrome. Eighty percent have a bicuspid aortic valve. The lesion is usually distal to the left subclavian artery. In the neonate the lesion is usually pre-ductal and may cause total aortic occlusion presenting with cardiac failure. Collateral blood vessels form via the thyrocervical trunk and retrograde flow occurs through the intercostal vessels causing rib-notching which may be seen on the CXR after the age of six. High proximal pressures cause upper body hypertension, whilst lower distal pressures decrease renal perfusion which may lead to systemic hypertension, even after correction of the lesion. A widespread mid to late systolic murmur is heard over the upper chest and back and there may be a delayed, weak femoral pulse. A different BP may be found in the left and right arms depending on the site of occlusion. Correction is via a left thoracotomy, although percutaneous balloon angioplasty under general anaesthesia is sometimes sufficient for small coarctations. Despite correction there is an increased incidence of hypertension, ischaemic heart disease, aortic valve disease, stroke and premature death.

4.   *Tetralogy of Fallot.*   The VSD, right ventricular outflow tract obstruction, overriding aorta and right ventricular hypertrophy result in cyanosis. The size of the right-to-left shunt depends on a balance between the degree of stenosis and pulmonary and systemic vascular resistances. Children present with cyanosis and dyspnoea worsened by exercise. This is relieved by squatting which increases systemic vascular resistance and hence increases pulmonary flow and decreases the venous return of desaturated blood from the legs. An ejection systolic murmur is present over the pulmonary area. The second heart sound has no splitting. Finger clubbing and polycythaemia may be present by one year. The CXR shows oligaemic lung fields and a 'boot'-shaped heart. Cardiac catheterization allows the shunt, pressures and anatomy to be defined. An early palliative systemic to pulmonary shunt (e.g. Glenn or Blalock–Taussig) does not require bypass, but later formal correction does. Correction within the first 12 months is becoming more common, and diminishes the secondary damage from chronic hypoxia.

5. *Transposition of the great arteries.* Failure of spiralling of the trunco-conal septum causes the aorta to arise from the right ventricle and pulmonary arteries from the left. This creates two independent parallel circulations that are incompatible with life unless mixing occurs via a patent ductus arteriosus, foramen ovale, VSD or ASD. It presents early in life with cyanosis and the CXR shows an 'egg'-shaped heart with plethoric lung fields. Early atrial balloon septostomy may be life saving (Rashkind procedure). Formal correction consists of switching the great vessels and re-implantation of the coronary arteries.

Further reading

Burrows FA. Anaesthetic management of the child with congenital heart disease for non-cardiac surgery. *Canadian Journal of Anaesthesia* 1992; **39:** R60–70.
Findlow D, Doyle E. Congenital heart disease in adults. *British Journal of Anaesthesia* 1997; **78:** 416–430.

Related topics of interest

Air embolism (p. 9); Cardiac surgery (p. 65); Inherited conditions (p. 136); Neonatal surgery (p. 164); Paediatric anaesthesia – practical (p. 196)

CPR

In adults the commonest primary arrhythmia at the onset of cardiac arrest is ventricular fibrillation (VF) or pulseless ventricular tachycardia. The definitive treatment of these arrhythmias – defibrillation – must be administered promptly. Survival from VF falls by 7–10% for every minute after collapse. Advanced life support (ALS) is the process that attempts to deliver the definitive treatment for the underlying rhythm. Basic life support (BLS) extends the interval between the onset of the collapse and the development of irreversible organ damage.

Basic life support

Basic life support refers to maintaining airway patency, and supporting breathing and the circulation without the use of equipment other than a protective mouth shield. It consists of the initial assessment, airway maintenance, expired air ventilation (rescue breathing) and chest compressions. Failure of the circulation to deliver oxygenated blood to the brain for 3–4 minutes (less if the patient was initially hypoxic) will lead to irreversible cerebral damage. The purpose of BLS is to maintain adequate ventilation and circulation until the underlying cause of the cardiac arrest can be treated.

During two-person CPR 5 chest compressions (rate 100 min^{-1} with 4–5 cm sternal depression) are given for each breath of 400–600 ml.

Advanced life support

A universal adult ALS treatment algorithm has been developed. After the initial assessment it divides into two pathways; arrest in VF/VT and other rhythms. Each step in the algorithm assumes that the previous step was unsuccessful. When using the algorithm it is essential to remember that early defibrillation, adequate oxygenation and ventilation through a clear airway, and chest compressions, are always more important than the administration of drugs.

Above all, *treat the patient, not the monitor.*

Defibrillation

The initial three shocks in the treatment sequence of VF/VT should be delivered at 200 J, 200 J and 360 J. Thereafter each shock should be at 360 J. If VF/VT recurs after a period of spontaneous circulation, the first and second shocks should be delivered at 200 J. Defibrillators should always be charged with the paddles held against the patient's chest wall or whilst housed in the defibrillator. They should never be charged with the paddles held in the air. The most commonly used transthoracic defibrillators deliver energy as a damped sinusoidal waveform. Newer defibrillators using a biphasic waveform reduce the energy requirement for successful defibrillation. Automated defibrillators that deliver a current based shock appropriate to the measured transthoracic impedance (impedance compensation) are also available.

Vasopressor agents

Epinephrine (adrenaline) improves myocardial and cerebral blood flow and resuscitation rates in experimental animals. There is no clinical evidence that epinephrine (adrenaline) improves neurological outcome in humans. It remains, however, the only recommended pressor agent in adult cardiac arrest. Caution should be exercised before administering adrenaline in patients whose cardiac arrest is secondary to solvent or cocaine abuse.

Antiarrhythmic drug therapy

Haemodynamically significant bradycardias should be treated with atropine. A single dose of 3 mg Iv is sufficient to block vagal activity in fit adults with a cardiac output.

There is incomplete evidence to make firm recommendations on the use of any antiarrhythmic during VF/VT. Lidocaine (lignocaine), bretylium and amiodarone all have their proponents but defibrillation remains the treatment of choice for these rhythms.

Buffer agents

If effective BLS is performed arterial blood gas analysis does not show a rapid development of acidosis during cardiopulmonary resuscitation. A prospective randomized controlled trial of the use of a buffer in patients suffering out-of-hospital cardiac arrest failed to show an improvement in outcome. The judicious use of buffers is advocated in severe acidosis (pH < 7.1, base excess < −10) and in cardiac arrest associated with hyperkalaemia or following tricyclic anti-depressant overdose.

The denervated heart

A denervated heart (as occurs following heart transplantation) is exquisitely sensitive to the actions of adenosine. Supraventricular tachyarrythmias in a denervated heart should not be treated with adenosine. In the presence of severe bradycardia that does not respond to atropine or pacing, an adenosine antagonist (e.g. aminophylline) should be considered.

Return of spontaneous circulation (ROSC)

Patients who are successfully resuscitated should be referred immediately for post resuscitation care.

Further reading

Craft TM. Post resuscitation care. *Clinical Intensive Care*, 1999; **10**: 169–173.
Robertson C *et al.* The 1998 European Resuscitation Council guidelines for adult advanced life support. *Resuscitation*, 1998; **37**: 81–90.

Related topics of interest

Cardiac arrhythmias (p. 50); Cardiac pacemakers (p. 62); Organ transplantation (p. 187)

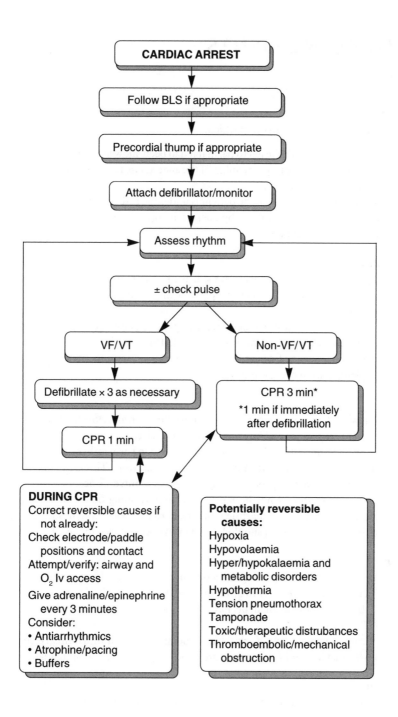

CARDIAC ARREST

↓

Follow BLS if appropriate

↓

Precordial thump if appropriate

↓

Attach defibrillator/monitor

↓

Assess rhythm

↓

± check pulse

VF/VT

Non-VF/VT

Defibrillate × 3 as necessary

CPR 3 min*

*1 min if immediately after defibrillation

CPR 1 min

DURING CPR
Correct reversible causes if not already:
Check electrode/paddle positions and contact
Attempt/verify: airway and O_2 Iv access
Give adrenaline/epinephrine every 3 minutes
Consider:
• Antiarrhythmics
• Atrophine/pacing
• Buffers

Potentially reversible causes:
Hypoxia
Hypovolaemia
Hyper/hypokalaemia and metabolic disorders
Hypothermia
Tension pneumothorax
Tamponade
Toxic/therapeutic distrubances
Thromboembolic/mechanical obstruction

CRITICAL INCIDENTS

Richard Struthers

Definition

A critical incident is an event which:

- led to or could have led to harm if it had been allowed to progress.
- involves an error by a member of the anaesthetic team or a failure of equipment to function properly.
- occurs at a time when the patient is under the care of the anaesthetist.
- is described in clear detail by a person involved in the incident.
- is clearly preventable.

Background

The study of critical incidents in medicine has developed from work in areas where there are interfaces between people, machines and the environment – especially aviation.

Systematic critical incident reporting in anaesthesia was pioneered by the Australian Incident Monitoring Study (AIMS) in the early 1990s. In the UK the Royal College of Anaesthetists introduced a system in 1998 with a view to the implementation of a national scheme.

Aim

The aim of critical incident reporting is to allow appropriate measures to be taken to prevent recurrence and improve quality of service.

By including all incidents that could have led to harm rather than those leading to morbidity or mortality the number of reports increases. This raises the possibility of uncovering errors in processes before an adverse outcome occurs.

Reporting should not be regarded as apportioning blame or criticism. While events occurring in a department may be hard to report anonymously any data sent outside the department should have identifying features removed.

Findings

In several studies reporting rates of around 30% have been found. More serious incidents are more likely to be reported than those perceived as minor.

In studies critical incidents have been reported as occurring in between 0.28 and 6.7% of anaesthetics.

Approximately 75% of critical incidents are associated with human error. It is suggested that in 30% of cases events are associated with violation of standard practice.

Prevention

The Royal College of Anaesthetists has a scale of preventibility:

- Probably preventable within current resource (e.g. failure to do a pre-op check).
- Probably preventable with reasonable extra resource (e.g. detection of oesophageal intubation by the use of a capnograph).

- Possibly preventable within current resource (e.g. pneumothorax during CVP insertion by better training and supervision).
- Possibly preventable with reasonable extra resource (e.g. an anaesthetist who is unwell might be replaced if there were more cover).
- Probably not preventable by extra resource (e.g. electricity grid failure).

If critical incident reports are studied over a period of time the reporting of those events due to hidden errors in the system of anaesthesia reduce. There is, however, no change in the rate or type of other critical incidents reported.

Further reading

Gaba D. Anaesthesiology as a model for patient safety in health care. *British Medical Journal*, 2000; **320:** 785–788.
Royal College of Anaesthetists at   http://www.rcoa.ac.uk/critincident/ciweb.html

Related topics of interest

Anaesthetic records (p. 21); Audit – national (p. 30); Ethics and duty of care (p. 115); Governance (p. 121)

DAY SURGERY

A surgical day case is a patient who is admitted for an investigation or operation on a non-resident basis but who also requires facilities for recovery. The British definition of a day case is one who does not stay overnight (other countries accept a definition that comprises less than 24 hours spent in hospital). Accurate selection of both patients and procedures is the key to safe and effective day case surgery. Once accurate selection is assured the potential benefits of day surgery may be attained. These include: lower medical costs, patient convenience and psychological benefit, reduced in-patient workload and increased hospital efficiency, staff benefits (social hours and lower staffing levels), reduced incidence of hospital-acquired infection, and early mobilization (fewer DVTs).

Potential difficulties arising from day surgery include: less time for preoperative communication and psychological preparation, limited patient and operation suitability (though the limits are constantly being expanded), a need for rapid recovery from anaesthesia, postoperative hospital admission must be possible, limited care may be available to the patient after discharge.

Selection criteria

1. Operation suitability. Surgery should be predictable and take less than 1 hour. The complication rate should be low, blood loss negligible, and postoperative pain easily controlled.

2. Patient selection. ASA I and II with medically stable ASA III patients being increasingly accepted. Age limits set at arbitrary levels are meaningless. The older the patient, however, the greater the need for a thorough assessment of medical fitness and social arrangements postoperatively. The patient should have a responsible adult to escort them home and remain with them for the first night. Their journey time should be reasonable (e.g. < 1 h), and they should live in reasonable social circumstances (sanitation, stairs, access to a telephone, etc.). Patients should be generally fit and ambulant. They should not be grossly obese (e.g. BMI > 35). Patients may be screened in the surgical clinic, an anaesthetic assessment clinic, by telephone, by postal questionnaire or on admission to confirm suitability for day surgery. No investigations are required as a matter of routine. Certain investigations may be required on establishing the patient's medical history.

Investigations

1. Haemoglobin (Hb). Studies have shown that less than 0.5% of patients are found to have a Hb less than 11 g/dl when tested routinely and those that did could have been predicted by their history. A history suggesting a risk of anaemia may include renal disease, menorrhagia, or GI blood loss.

2. ECG. Whilst some units perform an ECG on all those over a given age, others reserve them for those with a history of cardiorespiratory disease.

3. Chest X-ray. Patients thought to require a chest X-ray to assess suitability for day surgery are almost certainly not suitable. The pick up rate of clinically significant abnormalities on a chest X-ray in asymptomatic patients is extremely low.

Anaesthetic management

Premedication with small doses of anxiolytics or short-acting opioids does not delay recovery in the majority. Gastric prokinetic agents, antiemetics and H_2 antagonists should be administered to patients at high risk of postoperative nausea and vomiting and considered for all.

The patient usually walks to the anaesthetic room. Monitoring should be identical to that for in-patients.

1. Regional anaesthesia. The problems of general anaesthesia are avoided but prolonged block may delay discharge, e.g. urinary retention following caudal, spinal or epidural blocks. Individual nerve blocks and local infiltration have fewer side-effects. Intravenous sedation with propofol or midazolam may be required.

2. General anaesthesia. Short-acting agents should be used. Local anaesthetic wound infiltration may be used to provide postoperative analgesia. NSAIDs have a morphine-sparing effect and are frequently used. Suxamethonium and intubation should be avoided if possible (producing myalgia and sore throat, respectively). A regional technique may be combined with light general anaesthesia.

- *Postoperative morbidity.* Nausea and vomiting is more common in female patients, those receiving their first general anaesthetic and following prolonged procedures. The incidence varies with the agents used and the operation site. Drowsiness, headaches, sore throat, myalgia, weakness and postoperative pain are also common problems.
- *Discharge criteria.* The patient should be orientated and have stable vital signs. They should not be suffering from nausea or vomiting and they should be mobile, able to drink and to pass urine. Psychometric tests to assess recovery may be used (e.g. the critical flicker fusion threshold test or reaction timing devices). Pain must be controllable with oral medication and there should be no surgical complications. Clear instructions should accompany any analgesics given to the patient to take home. A responsible and capable adult must accompany the patient home, and care for them for 24 hours. Instructions should be given to contact the hospital in case of problems. The patient should be told to avoid alcohol, driving and using machinery for 48 hours as the time to recovery of full psychomotor function varies between individuals and the anaesthetic agents used.

Improving day care surgery

As with inpatient surgery all units undertaking day surgery should, as a matter of routine, monitor and record their effectiveness. All aspects of the episode of care should be included. This means constant monitoring of the suitability of the surgical procedures chosen for day cases, the patient selected to undergo them, the occurrence of critical incidents during the procedure, and the incidence of postoperative complications. This latter should include follow-up of the patient once they have gone home. Such follow-up should be proactive (i.e. contact the patient directly) rather than simply asking the patient to return a questionnaire once they have gone home. Attention to any shortcomings revealed by a continuous audit of practice will lead to the development of yet safer day surgical care for increasing numbers of patients undergoing an ever broadening spectrum of procedures.

It is a stated political aim of the current government to see 50% of all surgery in the UK undertaken on a day-case basis.

Further reading

Guidelines for day case surgery. Royal College of Surgeons of England. London,1992.

Millar JM, Rudkin GE, Hitchcock M. *Practical Anaesthesia and Analgesia for Day Surgery.* Oxford: BIOS, 1997.

Related topics of interest

Obesity (p. 173); Pain relief – acute (p. 199); Sequelae of anaesthesia (p. 232); Vomiting (p. 279)

DENTAL ANAESTHESIA

Despite the recommendations of the regulatory changes of the General Dental Council (GDC), each year 2 or 3 patients, usually children, die as a result of receiving general anaesthesia in the dental chair in the UK. For this to change there needs to be a cultural change amongst patients that accepts that general anaesthesia is not necessary for the vast majority of dental procedures. Dental practitioners need to stop referring patients for treatment under general anaesthesia unless there is a clear over-riding reason. Such reasons would include mental or physical handicap, absolute dental phobia, and *some* children. In such circumstances special arrangements will be necessary and the treatment will not be suitable for the dental chair. Even when carried out in a hospital setting, dental anaesthesia carries particular challenges.

The GDC have ruled that general dental anaesthesia may only be administered by those on the specialist register of the GMC as an anaesthetist.

Problems

- Those of day case anaesthesia (q.v.).
- Competition for the airway.
- Patients are often children.
- Mentally handicapped patients frequently undergo dental surgery under general anaesthesia. They may be institutionalized and pose a higher hepatitis B risk.

Techniques

1. Local anaesthesia. This is usually administered by the dental practitioner. Agents with or without adrenaline are injected into the buccal fold of the gum adjacent to the tooth to be treated. Lingual and mental nerve blocks may also be performed intraorally to provide more extensive anaesthesia to the lower incisors. Infraorbital nerve blocks will anaesthetize the upper jaw.

2. Sedation. This may be achieved with drugs administered via the following routes.

- Oral, e.g. benzodiazepines.
- Inhalational, e.g. N_2O in O_2 in concentrations from 10 to 50% (relative analgesia).
- Intravenous. Diazepam (0.1–0.2 mg/kg) is now less popular due to pain and thrombophlebitis on injection. Diazemuls is devoid of these side-effects but requires 20% more drug to achieve equipotency. It also has active metabolites and recovery may be prolonged.

  Midazolam has a half-life of 1.5–2.5 hours and is suitable for use in the dental surgery. It does, however, lower the blood pressure to a greater extent than diazemuls. Incremental methohexitone has also been used for dental sedation. Patient controlled sedation using propofol has been used successfully in the dental chair.

3. General anaesthesia.

Anaesthetic management

The same principles apply to dental anaesthesia as apply to day case anaesthesia. All sites at which dental anaesthesia is given should be equipped with resuscitation and monitoring equipment. These include an ECG monitor, pulse oximeter, automatic blood pressure machine, defibrillator and resuscitation drugs. If tracheal intubation is contemplated then means of assessing the expired CO_2 should also be provided. Members of the dental surgical team should be trained in cardiopulmonary resuscitation. Extremely anxious patients may benefit from oral premedication with a benzodiazepine.

Mentally handicapped patients provide a further challenge. Their dental hygiene is often poor. Communication with the patient may be difficult or impossible. There may be associated physical problems including a large tongue, short neck and cardiovascular abnormalities. The patient may be frightened and struggle during induction and emergence. They are often uninhibited and physically very strong.

Induction may be inhalational or intravenous. Inhalational induction is associated with a higher incidence of cardiac arrhythmias. Enflurane and isoflurane anaesthesia results in an incidence of ~10%, whilst the incidence with halothane is ~30%. It has been suggested that sevoflurane may be the inhalational agent of choice for dental anaesthesia but economic reasons prevent its widespread adoption. Episodes of airway obstruction also increase the incidence of arrhythmias. A recent viral infection with coxsackie B virus may predispose to arrhythmias in the dental chair, possibly as a result of asymptomatic myocarditis.

Intravenous lidocaine (lignocaine) (1 mg/kg) may offer some protection against arrhythmias.

Maintenance of anaesthesia during dental surgery requires the provision of a clear airway. A nasal mask may be held in place and the anaesthetist's fingers support the lower jaw. A mouth pack is inserted to prevent mouth breathing and thus lightening of anaesthesia and to prevent airway soiling. The laryngeal mask airway (LMA) has become increasingly popular for longer cases. Close co-operation between the dentist and the anaesthetist is necessary to ensure unobstructed respiration. The pharynx should be cleared of secretions and debris by suction at the end of surgery and the patient turned into a full lateral recovery position. A slight head-down tilt may be employed to ensure blood and secretions drain away from the vocal cords. Trained recovery staff must remain with the patient until they are fully conscious.

Extraction of impacted molars

This is now frequently performed on a day case basis. Tracheal intubation (whether oral or nasal) is no longer mandatory for this operation. The flexible LMA permits surgical access to the mouth whilst allowing maintenance of a clear airway. As with all day surgery, control of postoperative symptoms (pain and swelling) is essential to permit discharge of the patient. Swelling may be reduced by the intravenous administration of dexamethasone. Analgesia may be provided by intravenous opioids, antiprostenoids (NSAI), including rectal diclofenac, and infiltration with local anaesthetic agents.

The guidelines for postoperative care of those undergoing day case anaesthesia apply to patients receiving general anaesthesia in the dental chair.

Further reading

Cartwright DP. Death in the dental chair. *Anaesthesia*, 1999; **54:** 172–4.

Worthington LM, Flynn PJ, Strunnin L. Death in the dental chair: an avoidable catastrophe? *British Journal of Anaesthesia*, 1998; **80:** 131–2.

Related topics of interest

Airway surgery (p. 12); Day surgery (p. 80)

DEPTH OF ANAESTHESIA

Consciousness and unconsciousness during anaesthesia probably exist at either end of a continuum. At low brain concentrations of anaesthetic agent patients will respond to verbal commands and have explicit memory (recall) of the event. At higher concentrations patients may still recall events if given a prompt (cued conscious recognition). As concentrations increase further still, the ability for explicit memory is lost but information may still be retained as implicit memory. Such memory may only be accessed using psychological techniques (e.g. hypnosis). Finally, at adequate levels of anaesthesia neither explicit nor implicit memory is possible. Awareness during anaesthesia is a modern problem. In the mid-nineteenth century when only di-ethyl ether, N_2O and chloroform were available to induce and maintain general anaesthesia, a state of unconsciousness was reached before the surgical planes of anaesthesia. Imbalance of one or more of the components of the triad of modern anaesthesia (unconsciousness, analgesia and muscle relaxation) will predispose to awareness and recall. Such an imbalance is more likely at induction of anaesthesia and following the completion of surgery when anaesthesia may be lightened. Anaesthetic techniques which employ a high inspired concentration of O_2 in N_2O with low concentrations of volatile agent (e.g. Caesarian section under general anaesthesia) are also associated with a higher incidence of awareness. Spontaneous recall of intraoperative events may be associated with memory of pain and result in long-term post-traumatic neurosis. A patient's attitude towards an episode of recall will be considerably influenced by whether or not they were also in pain. The administration of intravenous benzodiazepines following a suspected episode of awareness does not guarantee retrograde amnesia and thus a lack of recall.

Monitoring depth of anaesthesia

1. *Clinical signs.* Guedel (1937) described signs of anaesthesia, divided into stages and planes, under spontaneously breathing ether anaesthesia.

- First stage – analgesia. From the beginning of induction to loss of consciousness. Respiration is regular, the pupils and muscle tone are normal, the eyelash reflex is lost at the end of this stage.
- Second stage – excitement. From the loss of consciousness to the onset of automatic breathing. There may be struggling, breath holding, vomiting, coughing, or swallowing. The pupils dilate and the eyelid reflex is lost.
- Third stage – surgical anaesthesia. From the onset of automatic respiration to respiratory paralysis.

  Plane 1   To the cessation of eyeball movement.
  Plane 2   To the commencement of intercostal paralysis.
  Plane 3   To the completion of intercostal paralysis.
  Plane 4   To the onset of diaphragmatic paralysis.

- Fourth stage – overdosage. From the onset of diaphragmatic paralysis to apnoea and death. All reflex activity is lost and the pupils are widely dilated.

  This classification is of limited use following intravenous induction as the third stage is rapidly reached. Premedication with opioids or anticholinergics may modify the pupil size.

2. *Clinical scoring.* Heart rate, blood pressure, and the presence or absence of sweating and lacrimation have been used in a scoring system to measure the depth of anaesthesia; the higher the score, the more lightly anaesthetized the patient.

3. *Population parameters.* Minimum alveolar concentration (MAC) has been employed as a means of predicting adequate levels of anaesthesia. As well as showing considerable interindividual variation, MAC is affected by a number of variables including age, temperature, the presence of other agents used for preoperative medication and intraoperatively, and changes in CSF sodium concentration. Minimum infusion rate (MIR) is the intravenous equivalent of MAC.

4. *Instrumental monitoring.*
- Skin conductance is a quantification of sweat gland activity and decreases with increasing depth of anaesthesia. It is affected by drugs such as atropine and anticholinesterases.
- Heart rate variability may be analysed during anaesthesia and be used to suggest trends in the depth of anaesthesia.
- Electroencephalogram (EEG). This is not widely used as a monitor of anaesthesia as it is difficult to interpret and different agents produce different effects. Cerebral function monitors (CFM) use a bi-parietal trace to produce frequency plots which provide a crude index of the EEG. The frequency and amplitude of blocks of EEG data have been subjected to Fourier analysis to produce trends in the fundamental frequencies and harmonics (CFAM). Bispectral analysis (BIS) is a technique of mathematical signal processing that quantifies the degree of phase coupling between different frequency components of an EEG signal. There is some correlation between this information and cerebral hypoxia and possibly depth of anaesthesia and BIS monitors are being assessed in clinical practice.
- Electromyograms of spontaneous activity of muscles such as the frontalis have been used to indicate depth of anaesthesia but accurate monitoring of neuromuscular blockade is essential.
- In the isolated forearm technique the forearm circulation is isolated by a tourniquet applied before muscle relaxants are given. Considerable skeletal muscle activity can be demonstrated during apparently adequate anaesthesia and indeed patients may respond to instructions to move their arm during anaesthesia. Little correlation exists, however, between patients responding to instructions and those able to recall intraoperative events in the postoperative period.
- Evoked potentials from somatosensory, auditory, and visual modalities have been studied during anaesthesia. Cortical evoked potentials are more susceptible to depression than brain stem evoked potentials as there are more synapses involved in the former. A high degree of skill is required for the interpretation of these data but middle latency auditory evoked potentials have been shown to reflect the level of anaesthesia using a wide range of drugs.
- Lower oesophageal contractility is a measure of smooth muscle activity and as such is not affected by neuromuscular blocking agents. The

frequency of contractions may correlate with the depth of anaesthesia. Spontaneous contractions are nonpropulsive and occur in the lower third of the oesophagus approximately five times per minute. Their frequency is increased by stress and suppressed by anaesthesia. Contractions may also be provoked, the amplitude of such contractions being inversely related to the depth of anaesthesia.

A parameter that relates directly to the state of consciousness of an individual has yet to be defined. A universally applicable depth of anaesthesia monitor does not therefore exist. Observing the patient's response to noxious stimuli (surgery) is still the best way of assessing depth of anaesthesia clinically.

Further reading

Heier T, Steen PA. Assessment of anaesthesia depth. *Acta Anaesthesiologica Scandinavica,* 1996; **40:** 1087–100.
Thornton C, Sharpe RM. Evoked responses in anaesthesia. *British Journal of Anaesthesia,* 1998; **81:** 771–81.

Related topics of interest

Breathing systems (p. 42); TIVA (p. 264)

DIABETES

Diabetes is a disorder of sugar metabolism resulting in a fasting plasma glucose of >7.0 mmol/l. It is associated with multi-system disease, the severity of which depends on the quality of blood sugar control and the duration of disease. The prevalence of diabetes is 2%. Diabetics with some insulin function are predominantly older and more obese (type II), whilst those with an absence of endogenous insulin are younger (type I), although there is overlap. Diabetes may also be a feature of other associated conditions. Medical management includes the control of dietary sugar intake together with weight loss in the obese. Type I patients usually require exogenous insulin whilst type II patients may often be managed with oral hypoglycaemic agents such as metformin, acarbose and sulphonylureas. Surgery is often related to the complications of diabetes, particularly sepsis, skin ulceration, and peripheral vascular disease.

Problems

1. Perioperative control of blood sugar. There is a risk of intraoperative hypoglycaemia in those taking long acting oral hypoglycaemic agents (metformin) or insulin. Equally, blood sugar control should be continued through the operative period and hyperglycaemia avoided. Inhalational anaesthetic agents increase the blood sugar. The endocrine response to hypoglycaemia (glucagon, epinephrine (adrenaline)) is reduced during anaesthesia. β-blockade may allow prolonged, undetected hypoglycaemia to occur as the signs are masked.

2. Complications of diabetes. Intensive control of blood glucose decreases microvascular complications, but not macrovascular disease or diabetes related mortality.

- Vascular disease (15–60%) – IHD and cerebrovascular complications are increased. Hypotension is poorly tolerated. Mortality rates of diabetics are twice those of non diabetics undergoing CABGs.
- Hypertension (30–60%). This is the strongest correlate of autonomic neuropathy which results in sudden tachycardia, hypotension and unexpected cardiac arrest. It also causes delayed gastric emptying, increasing the risk of aspiration. Controlling BP to less than 150/85 decreases risk of death and complications of diabetes.
- Cardiomyopathy – leading to ventricular dysfunction. Patients may require CVP or PAOP monitoring.
- Nephropathy. Glomerulonephritis and renal papillary necrosis increase the risk of acute renal failure and urinary tract infection. Microalbuminuria is a sensitive indicator of diabetic microvascular disease. ACE inhibitors delay the development of nephropathy in diabetes.
- Infection. Sepsis is a major cause of perioperative morbidity.
- Respiratory – there is a decreased FEV_1 and FVC with the onset of diabetes. Poor blood glucose control impairs pulmonary function. The incidence of chest infection and chronic obstructive airways disease is increased particularly in obese patients.

- Retinopathy. There is a risk of vitreous haemorrhage during hypertensive manoeuvres, e.g. intubation.
- Atlanto-occipital disease. Juvenile onset diabetics may have reduced neck movement making intubation difficult.

3. **Medical conditions associated with diabetes.** Hyperpituitarism, hyperthyroidism, hyperadrenalism, phaeochromocytoma, pancreatic α-cell tumour, obesity, stress and pregnancy.

4. **Diabetes may be associated or aggravated by drug therapy.** Incriminated agents include corticosteroids, thiazide diuretics and the combined oral contraceptive pill.

Anaesthetic management

1. **Assessment and premedication.** All except life-saving emergency surgery in the poorly controlled diabetic should be delayed until hyperglycaemia, dehydration and acidosis are corrected (diabetic acidosis may mimic an acute abdomen). The patient is assessed with particular reference to the problems given above. Postural hypotension and reduced heart rate response to the Valsalva manoeuvre suggest autonomic neuropathy. Assess the likely catabolic response to surgery and the duration of starvation.

All patients requiring major surgery should be controlled on insulin, glucose and potassium intravenous infusions preoperatively. Record the insulin usage, the glucose administration and the blood glucose. Type II diabetics requiring minor surgery (starvation of short duration) should omit their morning oral agent and have their blood glucose measured regularly throughout the day of operation. Type II patients treated with metformin have less diabetes related complications, fewer deaths and less myocardial infarctions. These facts may increase the usage of this long-acting biguanide. Lactic acidosis is a recognized complication, and metformin should be discontinued several days preoperatively.

Insulin-requiring patients should not be given any of their long-acting insulin on the day of surgery but should be managed with subcutaneous or intravenous insulin on a sliding scale. The blood glucose should be monitored regularly and insulin or glucose given as required. The ideal is for the patient to present for surgery with a normal blood sugar and normal glycogen stores. Whenever possible, diabetic patients should be operated on at the beginning of a surgical list to prevent them becoming hyperglycaemic with depleted glycogen stores. Premedicants should be given as usual.

Diabetic ketoacidosis is treated with large volume fluid resuscitation with normal saline (750–1000 ml in the first hour then according to the deficit). An intravenous insulin infusion administered according to a sliding scale is commenced. The CVP, urine output, acidosis, potassium and blood sugar are initially monitored hourly. When the blood sugar falls to 10 mmol/l, 5% glucose is commenced at a rate of 100 ml/h. Although the initial potassium is high the total body store is depleted and large amounts of potassium may need to be given as it enters cells together with glucose. If emergency surgery is required, start treatment and allow surgery to proceed when a biochemical improvement is seen. (Some surgical conditions must be treated to allow control of the ketoacidosis, e.g. sepsis.)

2. *Conduct of anaesthesia.* If gastric stasis is suspected a rapid sequence induction should be performed. Lactate containing intravenous fluids (Hartmann's, Ringers) are avoided as lactate is converted to bicarbonate. Regional techniques decrease the stress response but any peripheral neuropathy should be documented prior to their use. Hypotension and myocardial depression should be avoided. Mild hyperventilation may be beneficial. The blood sugar should be kept within the normal range (cerebral injury associated with cardiac standstill is increased in the presence of hyperglycaemia). Separate insulin and glucose infusions are often used rather than combined glucose, insulin and potassium regimes.

3. *Postoperatively.* Continue monitoring the blood sugar until the normal routine is established.

Further reading

McAnulty GR, Robertshaw HJ, Hall GM. Anaesthetic management of patients with diabetes mellitus. *British Journal of Anaesthesia*, 2000; **85**: 80–90.
UK Prospective Diabetes Study Group. Effect of intensive blood-glucose control with metformin on complications in overweight patients with type 2 diabetes (UKPDS 34). *Lancet*, 1998; **352**: 854–865.
www.diabetes.org.uk

Related topics of interest

Phaeochromocytoma (p. 203); Preoperative preparation (p. 209); Thyroid surgery (p. 261); Vascular surgery (p. 273)

DIATHERMY

Steve Hill

The first documented use of surgical diathermy was by Riviére in 1900. Diathermy is used to coagulate blood vessels or cut tissues during surgery.

Physics

Radio frequency (RF) alternating current, usually 500 kHz (range 100 kHz–5 MHz), is used in diathermy. The human body and especially the cardiac conducting system is very sensitive to low frequency electrical stimulation (50 Hz). High frequency alternating currents (>10 kHz) do not, however, cause depolarization of skeletal or cardiac muscle or cause pain. High voltages (peak 2000 V) can therefore be applied safely during surgical operations. Muscle does contract when cut with diathermy but this is as a result of local mechanical and thermal stimulation.

Electrical currents produce heat when passing through a resistor. The contact area between a diathermy electrode and tissue is relatively small and therefore has high resistance. Local heating thus occurs when the current flows.

The return current flows though the *dispersive electrode*. This has low resistance due to its large surface area and a layer of conductive gel. Thus little or no heating occurs at the dispersive electrode, which is usually attached to the patient's leg. The production of heat is due to the concentration of current over a small area, this is called *current density*.

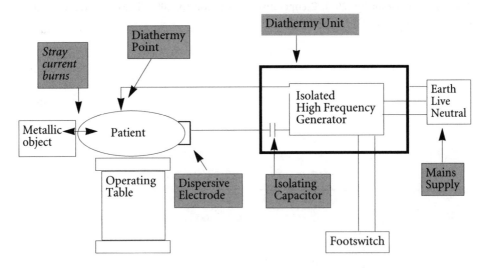

Clinical effects

The effect of diathermy on tissues varies according to the waveform used. *Cutting diathermy* uses a constant sine wave, creating a continuous arc. This vaporizes the tissues at the point where the arc makes contact, due to high current density.

Coagulation is performed with interrupted bursts, typically on for 5 microseconds and off for 20 microseconds. New arcs form with each burst, so that multiple heating points occur. This more dispersed current pattern results in lower heating effect over a wider area. This coagulates blood vessels without causing extensive tissue damage. The two types of waveform can be blended together so that cutting and coagulation occur simultaneously.

Hazards

1. **Electrocution** can occur as a result of faults in the diathermy machine. All modern machines are earth isolated and include monitors to check this. Earth isolation reduces risks of micro or macro shock from any source. The patient is connected to the diathermy machine via a relatively small capacitor, this allows radiofrequency currents to flow though the circuit but has high resistance to mains frequency (50 Hz) and DC voltages.

2. **Burns** can occur due to inadequate contact with the dispersive electrode. Reduced contact area can lead to local heating. Creases or indentations on the electrode may cause hot spots where the current is concentrated. Modern diathermy machines monitor the quality of the dispersive electrode contact and alarm if it is inadequate. Burns can also occur if the patient is touching a metal object, which can act as a capacitor. Quite large currents and hence burns occur due to the high frequency voltage charging and discharging of this capacitor. Stray currents of this type can also occur if the patient is connected to earth, e.g. via a faulty ECG machine or other electrical device not designed to withstand RF currents.

3. **Accidental operation** of the diathermy machine can result in burns if the diathermy point is near to the patient e.g. resting on the surgical drapes. The voltage generated is sufficient to make an arc 1 cm long so there is also a risk of igniting the drapes. It is important, therefore, that the diathermy point is kept in an insulated quiver when not in use.

4. **Neuromuscular stimulation** should not occur at normal diathermy frequencies. However it is not unusual to see muscle stimulation especially during transurethral prostate resection. This may be due to low frequency components in the diathermy signal or tissue response to high currents.

5. **Fire or explosions** occur due to spark ignition of drapes or volatile skin preparation solutions. Other risks include flammable anaesthetic agents, intestinal gas and hydrogen/oxygen gas bubbles due to electrolysis of water in the bladder.

6. **Radiofrequency interference** can affect monitoring equipment as well as pacemakers and infusion pumps.

Bipolar diathermy

These problems can be reduced by using a bipolar diathermy. Bipolar diathermy is applied using special forceps. Current passes between the two points of the diathermy forceps and heats the tissue held in the points. No heating occurs elsewhere and this makes bipolar diathermy preferable for work on delicate tissues, e.g. the eye and where convention diathermy might coagulate the artery supplying the area e.g. penis or testicle. Bipolar diathermy produces much less radiofrequency interference and is preferable if the patient has a pacemaker. There are limitations to the use of bipolar diathermy; it has relatively low power and cannot be used for cutting. It cannot be used for transurethral resection of the prostate gland.

Further reading

Langton JA. Electrical safety. *Royal College of Anaesthetists Newsletter*, Jan 2000; issue 50: 290–292.

Related topics of interest

Cardiac pacemakers (p. 62); CPR (p. 75)

DROWNING

Drowning is the third most common cause of accidental death in children in the UK (1500 deaths p.a.) after road traffic accidents and burns. It occurs even more frequently in less temperate climates with water-oriented societies (Australia, USA). Children who arrive in hospital following a submersion incident (near drowning) have a high survival rate. A poor outcome is predicted by fixed dilated pupils on arrival. These children either die or are left with a neurological deficit. Because of the potential for neurological improvement in some children and the high survival rate amongst others, all children should have full cardiopulmonary resuscitation after severe submersion incidents. This should not be abandoned until they are rewarmed to at least 33°C.

Effects of immersion

The majority of deaths from drowning occur within 10 metres of a safe refuge. It has therefore been suggested that the initial immersion is associated with a physiological disturbance which is responsible for further incapacitation.

1. *Initial immersion.* This may be due to temporary loss of consciousness or intoxication. Falling into water may injure the victim and make further immersion more likely.

2. *Cold-shock response.* The increase in sympathetic outflow to the heart and increase in vasomotor tone which rapidly follow cold immersion may cause acute myocardial embarrassment and infarction in an ischaemic heart. Even competent swimmers appear unable to swim in very cold water (5°C) unless they are accustomed to it. Hypothermia alone cannot explain their incapacitation.

3. *The diving reflex.* This is more pronounced in children than adults and accounts for the ability of certain diving mammals to remain submerged for up to 30 minutes. The reflex is triggered by the ophthalmic branch of the trigeminal nerve. It comprises a shut down of the peripheral circulation with a profound vagally mediated bradycardia. The brain selectively receives most of the cardiac output. The rapid fall in body temperature reduces metabolic demands and the reflex overrides chemoreceptor and baroreceptor function. The protective effect of hypothermia is more pronounced in children than in adults because of the greater surface area : body weight ratio of the former. Ten to twenty per cent of drowning victims appear to die without evidence of aspiration. This may be due to glottic spasm as a result of parasympathetic stimulation.

Fresh water versus salt water drowning

Animal experiments with dogs have shown a theoretical difference between drowning in salt water and fresh water. Large volumes of water were introduced into the lungs of the animals. Alveolar surface tension fell particularly in the animals drowned in fresh water. These dogs also showed a rapid transfer of hypotonic fluid to the bloodstream. This resulted in massive haemolysis and ventricular fibrillation which was not seen in dogs drowned in salt water. The volume of water inhaled in fatal human drownings is considerably less than that used in the experiment. No significant differences have been found in the serum sodium, potassium, chloride, haemoglobin or the haematocrit of humans drowned in fresh water compared with salt water. Aspiration of as little as 3 ml of water per kg body weight produces marked hypoxia, pulmonary shunt (75%) and acidosis. Aspiration of more than 22 ml of water per kg body weight is invariably fatal.

Management of near drowning

Treatment is aimed at the restoration of adequate ventilation and circulation. The usual pattern of ABC of resuscitation is followed. Almost all comatosed near drowned children require intubation, airway toilet and suction, with positive pressure ventilation, a high inspired oxygen concentration and PEEP. Usually, more water is swallowed than inhaled. A nasogastric tube must be passed and the stomach emptied. As well as arterial gas analysis the plasma osmolality, clotting function and U+E should be measured. Urine should be examined for haemoglobin and an ECG performed to exclude cardiac conduction abnormalities. Profound acidosis with a pH of 7.1 or less may require the administration of bicarbonate. The use of frusemide to reduce pulmonary oedema and intracranial water is controversial. Rewarming should occur slowly (1°C per hour) if the patient is cardiovascularly stable. Humidified inspired gases, warmed Iv fluids and forced warm air blankets are used. If more rapid warming is required, peritoneal dialysis or extracorporeal warming can be used. If cardiopulmonary arrest occurs, emergency cardiopulmonary bypass can be instituted. Resuscitation efforts should continue until a core temperature of 33°C is achieved.

Problems

- Cerebral oedema.
- Pulmonary infection and septicaemia, often with exotic marine or sewage organisms. Prophylactic antibiotics are not recommended.
- Renal failure.
- ARDS.
- Disseminated intravascular coagulopathy.

Further reading

Golden FS, Tipton MJ, Scott RC. Immersion, near-drowning and drowning. *British Journal of Anaesthesia* 1997; **79:** 214–225.
Wyatt JP, Tomlinson GS, Busuttil A. Resuscitation of drowning victims in south-east Scotland. *Resuscitation* 1999; **41:** 101–104.

Related topics of interest

DRUGS OF ABUSE

Dave Pogson

This topic covers the commoner drugs of abuse encountered in UK anaesthetic practice. The incidence of drug abuse is increasing in the UK and world wide, but the pattern of abuse differs between countries.

In general, abuse of cannabis and amfetamines (particularly ecstasy) tends to occur amongst young adults. Occasional drug use may not affect general health. Chronic abuse can result in deterioration in diet and social conditions, leading to cachexia, anaemia, liver function abnormalities and lung pathology in all abusers.

Owing to the CNS effects of abuse or the drugs themselves, patients may be abusive, uncooperative or combative. They may also be suffering from manifest withdrawal. Chronic abusers who inject drugs have a higher incidence of Hepatitis B and HIV infection, particularly amongst the prison population. Among drug abusers, polyabuse is extremely common. A history of drug and alcohol use should be sought in young adults and trauma victims requiring anaesthesia. General toxicology screening of 30 ml of sterile urine will detect most recreational drugs.

Amfetamines

Amfetamine use in the UK has risen greatly with the popularity of ecstasy (MDMA = 3,4-methylenedioxymethamfetamine) among young adults. Around 500 000 people use this drug every weekend. Amfetamines cause sympathetic stimulation by catecholamine release from adrenergic nerve terminals. Chronic use may deplete catecholamines.

Central 5HT release occurs and there is central dopamine agonism. Amfetamines cause MAO A inhibition.

Patients presenting with acute amfetamine intoxication may exhibit raised HR and BP, arrhythmias, metabolic acidosis, CNS agitation and hyperthermia. Rhabdomyolysis can occur. Excessive thirst has led to water intoxication resulting in dilutional hyponatraemia and cerebral oedema.

Anaesthetic management of acute abuse may require short acting beta blockade to reduce the risk of arrhythmia and the hypertensive responses of laryngoscopy and surgery.

Cerebral blood flow and cerebral metabolic rate will be increased, raising the MAC of volatile anaesthetics. The myocardium is sensitised to catecholamines therefore halothane should be avoided. Hyperpyrexia under anaesthesia may be due to amfetamines and dantrolene may be indicated. In chronic abuse catecholamine depletion obtunds the CVS response to stress and CVS collapse may occur. MAC is reduced. Use of epidurals in these patients has led to profound fall in BP.

Cannabis

Derived from *Cannabis sativa*, this is the commonest abused drug after alcohol and nicotine. Use among young adults is widespread with 10% of medical students admitting regular consumption.

The most studied active ingredient is delta-tetrahydrocannabinol. Bioavailability is higher (20%) when smoked than when ingested (4%). Selective plant breeding has led to higher dosages of the drug. Highly lipid soluble, the elimination half-life is prolonged and urinary screening may detect the drug at 20 days.

Cannabis modulates neuronal activity via cannabinoid receptors, with effects on calcium and potassium transport. There are complex interactions with many neurotransmitter systems particularly in the frontal cortex. Motor function, co-ordination and visual tracking are impaired, increasing the risk of accident. Cannabis toxicity does not occur. Most of the adverse effects occur because of smoking. In terms of bronchitis and epithelial damage, a single cannabis joint is equivalent to five tobacco cigarettes. This is because more smoke particles are inhaled more deeply to enhance the drug effect, resulting in higher levels of carboxyhaemoglobin. Oxygen carrying capacity and delivery to tissues are reduced.

The CNS depressant effects of cannabis mean that MAC of volatile anaesthetics is reduced. The actions of ketamine and thiopentone are prolonged. Withdrawal effects in chronic users may increase analgesic requirements due to anxiety.

Cocaine

The use of cocaine is far less in the UK than the US, where up to 5% of the population may be regular users. Most cocaine is inhaled nasally. Crack cocaine is the alkaline form of the drug. Crack is a very pure and highly addictive preparation, which is smoked.

Cocaine has several effects. Blockade of sodium channels confers a local anaesthetic action. Inhibition of 5HT re-uptake results in euphoria and alertness. Cocaine inhibits the re-uptake of catecholamines at presynaptic receptors. This results in profound sympathetic stimulation with hypertension, tachycardia and agitation.

Acute abuse may precipitate arrhythmias or myocardial infarction in patients with myocardial disease. Myocardial oxygen demand rises but coronary vasoconstriction occurs. Sodium channel block prolongs cardiac repolarisation thereby increasing the risk of arrhythmia. Chronic abuse leads to depletion of catecholamines.

Cocaine promotes the release of thromboxanes, increasing platelet aggregation and thrombus formation.

Abusers often present with airway complications such as septal perforation and sinusitis. Pulmonary oedema may occur. Abuse in pregnancy may mimic the signs of pre-eclampsia.

Cocaine overdose is usually fatal. Sudden death is commoner in abusers who are forcibly restrained.

The effects of cocaine last only 10 minutes, but the plasma half-life is about 1 hour. It can be detected in urine up to 6 hours post dose, with the metabolites measurable for far longer. Anaesthetic mortality in cocaine abusers usually occurs due to cardiovascular problems related to co-administration of vasopressors. The pressor response to intubation can be controlled with alfentanil, nitrates or calcium channel blockade. Beta blockade may lead to unopposed alpha stimulation and hypertension. Labetolol and esmolol have been used. Lidocaine is best avoided as the seizure threshold is reduced. Ketamine causes sympathetic stimulation and should be avoided. Similarly, halothane should not be used. The MAC of volatiles is probably increased. Isoflurane and enflurane have been used safely. Sufficient depth of anaesthesia will reduce the sympathetic effects of cocaine abuse. Cocaine is metabolised by pseudocholinesterase. The actions of suxamethonium and mivacurium may be prolonged. Epidural and spinal blockade have produced profound hypotension, especially in pregnancy. Incremental doses of local anaesthetic should be used. The response to ephedrine is preserved. Close postoperative monitoring of ECG and blood pressure are necessary as the risk of arrhythmia is prolonged.

Heroin

Heroin (diamorphine) is abused regularly by over 60 000 people in the UK. It is sold out with agents such as phenobarbitone, talc and starch. UK street heroin has around 30% purity. Daily usage varies some taking up to a gram. Intravenous injection is common, nasal and sublingual routes less so. Polyabuse of benzodiazepines and barbiturates is especially common.

The clinical effects of heroin include euphoria, unconsciousness, coma, miosis and respiratory depression. Preassessment of the heroin abuser should include a dosage history and the current state regarding withdrawal. Physical examination may identify malnutrition, signs of cardiomyopathy, endocarditis and liver disease. Sites suitable for venous access should be found. Skin sepsis is common among IV abusers.

Full blood count (25% of addicts are anaemic), electrolytes and glucose should be measured. Abnormal liver function is common and can result from cutting agents or viral hepatitis. CXR may reveal evidence of aspiration. Hilar lymphadenopathy is common. ECG is abnormal in around half of cases, commonly with prolonged QT interval. If polyabuse is suspected, urinalysis should be performed for other drugs. Heroin addicts account for 25% of cases of hepatitis B and 14–55% of HIV cases. HIV is commoner among IV heroin abusers in Scotland than in the rest of the UK. The patient's usual total daily dose of heroin should be ascertained and regarded as the background requirement. Analgesia with opioids can be added above this level. Addicts may exaggerate their usual dose to obtain more opiates, resulting in overdose. The timing of the addict's last dose should be known. The half-life of diamorphine is 4–6 hours. On the day of operation the patient's normal requirement can be given intramuscularly. Infusion or PCA can control postoperative pain above the background requirement, avoiding peaks and troughs. If spinal or epidural opiates are used the requirement will also be raised. Only one route of administration should be used to prevent delayed respiratory depression.

Regional techniques are desirable if the patient is co-operative. Any peripheral neuropathy should be documented.

The postoperative period is not the time to encourage withdrawal. The occurs 8–12 hours after the last fix, with piloerection, fatigue, weakness, fever and sympathetic overactivity. This continues for up to a week. It has been treated with methadone and clonidine to combat the sympathetic activity. Methadone is equipotent with heroin and is given daily with a half-life of 90 hours.

Further reading

Ashton C. Adverse effects of cannabis and cannabinoids. *British Journal of Anaesthesia*, 1999; **83:** 637–649.
Cheng D. The drug addicted patient. *Canadian Journal of Anaesthesia*, 1997; **44:** R101–R106.
Henry JA. Metabolic consequences of drug misuse. *British Journal of Anaesthesia*, 2000; **85:** 136–142.

Related topics of interest

AIDS and hepatitis (p. 7); Alcohol (p. 16); Liver disease and anaesthesia (p. 151); Smoking – tobacco (p. 239)

DVT and PE

Virchow's triad describes the predisposing factors for the development of a deep venous thrombosis (DVT). They are (i) stasis of blood flow, (ii) damage to blood vessels and (iii) abnormal coagulation. Pulmonary embolism (PE) is the most serious complication of DVT.

Patients at high risk include:

1.   Inherited.   Antithrombin III deficiency, protein C deficiency, protein S deficiency, dysfibrinogenaemias.

2.   Acquired.   Lupus disease, nephrotic syndrome, malignancy, low cardiac output states, polycythaemia, obesity, advancing age, oestrogen therapy, sepsis, stroke (75% incidence of DVT in paralysed leg), peripheral vascular disease.

3.   Surgical.   Orthopaedic patients represent the highest risk group with those undergoing hip or knee reconstructive surgery being at particular risk. Other operative risks include gynaecological surgery, surgery for malignancy, prolonged surgery, poorly fitted antiembolism stockings, poor operative positioning, pressure point compression of the legs, and hypotensive anaesthesia. Surgery causes a rise in circulating acute phase reactants and fibrinogen and changes in platelet function.

Clinical diagnosis of a DVT is often incorrect. Both false positives and false negatives occur. Venography or radio-labelled [^{125}I] fibrinogen uptake scans are required for the accurate diagnosis of a DVT.

Prevention

1.   General measures.   Patients at high risk scheduled to undergo elective surgery should have their risks reduced wherever possible. Obese patients should lose weight and patients with heart failure or active infection should have their conditions treated. Women taking the oral contraceptive pill, and who have a second risk factor (e.g. prolonged surgery or over the age of 40) should have their medication withdrawn. A period of 4 weeks should elapse between stopping the pill and undergoing surgery as there is an initial hypercoagulability after the withdrawal of exogenous oestrogens. Advice regarding alternative contraception must be given where appropriate. Hormone replacement therapy (HRT) is not associated with an increased incidence of DVT.

Surgical patients should be encouraged to perform regular leg exercises whilst in bed in the perioperative period. Early postoperative mobilization is advised.

2.   Specific therapy.
- Mechanical methods. Elastic compression stockings and intermittent calf compression devices have both been shown to reduce the incidence of DVT, although a reduction in the incidence of pulmonary embolism has not been shown clearly. Mechanical techniques have the advantage of not increasing the risk of haemorrhage.
- Pharmacological methods.

(a) Heparin enhances the effects of antithrombin III (which itself accelerates the inactivation of activated factors IIa and Xa). A preoperative dose of 2500 IU subcutaneously and 5000 IU at least as often as 12 hourly for 5 days following surgery has been shown to more than halve the incidence of DVT and reduce the risk of fatal pulmonary embolism by two-thirds in surgical patients. Low molecular weight heparin is at least as effective at preventing DVT as conventional heparin. The risk of major bleeding is the same with both. Low molecular weight heparin has advantages over unfractionated heparin. These include greater bioavailability when given by subcutaneous injection, more predictable anticoagulant effects (permitting the administration of a fixed dose and removing the need for laboratory monitoring), and an increased duration of action. The use of LMWH results in less heparin-induced thrombocytopenia, osteoporosis, and bleeding.

(b) Dextran 70 appears to coat vessel walls and have an antiplatelet action. It has been shown to reduce the incidence of fatal pulmonary embolus in women undergoing gynaecological surgery. The effect on the incidence of calf DVT was, however, less clear.

(c) Regional anaesthesia may contribute to a reduced tendency to form thromboses in the lower limb veins. Possible mechanisms for this include peripheral vasodilatation, and the reduction in blood viscosity associated with fluid loading. Extradural anaesthesia reduces fibrinolysis and the activation of clotting factors.

Pulmonary embolism

Pulmonary emboli almost always result from thromboses of the lower limbs, deep pelvic veins, or inferior vena cava. The mortality of patients with PE is lower in those who are treated than in those who are not or in whom the diagnosis was not suspected.

Clinical presentation

PE may present with one of three clinical syndromes:

- Pulmonary infarction/haemorrhage (60% of diagnosed cases of PE).
- Isolated shortness of breath (25% of diagnosed cases of PE).
- Sudden circulatory collapse (10% of diagnosed cases of PE). One third of these patients die within a few hours of presentation.

The three most common symptoms are dyspnoea, tachypnoea and pleuritic chest pain.

There may be little in the way of positive clinical signs. Those that are present are usually non-specific and at best support the diagnosis. They include signs of right heart strain, pulmonary hypertension and DVT. The ECG may show non-specific ST segment changes, axis changes, or rarely, and only in the case of a large PE, an S wave in lead I, a Q wave and T wave inversion in lead III ('S1, Q3, T3'). The CXR often shows a parenchymal abnormality (e.g. atelectasis). There may also be an elevated hemidiaphragm. The patient may have a mild pyrexia and elevated white cell count. The finding of a low PaO_2 also supports the diagnosis.

Specific investigation

The most useful investigation is probably a combination of a pulmonary ventilation/perfusion (V/Q) scan and measurement of the plasma D-dimer levels. D-dimer is formed when plasmin digests cross-linked fibrin. A low D-dimer level is strong evidence against the diagnosis of a PE.

V/Q scan

Pulmonary perfusion scans are usually performed using intravenous albumin labelled with technetium-99m. A ventilation scan is performed following the inhalation of xenon-133. A pulmonary perfusion scan which is interpreted as showing a high probability of a PE is no less sensitive a predictor of PE than a combined V/Q scan. If the result of the perfusion scan is of intermediate probability a subsequent V/Q scan may change the interpretation to a more definitive probability. The Prospective Investigation of Pulmonary Embolism Diagnosis (PIOPED) study defined five categories for V/Q scans; high, intermediate, low, very low probability, and normal.

Leg studies

A patient with a non-diagnostic V/Q scan requires further investigation. A venogram or compression ultrasound will determine the presence of a DVT. The finding of a DVT guides therapy since the treatment of PE and DVT is the same.

Pulmonary angiography

This remains the diagnostic standard for PE. The finding of an intraluminal filling defect is specific. Fewer than 2% of patients suffer serious adverse effects during pulmonary angiography.

Contrast-enhanced spiral CT

Early evidence suggests that this imaging technique may be of high specificity and selectivity if the PE is in the central pulmonary vessels. Its value in diagnosing PE in more peripheral vessels is less clear and the true role of contrast-enhanced spiral CT in the investigation of possible PE has yet to be fully defined.

Management

1.   Anticoagulation.   Patients with an uncomplicated PE should be treated with heparin to maintain the APTT (activated partial thromboplastin time) at 1.5–2 times the control. Oral anticoagulation may be commenced at the same time or shortly after starting heparin. There should be a 5 day overlap with both therapies and the INR maintained at approximately 2–3 times normal before the heparin is stopped. Some centres now manage uncomplicated DVT and PE with administration of LMWH and commencement of oral anticoagulation at home, thus avoiding hospital admission altogether. Early follow up of patients managed in this way has shown comparable rates of fatal and non-fatal PE compared with patients treated with unfractionated heparin.

2.   Inferior vena cava (IVC) filters.   IVC filters should be inserted in patients with a proximal DVT or PE in whom anticoagulation is contraindicated or if PE has recurred despite adequate anticoagulation. A caval filter may also be inserted if the PE is severe (hypotension or right ventricular failure) or if recurrent PE is likely to be fatal. IVC filters are inserted percutaneously.

3. _Thrombolytic therapy._ Lysis of PE occurs more rapidly when thrombolytics are given than with anticoagulation alone. In patients who have not had a massive PE, long-term survival is the same for both groups, however. Thrombolysis has been shown to alter outcome in patients with a massive PE. They had a lower in-hospital mortality and rate of PE recurrence but higher incidence of major haemorrhage than similar patients treated with anticoagulation alone.

4. _Pulmonary embolectomy._ Patients who have suffered a massive PE, and are shocked despite resuscitative measures and thrombolysis, may benefit from open embolectomy. Mortality remains high even in patients offered surgery.

Further reading

Cochrane Database Systematic Review. 2000; **2.** CD000305

Wheatley T, Veitch PS. Recent advances in prophylaxis against deep vein thrombosis. *British Journal of Anaesthesia,* 1997; **78:** 118–120.

Related topics of interest

Positioning (p. 207); Sequelae of anaesthesia (p. 232); Spinal and epidural anaesthesia (p. 241)

ECT

'Electric shock treatment' commenced in the 1930s without anaesthesia. With the introduction of antidepressants in the 1950s its popularity waned. More recently with further research and modern anaesthetic techniques, it has experienced a resurgence. ECT (electroconvulsive therapy) is generally more efficacious for acute affective disorders than for chronic thought or movement disorders. ECT may be life saving, and there are therefore no absolute contraindications. The risk–benefit argument must be examined in each case. ECT produces synchronous depolarization of cell membranes and allows propagation of seizure activity. The therapeutic action is related to the seizure, by its duration, intensity and characteristics. It is suggested that ECT enhances dopaminergic transmission, and patients with Parkinson's disease can be clinically improved. Numbers of 5-HT_2 and muscarinic cholinergic receptors fall. During a seizure, blood pressure rises with increased cerebral blood flow and increased oxygen and glucose metabolism. Intragastric, intraocular and intracranial pressures all rise. The degree of autonomic stimulation correlates with seizure duration and intensity.

Problems

1. Isolated site. The Royal College of Psychiatrists published guidelines in 1995. The service should be consultant based, with qualified anaesthetic assistance and recovery personnel. Anaesthetic, resuscitation and monitoring equipment should match 'in hospital' standards.

2. Memory impairment. This is more likely if the patient has pre-existing confusion, and a bilateral prolonged fit is induced. Discrete memory gaps can occur.

3. Trauma. Dental damage, fractures and dislocations.

4. Mortality. This is quoted at 0.02–0.04%.

Anaesthetic management

1. Assessment and premedication. The preparation of the patient should be the same as for any other patient requiring general anaesthesia. This includes starvation, history, examination, consent, and investigations. Care must be taken over concurrent medications, particularly older monoamine oxidase inhibitors (hypertensive crises) and lithium (prolonged neuromuscular block). Premedications are not normally used as benzodiazepines can attenuate seizure activity. Relative contraindications to ECT include recent MI, raised ICP, cerebral aneurysm, cervical instability, pregnancy and muscle diseases. High risk patients should be transferred to, and treated in, a facility with appropriate backup such as an ITU.

2. Conduct of anaesthesia. Intravenous access is secured and i.v. induction of anaesthesia is performed with or without preoxygenation. Methohexitone is commonly used as propofol decreases seizure duration and recovery is no quicker in the postictal patient. However, during 1999 and 2000 there has been no methohexitone produced, and its use longer term may wane. A rapid sequence induction is performed if appropriate and 100% O$_2$ is given. Hyperventilation prior to ECT lowers the seizure threshold and prolongs the seizure duration. A softbite guard is introduced prior to electrical stimulation. The skin impedance is decreased by cleaning with alcohol, and by using an electrode gel. An initial stimulus, in joules, of approximately a half of the patient's age is administered once maximal muscle relaxation has occurred following suxamethonium (0.5 mg/kg). For subsequent ECT the doses of methohexitone, suxamethonium and electricity are recorded and modified according to the witnessed responses. Atopine or glycopyrollate are often given to prevent bradycardia associated with suxamethonium and ECT. A seizure duration of between 30 seconds and 2 minutes optimizes therapeutic effect and minimizes cognitive impairment. If a prolonged fit occurs > 2 minutes, it should be terminated with a benzodiazepine.

3. Postoperatively. The postictal/anaesthetic patient should be recovered by appropriately trained staff in a suitably equipped area.

Further reading

Avramov MN, Husain MM, White PF. The comparative effects of methohexital, propofol and etomidate for electroconvulsive therapy. *Anesthesia and Analgesia*, 1995; **81:** 596–602.
Simpson KH, Lynch L. Anaesthesia and electroconvulsive therapy (ECT). *Anaesthesia*, 1998; **53:** 615–617.

Related topics of interest

Cardioversion (p. 70); Day surgery (p. 80); Dental anaesthesia (p. 83); Epilepsy (p. 113); MRI (p. 156); Preoperative preparation (p. 209)

ELDERLY PATIENTS

Increasing numbers of increasingly old people present for increasingly complicated surgery. The anaesthetist may face both the problems of ageing of all body systems and of the specific diseases which become more prevalent with increasing age. Chronological age does not equate with physiological age. Anaesthesia should not be refused, despite high risk, if the patient is aware of the risks and 'quality' life may be prolonged or suffering relieved.

Problems

1. **Cardiovascular system.**   Decreasing vessel elasticity leads to a less compliant vascular tree (a raised SVR) with systemic hypertension, left ventricular strain and hypertrophy. Cardiac conduction time and stroke volume are reduced. Conduction defects may necessitate pacing. Cardiac output falls by 3% per decade, and arm–brain circulation time is increased. Baroreceptor sensitivity, sympathetic tone and the ability to increase the heart rate when required are reduced.

   Diseases: Hypertension, heart failure, IHD, valvular disease (especially mitral regurgitation and aortic stenosis) and peripheral vascular disease.

2. **Respiratory.**   Pulmonary elasticity, lung and chest wall compliance, FEV_1, FVC, vital capacity and inspiratory reserve are all reduced. The closing volume exceeds FRC in the supine position after the age of 45 years with resultant V/Q mismatch and hypoxaemia. The residual volume is increased. There is a reduced response to hypoxaemia and hypercarbia, and protective airway reflexes decrease in old age.

   Diseases: chronic obstructive airflow and emphysema.

3. **Central nervous system.**   Neuronal density (30% loss by 80 years), brain transmitters, cerebral blood flow, and $CRMO_2$ are all reduced. This lowers the dose of induction and volatile agents, sedatives, opioids, and local anaesthetics. Reduced peripheral nerve function leads to a reduction in afferentation and less sensitive sensory input. Autonomic neuropathy may occur.

   Diseases: CVAs, dementia, Parkinsonism and depression. Deafness and poor vision may make communication difficult.

4. **Renal.**   Renal blood flow, GFR and concentrating ability are all reduced. There is a 1% loss in function per year after 30 years. This leads to reduced renal clearance of drugs, a raised blood urea but a stable blood creatinine.

   Diseases: transitional cell malignancy, prostatic hypertrophy and malignancy.

5. **Hepatic.**   Hepatic blood flow and drug clearance are reduced. There is a 1% loss in function per year after 30 years.

6. **Metabolic/endocrine.**   Adipose tissue increases whilst muscle bulk and total body water are reduced. The BMR falls by 1% per year after 30 years, and thermo-regulation is impaired.

Diseases: diabetes (in 25% of over 85-year-olds), thyroid disease, osteoporosis and nutritional disorders.

7. *Pharmacology.* Altered drug absorption, protein binding, metabolism and excretion in combination with ageing body systems make drug effects more variable in the elderly. One third of over 75-year-olds take three or more drugs each day.

Anaesthetic management

1. *Assessment and premedication.* History and examination is followed by a FBC, U+E and ECG in all over 65-year-olds. Other investigations are performed as indicated. The elderly are often stoical but a small dose of anxiolytic may be helpful. Avoid hyoscine and large doses of depressant drugs.

2. *Conduct of anaesthetic.* Monitoring is as indicated by the systems pathology and planned surgery.

Regional anaesthesia avoids the problems of a general anaesthetic but with a poorly compliant vascular tree and reduced autonomic control, hypotension is common. All patients should receive supplementary O_2. Hypotension and hypoxaemia may lead to perioperative confusion.

For general anaesthesia consider preoxygenation. Intravenous agents should be given slowly and in small doses, being wary of a slow arm/brain circulation time. IPPV may cause a marked fall in blood pressure. Special care should be taken with respect to pressure points when positioning the patient. Hypothermia should be prevented and surgery should not be prolonged. Glycopyrollate should be used in preference to atropine, as it does not cross the blood–brain barrier to cause confusion.

3. *Postoperatively.* Supplementary O_2, intensive physiotherapy and early mobilization will reduce postoperative sequelae. Analgesia is titrated to effect when using opioids. PCA or regional techniques may also be used.

Further reading

Critchley LA. Hypotension, subarachnoid block and the elderly patient. *Anaesthesia* 1996; **51**: 1139–1143.
Dodds C, Allison J. Postoperative cognitive deficit in the elderly surgical patient. *British Journal of Anaesthesia*, 1998; **81**: 449–462.
Smith B *et al. Anesthesiology and Pain Control in the Geriatric Patient*, 2nd ed. McGraw-Hill Publishing Company, 2000.

Related topics of interest

Diabetes (p. 89); Hypertension (p. 131); Positioning (p. 207); Preoperative preparation (p. 209); Sequelae of anaesthesia (p. 232); Thyroid surgery (p. 261)

EMERGENCY ANAESTHESIA

Despite increases in the number of emergency anaesthetics administered by consultants, emergency procedures are still often undertaken by less experienced clinicians at night or weekends. The very nature of the emergency may mean that these patients have increased perioperative risks.

Problems

1. Limited time to prepare the patient for surgery and anaesthesia.

2. Hypovolaemia. This is common and may be related to poor fluid intake, haemorrhage, diarrhoea, vomiting, sweating, or abnormal fluid shifts. There may be associated electrolyte disturbance. Covert or overt haemorrhage may also be the cause of hypovolaemia.

3. Aspiration risk. Stomach emptying depends on a variety of factors such as the volume and the content of the last meal and the emotional state of the patient. Gastric motility is reduced by fear, pain, opioids and vagotomy. Disagreement thus exists as to when it is safe to assume the stomach is empty. A 6-hour rule is often applied from the ingestion of food to anaesthesia, but trauma victims have in some instances been found to have substantial food residues after 24 hours. The time from the ingestion of food to the time of trauma is useful in deciding the likelihood of gastric emptying having occurred (a solid meal taking ~6 hours).

4. Pain.

5. Premedication is often not possible.

6. Co-existing disease. Uncontrolled medical conditions may present at the same time as a surgical emergency. For example, diabetes, hypertension, cardiac failure, or atrial fibrillation, all of which may be further assessed and improved given sufficient time.

Anaesthetic management

All patients must be assessed prior to anaesthesia. Patients requiring emergency surgery are no exception to this. The risk of pulmonary aspiration, and the anticipated ease of intubation should be noted. The results of relevant investigations and the availability of blood and blood products should be checked. Results of necessary investigations should be available prior to anaesthesia unless there is an immediate threat to life, e.g. ruptured aortic aneurysm.

Fluid resuscitation should be initiated and hypovolaemia and electrolyte disturbance treated before anaesthesia is commenced. Diabetes, cardiac failure and other acute medical conditions should also be treated appropriately.

Premedication may be limited to an explanation of the proposed anaesthetic procedure and the control of pain. The need for antibiotic prophylaxis and the prevention of venous thrombosis should be considered. The planned management of the case should be discussed with senior staff and appropriate help requested.

Measures to empty the stomach (postpone operation, fasting, gastric suction, prokinetic agents), and acid prophylaxis to reduce the risk if regurgitation occurs should be considered.

The standard equipment checks should be made and appropriate monitoring should be established. Capnography must always be available at the site of administration of anaesthesia.

Emergency drugs such as vasopressors, atropine and adrenaline should, as always, be accessible. Ensure adequate intravenous access with a large bore cannula. Preoxygenate the patient with 100% O_2 for 3 min (or four vital capacity breaths).

A rapid sequence intravenous induction with thiopental, cricoid pressure and suxamethonium (unless contraindicated) is the method of choice for general anaesthesia. Induction agents should be administered with care in patients who are hypovolaemic. Ketamine and etomidate are associated with less hypotension following their administration.

A technique should be chosen which guarantees rapid return of protective airway reflexes. The aspiration risk is still present at extubation and this should only be performed after full return of these reflexes, when the patient is awake.

A regional anaesthetic may be appropriate.

Postoperatively, high dependency or intensive care should be considered if the patient remains unstable or requires further resuscitation.

Further reading

http://www.NCEPOD.ORG.uk/keyiss.htm
Vanner RG, Asai T. Safe use of cricoid pressure. *Anaesthesia*, 1999; **54**: 1–3.

Related topics of interest

Audit – national (p. 30); Cardiac assessment (p. 55); DVT and PE (p. 101); Preoperative preparation (p. 209)

EPIGLOTTITIS

Acute epiglottitis is an uncommon but dangerous bacterial infection of the throat. It is becoming increasingly uncommon following vaccination programmes in the developed world. It is usually seen in children aged less than 8 years with a peak incidence between 2 and 5 years. It may also occur in adults. The usual causative organism is *Haemophilus influenzae* type B but this is not invariable and β-haemolytic streptococci, staphylococci, or pneumococci may also be isolated, especially in adult cases. The differential diagnosis in children is acute laryngotracheobronchitis (croup) which is a viral infection occurring principally in those under 3 years. The mortality in adults is quoted to be as high as 6–7% but this is usually due to misdiagnosis and inappropriate treatment.

Problems

- Upper airway obstruction.
- Lethargy and exhaustion.
- Potential difficulty with intubation.

Diagnosis

The provisional diagnosis is made on the history and examination. Typically the history is short with a rapid deterioration. The patient presents with a sore throat, fever, muffled voice and dysphagia. Pain may exceed that expected from the brevity of the history. Inspiratory stridor develops rapidly and progression to complete respiratory obstruction may occur within 12 hours.

Children prefer to sit up and drool saliva from the mouth. Swallowing is avoided because of the extremely sore throat.

Indirect laryngoscopy should not be undertaken to confirm the diagnosis as this frequently precipitates airway obstruction, especially in children. Lateral neck X rays may confirm a swollen epiglottis but are not essential. A sick child should not be sent to the X-ray department without the continual presence of someone skilled in paediatric intubation. A child with suspected epiglottitis will invariably require an examination of their upper airway under anaesthesia and X-rays are frequently unnecessary. The airway can then be secured with a tracheal tube.

Management

The child is moved to a quiet induction area where all the necessary aids to a difficult paediatric intubation are readily to hand. The child is allowed to remain in an upright posture as sudden changes in position, especially lying down, may result in complete airway obstruction.

An inhalational induction of anaesthesia is usually preferred. Venous access can be obtained once the child is unconscious. Atropine may then be administered if required. In the presence of airway obstruction it may take more than 15 minutes before anaesthesia is deep enough to permit safe laryngoscopy.

Laryngoscopy will show a swollen 'cherry red' epiglottis. There is often associated swelling of the aryepiglottic folds. In severe cases the only clue to the glottic opening may be bubbles issuing from behind the epiglottis during expiration.

Once intubated the child should then be transferred to a critical care area. Blood cultures and throat swabs are taken for microbiological examination. Therapy is continued with intravenous rehydration, humidified inspired gases, airway toilet, and antibiotics.

The management of adult cases follows a similar course, although observation of the unintubated patient in a critical care environment has been recommended by some. The risk in this strategy is the possibility of death from sudden complete respiratory obstruction.

Antibiotics

Ampicillin and chloramphenicol are the usual 'best bet' antibiotics until the organism's sensitivities are known. Cefuroxime is an alternative.

Progress

Epiglottic oedema settles rapidly following commencement of the antibiotics and an increasing leak around the tracheal tube is expected. Once the patient is afebrile and appears well, extubation may be considered. This is usually within 24–48 hours. It is not necessary to re-examine the larynx prior to extubation.

Related topics of interest

Airway surgery (p. 12); Intubation – difficult (p. 141)

EPILEPSY

Epilepsy has a prevalence of 1:200. Surgical procedures are usually unrelated to epilepsy, but surgical excision of a seizure focus can be performed in those with medically intractable epilepsy. Uncontrolled epilepsy may necessitate intensive care with ventilatory support whilst therapeutic control is obtained (lorazepam may be best). Muscle relaxants may be required to prevent acidosis from the severe muscle activity associated with seizures. Sensory, motor, autonomic and higher centre function can be involved. Seizures represent a sudden alteration of nervous system function which can occur at any time and are usually associated with a full return of function. The electroencephalogram (EEG) shows abnormal discharges during attacks. There is usually a focal origin, but different patterns of epilepsy are seen, including grand mal, petit mal, focal, psychomotor and myoclonic epilepsy. Differing drug regimens are used for different patterns of epilepsy. These drugs aim to raise the electrical threshold for seizure activity. Carbamazepine, phenytoin and sodium valproate are first line drugs for generalized seizures. Other drugs include phenobarbitone, ethosuximide, vigabatrin, lamotrigine, topiramate and gabapentin. They are used for petit mal, myoclonic seizures or where control is difficult. Epilepsy may be caused by cerebral tumour or abscess, HIV infection, meningitis, cerebrovascular disease, drugs, metabolic disorder, a head injury or be idiopathic.

Problems
- Risk of further seizures.
- Drug therapy for epilepsy.
- Potential for anaesthetic agents to affect the EEG and predispose to seizures.
- Underlying aetiology of the epilepsy.

Anaesthetic management

1. Assessment and premedication. The pattern of epilepsy and the frequency of seizures is ascertained. Any underlying cause should be determined, and the current drug therapy with any associated side-effects noted. Anticonvulsants should not be omitted preoperatively. Premedication with a benzodiazepine is appropriate.

2. Conduct of anaesthesia. Any anaesthetic must prevent the precipitating causes of fits (see below). Drugs that induce, precipitate or exacerbate seizures should be avoided. These include methohexitone, ketamine, etomidate, propofol, ether and enflurane. An induction with thiopental and maintenance with opioids and isoflurane, with relaxants and ventilation if required is an acceptable anaesthetic technique.

3. Postoperatively. Provided no seizures have occurred, no special postoperative care is required and the normal anticonvulsant regimen should be recommended as soon as possible.

4. Fits during anaesthesia. Patients who suffer seizures during an anaesthetic are usually known epileptics. Children are more predisposed to fits than adults. Good anaesthetic technique will avoid most of the preventable precipitating factors.

If a seizure occurs *de novo*, without a clear cause, then investigations should be performed to determine the aetiology.

5. Causes

- Anaesthetic. Including hypoxia, hypercarbia, hypocarbia and 'light anaesthesia'.
- CNS disease or old head injury.
- Metabolic. A low blood sugar, sodium, magnesium or calcium, and uraemia lower the threshold for convulsions.
- Hyperpyrexia.
- Drugs e.g. local anaesthetic toxicity.
- Eclampsia.

6. Management. If a seizure occurs during anaesthesia the airway should immediately be protected and 100% O_2 given by controlled ventilation. Thiopental is usually the most available anticonvulsant and may be given to control the fit. Lorazepam, midazolam, clonazepam or diazepam are alternatives. The above list of causes will direct investigation and further management. The use of prophylactic anticonvulsants to prevent seizures in the postoperative period should be considered.

Further reading

Cheng MA, Tempelhoff R. Anesthesia and epilepsy. *Current Opinion in Anaesthesiology*, 1999; **12:** 523–528.
Antiepileptics. *British National Formulary*, 2000; **39:** 222–233.
http://www.druginfozone.org

Related topics of interest

ECT (p. 105); Neuroanaesthesia (p. 167); Neurological disease (p. 170)

ETHICS and DUTY of CARE

Adrian Walker

Morality is the personal, communal or cultural view about right and wrong which determines human conduct. Ethics describes the various ways of examining and understanding the moral life. Medical ethics is a practical application of ethics or moral philosophy which addresses the rights and wrongs of different areas of health care practice and develops general moral guidance for use in biomedical fields.

Elements of medical ethics

1. ***Principles.*** Principles derive from considered judgements in the common morality and medical tradition (Beauchamp and Childress). Principles are general guides that allow latitude for judgement in individual cases but provide a secure basis for the development of more detailed rules and policies.

- *Respect for autonomy* requires acknowledgement of, and action to promote a person's rights to make choices free from interference and from limitations that prevent intelligent decisions.
- *Non-maleficence* is associated with the maxim *primum non nocere*: above all do no harm. It asserts an obligation to avoid causing harm to patients as well as protecting them from risk of harm.
- *Beneficence* is expressed in the Hippocratic Oath: 'I will use treatments to help the sick according to my ability and judgement'. The benefit however should be patient centred and regarded by the patient as a worthwhile outcome, now or in the future.
- *Justice* is interpreted as fair, equitable and appropriate medical care in the light of what is due or owed to persons.

2. ***Rules and rights.*** These provide more precise action guides for specific situations. They may define the legal or moral claims and expectations of patients or express the obligations and responsibilities of the professional.

3. ***Virtues and character.*** The development of a professional role requires the cultivation of worthy character traits to complement professional practice. These virtues enhance motivation, colour judgement and form the basis of relationships with patients and colleagues.

Frameworks for assessing the moral life

A number of ethical theories have been developed which provide a framework for examining and resolving moral dilemmas in health care practice. There is no perfect or even best moral theory but each will contain a particular perspective and include a variety of strengths and weaknesses.

1. ***Monistic theories*** have one overriding principle which determines the method and conclusion of the theory as in:

- *Utilitarianism* – actions are right or wrong according to the balance of their good or bad consequences. There is a requirement to produce the greatest good for the greatest number.

- *Kantianism* (Immanuel Kant 1724–1804) – emphasizes the pre-eminence of duty and requires the development of morally acceptable rules which provide the direction of action.
- *Character ethics* – focuses on the agent who performs actions and makes choices. This follows in the tradition of Plato and Aristotle and suggests that an examination and promotion of human virtues will define and determine moral behaviour. Virtues such as compassion, integrity and discernment are particularly valued in the cultivation of a professional role.

2. Pluralistic theories are based on two or more non-absolute principles. Common morality ethics recognizes socially approved norms of conduct, which are universal standards. The principles within these shared moral beliefs are both binding and subject to revision (Beauchamp and Childress). Abstract principles must be defined to meet and address practical situations and judgements about the relative weight of principles; rules and rights are frequently necessary to resolve moral conflicts.

Duties of a doctor

Moral guidance for doctors has traditionally been enshrined in the Hippocratic Oath which placed certain obligations on those who followed the discipline of medicine.

The American Medical Association's first code of ethics (1847) was based on the teaching of the British physician Thomas Percival whose doctrine of medical ethics (1803) accorded priority to the principles of beneficence and non-maleficence over patient's rights or choices.

In the closing decades of the 20th century ethical debate and professional codes have emphasized the need to respect the autonomy of a patient. The opportunities of scientific and technological developments have raised many problems in the allocation of health care resources and other issues of distributive justice.

The General Medical Council (GMC) is the statutory body in the UK with powers granted by Parliament to regulate the medical profession. The GMC keeps and publishes the registers of those competent to practice. It controls the education standards of entry in the registers and removes doctors from the registers, temporarily or permanently, when they are deemed to have become unfit to practice.

Professional codes are statements of the role morality of members of the profession. They provide standards against which an individual doctor's fitness to practice may be judged. *Good Medical Practice* is published by the GMC (July 1998) and defines the duties and responsibilities of a doctor set by the regulatory body. 'All patients are entitled to good standards of practice and care from their doctors'. This requires:

- Practising and maintaining professional competence.
- Maintaining trust and professional relationships with patients and colleagues.
- Observing professional probity.

Further guidance on a number of issues raised in *Good Medical Practice* is published by the GMC including maintaining good medical practice; seeking patients' consent:

the ethical considerations; confidentiality; HIV and AIDS: the ethical considerations; advertising.

Further reading

Beachamp T, Childress J. *Principles of Biomedical Ethics*, 4th edn. Oxford University Press, 1994.
Campbell A, Charlesworth M, Gillet G, Jones G. *Medical Ethics*, 2nd edn. Oxford University Press, 1997.
Good Medical Practice. GMC 1998. http://www.gmc-uk.org

Related topics of interest

Audit – national (p. 30); Brain death and organ donation (p. 37); Critical incidents (p. 78); Evidence based medicine (p. 118); Governance (p. 121); Preoperative preparation (p. 209)

EVIDENCE-BASED MEDICINE
Alison Pickford

Evidence-based medicine is the conscientious, explicit and judicious use of current best evidence in making decisions about the care of individual patients or groups of patients. It means integrating individual clinical expertise with the best available external clinical evidence from systematic research.

Hierarchy of trustworthiness

Type	Strength of evidence for a therapeutic intervention (Gray 1997)
I	Strong evidence from at least one systematic review of multiple, well-designed Randomized Controlled Trials (RCTs).
II	Strong evidence from at least one well-designed RCT of appropriate size.
III	Evidence from well-designed trials without randomization, from single group pre- and postintervention, cohort, from time series or from matched case-controlled studies.
IV	Evidence from well-designed non-experimental studies from more than one centre or research group.
V	Opinions of respected authorities, based on clinical evidence, descriptive studies or reports of expert committees.

Types of evidence

1. Systematic reviews. The evidence is identified, appraised and conclusions drawn. The Cochrane Database of Systematic Reviews is a growing international collection of updated systematic reviews. However, in August 2000, only 9 out of 859 reviews were of direct relevance to anaesthesia.

2. Meta-analysis. This is a purely statistical technique to summarize several studies to provide a single estimate of the effect of an intervention.

3. Randomized controlled trials. Subjects are randomly assigned to either a study or control group (either placebo or, preferably, a currently accepted treatment). In some situations it may not be possible to randomize patients for either ethical or practical reasons. Evidence produced by non-randomized trials is less compelling, as statistical comparison of the groups may not be valid.

4. Cohort studies. Groups of people are chosen on the basis of differences between them and then followed over a period of time (usually years) to determine differences in either incidence of disease or disease progression (e.g. Doll and Hill's study on smoking and the incidence of lung cancer and death).

5. Case control studies. Patients with a particular condition are matched with controls and then both sets carefully questioned to determine if exposure to potential causative agents differ. This sort of study is often conducted to determine the aetiology of rare conditions and the main problem is in defining appropriate cases and controls. They can be viewed as retrospective as the investigator is looking backwards from the disease to a possible cause.

6. Cross-sectional studies. Information is collected from a population at a certain time. They are often prevalence surveys.

7. Case reports. The clinical history of one patient, or a series of patients, is used to highlight a particular problem.

Critical appraisal of clinical trials

Appraisal of the design and methodology of a trial must precede reading the results. Results from a poorly designed and conducted piece of research will be meaningless.

1. Trial design. The purpose of the trial must be clearly stated.

2. Subjects. Subjects should be described, including the source of recruitment, inclusion and exclusion criteria. These factors will determine whether the findings of the study can be applied to the whole population. All patients recruited to the trial should be accounted for in the paper. Analysis of treatment groups should reveal that subjects were similar in age, sex, height, weight, associated risk factor and disease severity characteristics. If they differ significantly statistical comparison of the two groups may not be valid.

3. Intervention. The intervention under investigation and the 'control' intervention should be carefully described. The patients should receive identical care in all other aspects of their treatment.

4. Controls. In a RCT this may be a placebo or a current, standard treatment (in an appropriate dose) given to a comparison group. The use of a placebo may be more likely to produce a statistically significant result but will not provide information on whether the new or standard treatment is more effective.

5. Outcome. This is the result of an intervention and should be objective and reproducible, using a method which is relevant to clinical practice. Ideally, one trained observer should take measurements. Unwanted effects should also be sought.

6. Bias. This is a deviation of results from the truth. Types of bias include detection, measurement, observer, performance, publication, responder, information retrieval or selection differences.

7. Randomization. Patients should be randomly assigned to one or other treatment groups, and the method of randomization described. Unequal group sizes suggest that randomization process was inadequate.

8. Blinding. Blinding of both investigator and patients (double blind) to the treatment group to which the patient is assigned reduces bias during assessment of outcome. With single blinding the patient is unaware of the group that they have been assigned to.

9. Intention-to-treat analysis. Analysis of subjects according to the group to which they were initially assigned, regardless of whether they were subsequently withdrawn from the trial, switched groups or were lost to follow-up. This will tend to reduce the difference between treatment groups.

10. *Study size.* This should be large enough to have a good chance of detecting as statistically significant a clinically important difference between intervention groups. The power of the study is its chance of detecting a true difference (this is usually 80–90%). A sample size or power calculation should be done before commencing the trial to ensure that it is not underpowered, which may lead to no difference being found when one exists (a type II error). This calculation requires a value for what is regarded as a clinically significant difference between the two intervention groups, and the mean and standard deviation of the primary outcome measurement. More subjects will be required if it is clinically worthwhile detecting a small difference between the intervention groups.

11. *Statistics.* Understanding the nature of the data that has been collected (continuous, discontinuous, normally distributed, etc.) and the assumptions made when using a particular statistical test are essential to ensure that appropriate statistical tests have been used.

12. *Probability and confidence.* The null hypothesis assumes that the intervention groups do not differ. The P value is the probability that the result occurred by chance and $P < 0.05$ is usually taken as indicating a statistically significant result, i.e. that the groups are different and the null hypothesis should be rejected. However, this result will occur by chance in 1/20 trials where there is no real difference between the intervention groups (a type I error). In addition, a statistically significant result may not be clinically significant if the difference between treatment groups is too small to be of clinical value. A negative result, where $P > 0.05$, may indicate that there is no difference between the groups, or that one exists but was not found because the sample size was too small (a type II error).

13. *Confidence intervals.* These give a measure of the precision of the trial findings. They estimate how likely the sample is to reflect the underlying population. The larger the sample the narrower the confidence intervals.

Further reading

Goodmann N. Anaesthesia and evidence-based medicine. *Anaesthesia*, 1998; **53:** 353–68.
Greenhalgh T. *How to read a paper. The basics of evidence based medicine.* British Medical Journal Publishing Group, 1997.
NHS Research and Development. Centre for Evidence-Based Medicine at: http://cebm.jr2.ox.ac.uk/

Related topics of interest

Audit – national (p. 30); Ethics and duty of care (p. 115); Governance (p. 121)

GOVERNANCE

Adrian Walker

Clinical governance was introduced in the Government white paper *The New NHS Modern–Dependable* (Dec 1997) and was defined as 'a framework through which NHS organizations are accountable for continuously improving the quality of their services and safeguarding high standards of care by creating an environment in which excellence in clinical care will flourish'.

The consultation document, *A First Class Service*, developed a strategy to deliver improved quality of care throughout the NHS and to remove unacceptable and substantial variations in performance and quality at all levels which were known to exist between and within Trusts.

NHS Trusts and Primary Care Trusts have a statutory duty (Health Act 1999) to monitor and improve the quality of care within and between their organizations. The development and delivery of clinical governance is at the heart of the quality agenda and central to the ability of Trusts to deliver these new responsibilities. The three elements of the model proposed in *A First Class Service* require:

Setting clear national quality standards

- A programme of evidence based National Service Frameworks to set out what patients can expect to receive from the Health Service in major care areas or disease groups.
- The National Institute for Clinical Excellence (NICE) to act as a nationwide appraisal body for new and existing treatments and to promote clinical and cost effectiveness through guidance and audit.

Ensuring local delivery of high quality services

All NHS organizations are required to promote clinical governance, reinforced by a new statutory duty of quality, supported by programmes of life-long learning and local professional self-regulation.

Monitoring delivery of quality standards

- A new NHS Performance Assessment Framework focuses on the quality and effectiveness of health care, as well as on efficiency.
- The Commission for Health Improvement provides an external assurance of the development of clinical governance through a rolling programme of Trust reviews.
- The statutory regulatory bodies for health professionals are involved in the development of arrangements for professional self-regulation.
- A national survey of patient and user experience.

Main components of clinical governance

'Clinical Governance – Quality in the New NHS'

1. ***Clear lines of responsibility and accountability*** for the overall quality of clinical care.

- The Chief Executive is responsible ultimately for assuring quality of services provided by NHS Trusts.
- A designated senior clinician is responsible for establishing and monitoring clinical governance.
- Formal arrangements for Trust Boards and Primary Care Groups to discharge their clinical quality responsibilities through a clinical governance committee.
- Board reports on quality to be given the same importance as financial reports.
- An annual report on clinical governance.

2. A comprehensive programme of quality improvement

- Full participation by all hospital doctors in local and national audit programmes and in the National Confidential Inquiries.
- Support for evidence-based practice and application in clinical care.
- Implementation of National Service Frameworks and NICE recommendations.
- Integration of workforce planning and development within the organization's service planning.
- Programmes of continuing professional development to meet the needs of individual professionals and the local service.
- Reviews of clinical care with high quality systems for record keeping and the collection of relevant information.
- Safeguards to govern access to and storage of confidential information.
- Processes to assure the quality of clinical care and integrated with quality programmes for the whole organization.
- Encouragement and support for relevant research and development activity.

3. Clear policies aimed at managing risks

- Controls assurance which promote self-assessment to identify and manage risk.
- Systematic clinical risk assessment and programmes of risk reduction.

4. Procedures for all professional groups to identify and remedy poor performance

- Reporting, investigating and learning from critical incidents.
- Review of complaints.
- Professional performance procedures which are understood by all staff, supportive to the individual and effective before patients are harmed.
- Support to staff in their duty to report any concerns about colleagues' professional conduct and performance and clear procedures to deal with these situations.

Clinical governance seeks to address the questions, 'Are we doing the right things?' and 'How well are we doing them?' Above all it is about changing organizations' values in a systematic and demonstrable way to develop an open and participative culture, a commitment to quality shared by clinicians and managers, an ethos of multidisciplinary team working and involvement of patients and the public.

Further reading

Department of Health. *Clinical Governance: Quality in the new NHS.* (HSC 1999/065). 16 March 1999.

The New NHS Modern–Dependable. Government White Paper. Her Majesty's Stationary Office. December 1997.

http://www.doh.gov.uk/public/wgpaper.htm   for White and Green Papers

Related topics of interest

Audit – national (p. 30); Ethics and duty of care (p. 113)

HEAD INJURY

Head injury accounts for approximately a third of all trauma deaths and is the leading cause of death and disability in young adults. However, severe head injury may still be compatible with a good outcome. Only preventative measures will help to address the primary brain injury. Secondary brain injury occurs sometime after the initial insult and is the result of cerebral hypoxia and ischaemia. Anaesthetists may be involved in the assessment and resuscitation of those with brain injuries, providing perioperative care to those undergoing surgery following such trauma, and the provision of critical care aimed at reducing the impact of secondary brain injury.

Causes of secondary brain injury and therapeutic aims

Cause	Aim
Hypotension	systolic blood pressure (SBP) > 120 mmHg (maintain cerebral perfusion pressure > 70 mmHg)
Hypoxia	$SpO_2 > 95\%$
Hypo/hypercapnia	$PaCO_2$ 4.5 kPa
Raised intracranial pressure (ICP)	ICP < 20–25 mmHg
Seizures	treat convulsions with diazepam and phenytoin
Hyperthermia	core temperature 35–37°C
Hyperglycaemia	blood sugar 4–7 mmol/l
Inflammatory mediator release	reduce release and impact of inflammatory mediators

Assessment and resuscitation

Initial resuscitation of patients with severe head injury should follow the ABCDE format. Hypoxia ($SpO_2 < 95\%$) and hypotension (SBP < 90 mmHg) independently increase mortality after severe head injury and must be treated aggressively. A rapid neurological assessment, including response to commands and any focal signs should be made before any sedative/paralysing drugs are given.

Airway

1. *Management of intubation.* Patients with head injuries should be sedated, paralysed, intubated and ventilated if there is airway compromise, ventilatory failure, a Glasgow Coma Score (GCS) < 9 or if warranted because of another injury. The airway should also be secured if there is any doubt that there may be airway compromise, or agitation may occur requiring sedation during a CT scan. It is appropriate to sedate and intubate patients with GCS scores of >8 to ensure optimal conditions for CT scanning and prevention of secondary brain injury. No head-injured adult or child should be sedated for a CT scan without control of the airway, even if this is to be reversed immediately afterwards.

An unstable cervical spine injury should be assumed until excluded. Oral tracheal intubation should follow a rapid sequence induction of anaesthesia and neuromuscular blockade with in-line stabilization of the cervical spine and cricoid pressure. Care should be taken to avoid hypotension during induction of anaesthesia as all intravenous anaesthetic agents are cardiovascular depressants.

Once intubated, sedation (with or without paralysis) should be maintained and an orogastric tube inserted. The oral route is preferred because of the risk of intracranial passage of a nasogastric tube in the presence of a base of skull fracture.

Breathing

All head injured patients requiring intubation will need ventilatory support. Ventilation should be monitored by arterial blood gas analysis and capnography.

In most cases the patient should be ventilated to normocapnia. In the early stages after head injury the patient should not be hyperventilated excessively because it induces vasoconstriction which results in a reduced cerebral blood flow (CBF). Long-term outcome has been shown to be worse following prolonged hyperventilation ($PaCO_2 < 3.4$ kPa) in adults with severe head injuries. If used, hyperventilation should be titrated against the ICP and jugular bulb oxygen saturation (SjO_2).

Circulation

Haemorrhage should be controlled by whatever means is required. Large-bore intravenous cannulae are inserted and the blood pressure maintained with i.v. fluid. Hypotonic solutions should be avoided. In the adult, BP should be maintained above 120 mmHg systolic (children > 90 mmHg systolic). A vasopressor may be needed to counteract the vasodilatory effects of anaesthetic drugs, once hypovolaemia has been excluded. In the multi-trauma patient persistent hypotension and tachycardia implies blood loss from extracranial injuries. Circulatory monitoring should include ECG, pulse oximetry, invasive blood pressure measurement, and urinary output. Severely head-injured patients should not be moved or transferred until life-threatening injuries are stable and an adequate mean arterial pressure has been achieved.

Disability

A rapid assessment of the GCS should be undertaken before anaesthesia is induced. An accurate assessment of the GCS and pupillary abnormalities takes a few seconds and has therapeutic and prognostic implications. See Scoring systems (p. 223).

Management of critically raised ICP

Critically raised ICP secondary to a CT proven or clinically suspected intracranial haematoma may be treated with a mannitol bolus (0.25–0.5 g/kg) and short-term hyperventilation. Mannitol is effective in lowering an acute rise in ICP but the hyperosmolality and dehydration may cause hypotension. Mannitol should be given as a bolus and not as an infusion. The use of hyperventilation or mannitol before ICP monitoring or CT scanning must be based on evidence of intracranial hypertension (pupillary dilation, motor posturing or progressive neurological deficit). Adequate sedation is essential. Serum osmolality may be used as a guide to mannitol therapy. The osmolality should not be allowed to rise above 310 mosmol/kg. Furosemide (frusemide) may be given instead of or in conjunction with mannitol.

Patients with severe head injury should be nursed approximately 30° head-up. This allows for adequate venous drainage and also reduces the risk of nosocomial pneumonia. A semi-rigid collar (if in place) should not be allowed to impede venous return and increase ICP.

Management of seizures

Seizures should be treated aggressively as they increase the cerebral metabolic rate and may lead to a critically raised ICP. The ABC sequence should be rechecked followed by a bolus of diazepam (0.1–0.2 mg/kg), thiopental or propofol. This is usually followed by a loading dose of phenytoin (15–20 mg/kg).

Identifying head-injured patients who require immediate life-saving neurosurgery

Patients who have an expanding intracranial haematoma and a critically rising ICP, as shown by a deteriorating level of consciousness and/or progressive focal signs, require immediate neurosurgery. If it is necessary to transfer the patient to another centre for neurosurgery, CT scan should not delay transfer if it can be performed more rapidly at the neurosurgical centre. Surgery may also be required for hydrocephalus and elevation of a depressed skull fracture.

Reducing cerebral metabolic requirements

If conventional therapy fails to control intracranial pressure adequately, an infusion of thiopental or propofol will reduce cerebral oxygen requirement ($CMRO_2$). Thiopental is given by infusion while monitoring the EEG to produce burst suppression. Increased temperature results in increased metabolic requirements and increased cerebral blood flow. Hypothermia to temperatures of around 33°C has been used and there is some evidence that suggests an improved outcome following severe head injury. Temperatures of less than 34°C are associated with coagulopathy which may have a negative effect on outcome, particularly in those patients with multi-trauma.

Computerized tomography

CT scanning is the most informative radiological investigation in the evaluation of head injury. CT scanning is needed to exclude lesions that require surgical intervention; the scans obtained have therapeutic and prognostic significance. The opportunity should also be used to scan the first and second cervical vertebrae and other areas of the cervical spine that are abnormal or inadequately seen on plain films. Adequate access to the patient, monitoring, and lack of movement must be ensured during CT scanning.

Monitoring

1. ICP monitoring   should be commenced in all patients with severe head injury who are being managed actively. The gold standard remains a surgically placed intraventricular catheter which also allows the removal of CSF to reduce ICP. Prolonged periods with ICP > 25 mmHg are associated with a poor outcome. Monitoring ICP allows cerebral perfusion pressure (CPP) to be measured (CPP = MAP–ICP). A

CPP < 70 mmHg is associated with a poor outcome. Therefore, CPP is maintained at >70 mmHg and it is usual for a vasopressor (e.g. noradrenaline) to be required to maintain this level.

2. SjO_2 is measured by a fibreoptic catheter placed retrogradely in the internal jugular vein at the level of the C1 vertebral body. Saturation measurements allow some assessment of global cerebral ischaemia or hyperaemia. Monitoring allows targeted hyperventilation, CPP management and osmotherapy. Saturations < 55% are associated with a poor outcome.

3. _Transcranial Doppler_ allows assessment of CBF velocity. A pulsatility index can be derived which with SjO_2 can be used to define the optimum CPP.

4. _Evoked potentials_ and the electroencephalogram (EEG) are used in selected patients to assess activity and gauge level of sedation in thiopental coma. Regular assessment of GCS is mandatory. Deterioration in the GCS and/or the onset of lateralizing signs necessitates urgent investigation.

Adjunctive therapy

Fluid balance should be carefully adjusted. Dramatic osmolar shifts, hyponatraemia and fluid overload should be avoided. Electrolyte disturbances are common in severe head injury patients as a result of fluid therapy, the stress response, osmotic and loop diuretics, and diabetes insipidus. Physiotherapy is important in preventing chest infection and limb contractures, but adequate sedation is required to prevent increases in ICP.

Prophylactic antibiotics are required only for invasive procedures. Prophylactic anticonvulsants are often commenced in severe head injury. However, there is little evidence that anticonvulsant therapy has an impact on the development of late seizures. The relationship of early seizures to outcome is unclear.

Early enteral nutrition reduces the incidence of gastric erosions, nosocomial chest infection and reduces the negative nitrogen balance that accompanies severe head injury. DVT prophylaxis should be initiated early. Compression stockings and calf compression devices may be used shortly after admission. Heparin therapy is often delayed because of the presence of intracerebral blood and the risk of further bleeding.

The future

Like all organs, the brain may be damaged by the effects of inflammatory mediators. A primary brain injury may result in the local release of mediators such as tumour necrosis factor α, interleukin-1β, and interleukin-6. These cytokines stimulate the restorative processes (gliosis). Gliosis may itself attract further cellular infiltration and perversely result in local ischaemia and cellular hypoxia. Circulating leucocytes are probably attracted to the site of injury by such mediators and encouraged to migrate through the capillary wall by raised concentrations of leucocyte adhesion substances. Attempts to produce drugs to influence this process have not thus far resulted in success. Until such time as they do, prevention of systemic hypotension, hypoxaemia and hypothermia together with optimization of cerebral oxygen delivery remain the mainstays of the management of acute head injury.

Further reading

Chestnut RM. Guidelines for the management of severe head injury. In: Vincent JL (ed). *Yearbook of Intensive Care and Emergency Medicine*, 1997. Berlin, Springer, pp. 749–765.

McKeating EG, Andrews PJD. Cytokines and adhesion molecules in acute brain injury. *British Journal of Anaesthesia*, 1998; **80**: 77–84.

Related topics of interest

Brain death and organ donation (p. 37); Epilepsy (p. 113); MRI (p. 156); Scoring systems (p. 223); Spinal injury (p. 245)

HISTORY OF ANAESTHESIA

The first demonstration of the use of anaesthesia for a surgical procedure was given at Massachusetts General Hospital, Boston, USA on 16th October 1846 (Ether Day). William Morton, a dentist, gave ether to a patient in a large amphitheatre now known as the Ether Dome. News of this travelled fast and in November of 1846 a demonstration of the anaesthetic properties of ether was given to a medical society meeting in London. Robert Liston, a surgeon at University College Hospital (UCH), London was present at the meeting and discussed it with William Squire, then a medical student at UCH. Squire had an uncle who was a pharmacist in Oxford Street and between them they conducted experiments with ether and developed apparatus for its administration. It was William Squire who, on 21 December 1846, administered ether for the first widely witnessed operation under anaesthesia in Europe. The amputation of a leg was performed in a crowded operating theatre at UCH by Liston on Frederick Churchill, a butler from Harley Street. The operation took place after the patient had breathed ether vapour for 2 or 3 minutes and was a great success.

The following year Simpson, professor of midwifery at Edinburgh University, overcame some of the technical difficulties of inhaling ether when he dropped chloroform onto a gauze held near the face. In 1853 John Snow gave chloroform to Queen Victoria at the birth of Prince Leopold. Royal approval thus led to the title chloroform à la reine for this practice.

Local anaesthesia was not described scientifically until 1884. Carl Koller accepted a suggestion in Vienna from his friend Sigmund Freud to assess further the actions of cocaine. This led to his description of the use of cocaine as topical analgesia in the conjunctival sac for ophthalmic surgery.

Milestone dates in the history of anaesthesia

1844   Horace Wells developed nitrous oxide inhalation for use during dental extraction.

1846   16th October. Morton gave the first ether anaesthetic for surgery, Boston, USA.

21st December. The first ether anaesthetic in Europe, given by Squire at UCH, London.

1847   Chloroform used by Simpson, Edinburgh.

1848   The first anaesthetic death from the effects of chloroform occurred in a 15-year-old girl just 11 weeks after its introduction into medical practice.

1853   Snow gave chloroform to the Queen at the birth of Prince Leopold.

1857   Claude Bernard demonstrated that curare acts at the neuromuscular junction.

1868   Nitrous oxide supplied in cylinders in the UK.

1872   Antisialagogue properties of atropine recorded.

1882   Synthesis of cyclopropane.

1884   Koller reported the local analgesic properties of cocaine.

1891   Quincke demonstrated lumbar puncture.

1894   Codman and Harvey Cushing in Baltimore, USA, advocated the keeping of anaesthetic record charts.

1898   Bier introduced spinal anaesthesia.

1901   Extradural caudal injection was developed in Paris.

1905   The first society of anaesthetists was founded. In 1945 it became the American Society of Anesthesiologists.

1909   Tracheal insufflation anaesthesia used in animals.

1910   Tracheal intubation performed in man.
McKesson introduced the first demand intermittent-flow gas and oxygen machine with calibration of the gases.

1917   Edmund Boyle described his portable nitrous oxide and oxygen apparatus.

1920   Guedel's paper on the signs of anaesthesia.

1923   Carbon dioxide absorption employed in man by Waters.

1928   Magill introduced blind nasal intubation.

1930   Sword produced a circle method of CO_2 absorption.

1933   Thiopentone introduced into clinical practice.
Ralph Waters appointed as the first professor of anesthesia in the USA.

1937   Robert Macintosh appointed Nuffield professor of anaesthetics in Oxford, the first chair of anaesthesia in Europe.

1941   Trichloroethylene advocated by Langton Hewer.

1942   The use of curare advocated by Griffith and Johnson.

1948   Griffith and Gillies introduced hypotensive anaesthesia.

1951   Halothane synthesized by Suckling in Manchester.

1952   Widespread use of IPPV with bag and tracheal tube during the polio epidemic in Copenhagen.

1953   The first examination for Fellowship of the Faculty of Anaesthetists of the Royal College of Surgeons of England.

1956   Halothane used clinically.

1966   Enflurane used in Denver, USA.

1984   Isoflurane introduced into clinical practice.

1985   Mandatory standards for minimal patient monitoring during anaesthesia adopted at Harvard, Boston, USA. ASA issued recommended standards the following year.

1986   Propofol introduced into clinical practice.
Laryngeal mask airway used in clinical practice.

1988   College of Anaesthetists established.

1992   Royal charter granted to the College of Anaesthetists.

1995   Sevoflurane introduced into clinical practice.

Further reading

Atkinson RS, Bolton TB. *The History of Anaesthesia*. Parthenon, 1989.
Rushman GB. *A Short History of Anaesthesia*. Butterworth Heinemann, 1996.

HYPERTENSION

Hypertension is the commonest indication in the Western World for chronic, lifelong treatment because of the incontrovertible evidence that such treatment reduces the risk of strokes. Of 315 patients with malignant hypertension studied with a median follow-up of 33 months 126 died within the study period. Of those patients 39.7% had renal failure, 23.8% suffered a CVA, 11.1% had a myocardial infarction (MI), and 10.3% had heart failure. In a meta-analysis of the impact of anti-hypertensive therapy comprising 9 trials including 43 000 patients with mild to moderate hypertension (diastolic pressure > 105 mmHg) there was a 38% reduction in fatal CVA and an 8% reduction in fatal MI in the treatment group. Similarly, in isolated systolic hypertension in the elderly (systolic pressure > 160 mmHg, diastolic pressure < 90 mmHg) treatment resulted in mean systolic pressures 11.1 mmHg lower. The treatment group had 36% fewer strokes and suffered 27% fewer MIs.

Problems
- Hypertensive patients may have associated medical problems (e.g. LVH [20–60% of hypertensives referred for hospital care], accelerated athero-sclerosis, reduced coronary vasodilatory reserve, altered autoregulation).
- Following induction of anaesthesia untreated hypertensives show a greater fall in blood pressure and episodes of perioperative myocardial ischaemia.
- Patients with hypertensive disease have increased perioperative cardiovascular risks.

Causes of perioperative hypertension
1. *Primary or essential hypertension.*

2. *Secondary*   (accounts for only 10% of hypertensives).
   - Renal, e.g. chronic pyelonephritis, chronic glomerulonephritis, renal artery stenosis, polycystic disease.
   - Endocrine, e.g. phaeochromocytoma, Cushing's syndrome, Conn's syndrome, acromegaly.
   - Pregnancy (pre-eclampsia, eclampsia) and the contraceptive pill.
   - Coarctation of the aorta.

3. *Related to anaesthesia:*
   - Hypoxia.
   - Hypercarbia.
   - Light anaesthesia/inadequate analgesia.
   - Fluid overload.
   - Drug interactions, e.g. monoamine oxidase inhibitors.
   - Surgical effects, e.g. aortic cross clamping.
   - Hypothermia.
   - Malignant hyperpyrexia.
   - Measurement errors, e.g. a too small blood pressure cuff or an underdamped arterial trace.
   - Raised intracranial pressure.

Hypertension and perioperative risk

- Hypertensive disease is associated with increased perioperative risk. This increased risk is probably mediated through target organ changes associated with hypertension. Hypertensive disease appears to be a risk factor for perioperative cardiovascular complications.
- The perioperative cardiovascular risks in an untreated hypertensive can be reduced by the use of pre-anaesthetic medication with a beta blocker.
- Elevated blood pressure in a non-hypertensive immediately preoperatively does not appear to be associated with increased perioperative risk.
- There is no evidence of an interaction between preoperative blood pressure and hypertensive disease i.e. the risks of a treated hypertensive patient with elevated preoperative blood pressure are those of a treated hypertensive patient without elevated pressure immediately preoperatively.

Perioperative management

A complete assessment of the patient will establish whether there is evidence of end organ damage due to hypertension. All patients on antihypertensive treatment should remain on their therapy throughout the perioperative period. As noted, hypertensives show exaggerated haemodynamic responses to anaesthesia and surgery. All general anaesthetic agents and sustained administration of, or high sensory blockade resulting from, local anaesthetics cause myocardial depression, hypotension, and changes in heart rate. Anticipation of these effects will permit a choice of anaesthetic technique to minimize their occurrence. In particular, attention to intravascular volume status is important. The combination of hypotension and tachycardia is most detrimental to the heart. Hypokalaemia requiring correction is common in those on long-term thiazide diuretic therapy.

Postoperative rebound hypertension is not uncommon amongst hypertensives and close monitoring should continue in the early postoperative period.

Further reading

Howell SJ, Sear JW, Yeates D et al. Hypertension, admission blood pressure and perioperative risk. *Anaesthesia*, 1996; **51:** 1000–1004.

Muir AD, Reeder MK, Sear JW, Foëx P. Preoperative silent ischemia has a relationship with hypertension. *British Journal of Anaesthesia*, 1988; **69:** 540.

Related topics of interest

Cardiac assessment (p. 55); Cardiac ischaemia (p. 58); Hypotensive anaesthesia (p. 133); Preoperative preparation (p. 209)

HYPOTENSIVE ANAESTHESIA

Deliberate hypotension was introduced in 1948 by Griffiths and Gillie and is now in common use. However, the need for, and the degree of, hypotension remain controversial.

Hypotensive anaesthesia improves the surgical field especially in major head and neck, ENT, plastic, vascular, orthopaedic, and microsurgical operations. It reduces blood loss by approximately 50% and therefore the need for transfusion. Major cancer surgery performed under controlled hypotension may increase survival. Hypotension may be essential during the clipping of an intracranial aneurysm, particularly if it has ruptured.

Contraindications to hypotension include hypertension, ischaemic or valvular heart disease, or a previous stroke. It should not be performed in hypovolaemia, pregnancy, anaemia, or if renal or hepatic disease is present. The latter two will be exacerbated by a reduction in organ blood flow. It is also contraindicated in those with glaucoma who are taking ganglion blocking drugs.

Problems

1. Cerebral. Autoregulation occurs between a mean arterial blood pressure (MABP) of 50 and 150 mmHg, but cerebral perfusion is the important factor. This is also affected by ICP and venous pressure. Normocapnoea should be maintained as the vasoconstricting effect of hypocarbia is lost below a MABP of 35 mmHg. Direct acting vasodilators (cf. ganglion blockers) allow autoregulation at lower pressures than usual. Awake normotensive patients tolerate a MABP as low as 35 mmHg.

2. Cardiac. Coronary perfusion is dependent on perfusion pressure, wall tension and the diastolic/systolic time ratio. Seventy-five per cent of coronary perfusion normally occurs during diastole.

3. Renal. Little perfusion and therefore filtration occurs if the MABP is <60 mmHg. Low perfusion pressures produce the potential for ATN and activation of the angiotensin/renin system. Mannitol is recommended for prolonged hypotension.

4. Pulmonary. Hypotension increases dead space, V/Q mismatching and reduces FRC. Some hypotensive agents may affect hypoxic pulmonary vasoconstriction.

Anaesthetic management

1. Assessment and premedication. Anxiolytic and sedative premedicants prevent tachycardia and hypertension prior to induction.

2. Conduct of anaesthesia. Premedication, patient position, good analgesia and the basic anaesthetic technique are the most important considerations. Propofol and remifentanil infusions or isoflurane can be used with the aim of maintaining cardiac output but lowering the peripheral vascular resistance and therefore the blood pressure. More profound hypotension can then be produced by interference with the homeostatic mechanisms of blood pressure control. Compensatory tachycardia may occur and require blocking to allow hypotension to develop.

Monitoring is commenced before hypotensive agents are given. Direct blood pressure measurements should be made via an arterial cannula if profound hypotension is required. An ECG is essential. Monitoring of the CVP is recommended if large blood losses are expected.

CNS monitoring during hypotension with EEG, CFM, CFAM and jugular venous O_2 content have all been advocated. The significance of changes is difficult to interpret and postoperative neuropsychological tests have not shown a correlation between impairment and hypotension. Renal function is monitored by urine output via a catheter. Blood gases should be taken for acid–base status. Pulmonary gas exchange during hypotension is monitored with capnography and arterial gases. Oximetry may be impossible if peripheral perfusion is low. Body temperature should also be measured. Anaesthetic techniques may induce hypotension by:

- Volatile agents reducing baroreceptor input to the brain stem.
- Anaesthetic agents affecting the brain stem vascular centre causing a fall in vasomotor tone.
- Epidural–spinal blockade reducing sympathetic outflow.
- Specific hypotensive drugs such as α- and β-blockers or trimetaphan (a ganglion blocker). Esmolol is a short acting β-blocker given by infusion.
- Direct vasodilators which act on resistance vessels. They include: hydralazine, isoflurane, nitroprusside, adenosine, glyceryltrinitrate, and the dinitrates. These drugs also have an effect on the capacitance vessels (venous) and are listed in ascending order of their potency at this site. Sodium nitroprusside achieves arteriolar and venous dilation which lasts for approximately 3 minutes. It is given by infusion, is light sensitive, exhibits tachyphylaxis and is metabolized to cyanide. The maximum dose is 10 mg/kg/min with a total dosage of 1.5 mg/kg given over several hours.

3. Postoperatively. Hypotension may persist postoperatively. Invasive monitoring and high depend-ency nursing should be available until the blood pressure is normal.

4. Complications of hypotension. Mortality related to hypotensive anaesthetic techniques is very low (< 1 in 2000). Non-fatal complications such as dizziness, delayed awakening, retinal thrombosis, DVT, anuria, oliguria and cerebral thrombosis or infarction can occur. The incidence of these serious side-effects is low, but a lower limit of a MABP of 60 mmHg is an appropriate safety precaution. When healthy patients were randomized to receive normotension or a MABP of between 50 and 60 mmHg, no morbidity, mortality or change in psychometric tests could be demonstrated in either group. The problems of drug interactions, retraction ischaemia and reactive bleeding need to be considered prior to undertaking a hypotensive technique.

Further reading

Hack H, Mitchell V. Hypotensive anaesthesia. *British Journal of Hospital Medicine*, 1996; **55**: 482–485.
Moss E. Cerebral blood flow during induced hypotension. *British Journal of Anaesthesia*, 1995; **74**: 635–637.

Related topics of interest

Cardiac surgery (p. 65); Cardiac valvular disease (p. 67); Hypertension (p. 131); Neuroanaesthesia (p. 167); Positioning (p. 207); Preoperative preparation (p. 209); Sequelae of anaesthesia (p. 232)

INHERITED CONDITIONS

Many genetic disorders cause minor anaesthetic problems but a few have serious implications. Some appear as individual topics, whilst others are discussed here.

Ankylosing spondylitis

A connective tissue disease that predominantly affects the sacroiliac joints and vertebral column. It occurs mainly in males (20–40 years) and with progressive ossification of joint and disc cartilages forms a fused kyphotic spine. The joints of the chest wall may be involved resulting in a fixed rib cage and a reduced vital capacity. It is associated with HLA B27, ulcerative colitis, uveitis, aortitis with aortic incompetence, apical fibrosing alveolitis, respiratory failure and general ill health. Anaesthetic implications are cardiovascular, respiratory and difficult intubation due to the fixed flexion deformity of the cervical spine. A fibreoptic intubation may be required. Spinal and epidural techniques may be impossible due to calcification of ligaments.

Downs syndrome

Trisomy 21 has an incidence of 1.5 per 1000 live births. Meiotic non-dysjunction is responsible for 90%, and is related to maternal age. The typical facial appearance is associated with a large protruding tongue, a small mandible, congenital heart disease (in 50%), mental retardation, epilepsy, scoliosis, atlanto-axial instability, immunological impairment, duodenal obstruction and cataracts. Surgery may or may not be related to the above, but their possible existence should be considered. An appropriate technique can then be selected. Sedative and antisialagogue premedicants are often used. Despite the anatomical abnormalities a difficult intubation is unusual.

Haemophilia

Haemophilia A is a recessive X-linked deficit of Factor VIII. The intrinsic clotting system is affected with a prolonged partial thromboplastin time (the bleeding time is normal). Plasma levels of Factor VIII vary between individuals resulting in differing severities of the disease. If the level is >10% of normal then abnormal bleeding is unlikely unless surgery is performed. Factor VIII concentrate is given to maintain levels at approximately 15% (an HIV risk in the past). A haematological opinion should always be sought prior to surgery, and levels approaching 100% ensured. DDAVP (desmopressin) raises Factor VIII levels. Careful planning of the procedure and the patient's perioperative care is vital. Intramuscular injections are not used. Increased care should be taken with the insertion of lines and patient positioning. Regional anaesthesia is not recommended. Factor VIII levels should be maintained for approximately 10 days postoperatively. PCA has been used to avoid I.M. injections and the risks of antiprostenoids.

Marfans syndrome

This connective tissue disease shows autosomal dominant inheritance and results in structural abnormalities. These include abnormal height, arachnodactyly, a high arched palate, upward displacement of the lens, a twisted sternum, hypermobility and muscle hypotonia. The CVS may be involved with aortic or mitral regurgitation, atrial septal defects and aortic aneurysms or dissections. Spontaneous pneumothorax and hernias are common. Surgery may be related to any of the above and careful preoperative assessment is essential. Anaesthetic problems relate to the potential difficult intubation, to cardiovascular and respiratory complications and to patient positioning.

Pierre Robin syndrome

Problems with the airway are common. Micrognathia, glossoptosis and cleft palate are seen. The syndrome may be part of more widespread congenital abnormalities. Airway obstruction and feeding difficulties occur which resolve as the infant grows. Nursing prone, a tongue suture or a tracheostomy may be required to prevent heart failure from chronic airway obstruction. A gastrostomy can be performed under local anaesthesia to overcome feeding problems. Intubation can be extremely difficult and sometimes impossible even with the use of fibreoptic instruments and other techniques. Tracheostomy may become necessary. A laryngeal mask may help in maintaining the airway. Senior staff should always be involved.

Further reading

Benumof JL. *Anesthesia and Uncommon Diseases*, 4th edn. Philadelphia: WB Saunders, 1997.
Mitchell V, Howard R, Facer E. Down's syndrome and anaesthesia. *Paediatric Anaesthesia* 1995; **5:** 379–384.
Schelew BL, Vaghadia H. Ankylosing spondylitis and neuraxial anaesthesia – a 10 year review. *Canadian Journal of Anaesthesia* 1996; **43:** 65–68.

Related topics of interest

Diabetes (p. 89); Intubation – difficult (p. 141); Myasthenia gravis (p. 158); Myotonia (p. 161); Obesity (p. 173); Porphyria (p. 205); Sickle cell disease (p. 235); Temperature-hyperthermia (p. 251); Temperature-hypothermia (p. 255)

INTUBATION – AWAKE

General anaesthesia is not essential in order to secure the airway with a tracheal tube. An awake intubation offers a number of advantages. Even when local anaesthetic agents are used in the airway the patient retains some ability to respond to a threat to the airway. Vomiting or regurgitation will produce coughing, retching or repeated swallowing despite the obtunded pharyngeal and laryngeal reflexes. Closing the mouth, gagging and swallowing will make the procedure more difficult. The degree of disturbance to the patient will depend upon the operator's skill, the psychological and pharmacological preparation and the advice that the patient has received. A tracheal tube can be passed nasally or orally using a fibreoptic bronchoscope. Alternatively it can be passed orally through an intubating laryngeal mask.

Indications

1. Potential upper airway obstruction. It is axiomatic to anaesthetic practice that muscle relaxants are not administered to patients with airway obstruction until it is clear that the airway can be maintained. Attempting intubation under deep inhalational anaesthesia can be hazardous, especially in the presence of a full stomach, and an awake intubation offers an alternative. However, airway obstruction can be precipitated by topical anaesthesia of the pharynx and larynx and attempted awake intubation for upper airway obstruction can result in total obstruction. Tracheostomy under local anaesthesia is therefore recommended if there is severe stridor with markedly abnormal laryngeal anatomy.

2. Predicted difficult intubation. Intubation of patients who are known or suspected to be a difficult intubation may be attempted awake with the knowledge that if a particular technique fails the patient is still breathing and in control of their airway. However, if a local anaesthetic block has been administered there is some loss of laryngeal reflexes, and there is a risk of aspiration despite being awake and breathing spontaneously.

3. Full stomach. This is more popular in the USA than in the UK.

4. Respiratory impairment. Patients are often *in extremis* and the use of cardiorespiratory depressant drugs in any amount may bring about their immediate demise.

Anaesthetic management

Assessment and premedication

A full assessment of the upper airway is made. A simple, unhurried explanation of the anaesthetic plan will help allay patient anxiety and is essential to secure co-operation. Antisialagogue premedication (atropine, hyoscine or glycopyrrolate) is recommended. A dry oropharynx will improve the view, reduce the patient's desire to swallow and increase the effectiveness of topical local anaesthetic agents.

Conduct of anaesthesia

Monitoring of the blood pressure, ECG and O_2 saturation should commence before undertaking an awake intubation. End tidal CO_2 should be available to assist confirmation of tube placement. Awake intubation may be performed orally, nasally, or via a retrograde route and either under direct vision or blind.

Local anaesthetic techniques

1. Topical anaesthesia. Thirty minutes prior to arrival in the operating department the patient may be given an amethocaine (tetracaine) or benzocaine lozenge to suck. This will anaesthetize the mouth and oropharynx. An alternative to the lozenge is to give nebulized lidocaine (lignocaine).

Surface anaesthesia of the nasal mucosae is obtained by packing the nose with ribbon gauze soaked in local anaesthetic solution or applying instillagel. Cocaine or oxymetazoline are used as potent vasoconstrictors. Lidocaine (lignocaine) 4% spray is administered progressively further down the airway as the operator advances by giving the solution down one of the channels of the fibreoptic endoscope. Care must be taken not to administer a toxic dose, as agents are readily systemically absorbed through mucosae that have a rich blood supply. Intubating fibreoptic endoscopes are at least 25 cm long and are available with small diameters e.g. 3 mm, although the field of view may be compromised.

Labat's syringe has a curved applicator and is used to drip local anaesthetic agents on to the glottis. The patient sits up and the tongue is held extended by the operator in a gauze swab. Local anaesthetic is then allowed to fall onto the vocal cords and through the larynx. Anaesthesia to the subglottic region may be further increased using a cricothyroid injection. A weal of local anaesthetic is raised in the skin over the cricothyroid membrane and a narrow gauge needle is inserted through it into the trachea. Correct placement is confirmed by the aspiration of air into the syringe. The patient is then asked to take a deep breath in. At the end of inspiration 2 ml of local anaesthetic are injected. This produces an explosive cough as the liquid hits the trachea and results in the local anaesthetic being sprayed onto the underside of the vocal cords and subglottic region.

2. Nerve blocks. Although these are described most operators prefer topical anaesthesia as it provides good conditions with limited risk. Sensation from the hard and soft palate, nasal mucosae and the nasopharynx is supplied by the second division of the trigeminal nerve (maxillary). The posterior third of the tongue, oropharynx and tonsillar area are supplied by the glossopharyngeal nerves.

The superior laryngeal nerve is a branch of the vagus nerve and gives rise to an external and an internal branch at the greater cornu of the hyoid bone. The external branch supplies the cricothyroid membrane whilst the internal branch serves the mucous membrane of the larynx down to the rima glottidis. Sensation below the rima glottidis is supplied by the inferior laryngeal nerves, the terminal branch of the recurrent laryngeal nerve.

- Maxillary nerve block. This is achieved by introducing a needle angled at 45° into the sphenopalatine canal via the greater palatine foraminae of the hard palate. A small volume of local anaesthetic (~2 ml) may then be deposited.
- A glossopharyngeal nerve block may precipitate airway obstruction following loss of tone at the base of the tongue. It is helpful, however, in patients with an active gag reflex. It is achieved by inserting an angled tonsillar needle behind the posterior tonsillar pillar and injecting 3 ml of local anaesthetic agent.
- Superior laryngeal nerve block. (i) Krause's method. The superior laryngeal nerve lies just below the laryngeal mucosa in the piriform fossa. A dental pledget soaked in anaesthetic solution and firmly held by a pair of Krause's forceps is held in the piriform fossa for about 1 minute on each side. (ii) Percutaneous block. The superior laryngeal nerve divides into internal and external branches at the greater cornu of the hyoid, a point at which it may be blocked. Both left and right nerves may be approached from a common midline point. A skin weal is raised over the thyroid cartilage in the midline and a needle advanced laterally and cephaladly onto the hyoid bone. The needle is walked off the hyoid at the greater cornu and 2 ml of local anaesthetic solution deposited. Passage to the cornu may be eased by gently pulling the hyoid bone to the left for a right nerve block and vice versa.

Sedation

Sedative agents including the benzodiazepines have been recommended to supplement local anaesthetic blocks for an awake intubation. It is important though that patient safety is not compromised by the use of such agents. Low dose TIVA and neurolept techniques (e.g. fentanyl and droperidol) have also been described.

Further reading

Hagberg CA. *Handbook of Difficult Airway Management.* Harcourt Publishers. 1999.
Shung J, Avidan MS, Ing R, Klein CD, Pott L. Awake intubation of the difficult airway with the intubating laryngeal mask airway. *Anaesthesia* 1998; **53:** 645–649.

Related topics of interest

Hypertension (p. 131); Inherited conditions (p. 136); Intubation – difficult (p. 141); Tracheostomy (p. 266)

INTUBATION – DIFFICULT

The following discussion of difficult intubation assumes that intubating conditions are optimal and that simple aids such as a gum elastic bougie are used. In particular, the patient's head should be correctly positioned. There should be anterior flexion of the lower cervical spine and extension of the atlanto-occipital joint ('sniffing the morning air'). This position results in the axial alignment of the mouth, pharynx and larynx. Attempts have been made to quantify difficult intubation with grading systems. Methods of predicting difficult intubation have also been developed. The incidence of difficulty with intubation is low (~1:65) with failure to intubate occurring in ~1:2000 patients (1 in 300 in obstetrics). Predictive tests must therefore be sensitive and specific. No single test is ideal. Anyone attempting an intubation must be familiar with a failed intubation drill.

Causes of difficult intubation

1. Congenital e.g. Pierre Robin syndrome, Down's, craniofacial dysostoses, etc.

2. Anatomical. Variants of normal anatomy, e.g. prominent teeth, short thick neck, deep protuberant or receding mandible, pregnancy.

3. Acquired e.g. trismus, soft tissue swelling, scarring, cervical rheumatoid arthritis, airway malignancy.

Grading difficult laryngoscopy

Cormack and Lehane graded obstetric laryngoscopy but this classification is now also widely used for non-obstetric intubations.

- Grade 1. Most of the glottis is seen and there is no difficulty.
- Grade 2. Only the posterior extremity of the glottis is visible and there may be slight difficulty. Pressure on the neck may improve the view of the larynx.
- Grade 3. The epiglottis can be seen but no part of the glottis is visible. There may be severe difficulty.
- Grade 4. Not even the epiglottis can be seen. Intubation is impossible without special techniques. This situation is rare if the anatomy is normal. It occurs with obvious pathology.

Patients with grade 4 intubations are usually detected in advance, and appropriate precautions, techniques and skills used to avoid morbidity and mortality. It is the unexpected grade 3 cases which give rise to the greatest risk.

Predicting difficult intubation

Methods of predicting difficulties with intubation have been developed and their reliability assessed using Cormack and Lehane's classification at laryngoscopy.

Mallampati described a predictive assessment made with the patient sitting opposite the assessor. It will only predict 50% of difficult intubations. The patient is asked to open their mouth and extend their tongue. The extent to which the structures are visible leads to a predictive classification.

- Class 1. The soft palate, faucial pillars and uvula are all visible.
- Class 2. The soft palate and faucial pillars are visible but the uvula is obscured by the base of the tongue.
- Class 3. Only the soft palate is visible.

Sansoon and Young later added Class 4 in which only the hard palate is seen.

The thyro-mental distance was used by Patil to predict the ease of intubation. If the distance was less than 6.5 cm or, more crudely, would not admit three fingers then a difficult intubation was predicted.

White and Kander retrospectively compared radiological measurements in those patients who had proved to be a difficult intubation with normals. The following were found to be useful predictors.

1. Ratio of mandibular length to posterior depth >3.6. Mandibular length is measured from the tip of the lower incisor to the posterior limit of the bone at its articulation with the temple. Posterior depth is the length of a perpendicular from the alveolar margin of the last molar tooth to the lower border of the mandible.

2. Increased anterior depth of the mandible (measured as a perpendicular from the tip of the most anterior incisor).

3. A reduced distance between the spinous process of C1 and the occiput (atlanto-occipital distance). This is a measure of the ability to extend the head during laryngoscopy.

Wilson *et al.* have produced a scoring system to predict the ease of intubation employing such factors as body weight, extent of movement of head, neck and jaw, the presence of a receding mandible and prominent teeth.

Management of difficult intubation

Attempts at intubating a patient known or predicted to be a difficult intubation should not be made without a suitably experienced anaesthetist with the skills to perform specialized techniques of intubation. Initially simple aids such as a gum elastic bougie with the tracheal tube railroaded over it may be used. More complex techniques may include cricothyroid puncture and retrograde intubation, intubation through a laryngeal mask, the use of difficult laryngoscopy blades e.g. a McCoy blade or the Bullard fibre-optic laryngoscope, or an awake intubation. A fibreoptic scope with a size 6 tracheal tube railroaded on its shaft can be passed down a size 3, 4 or 5 laryngeal mask and through the cords. The tracheal tube is then advanced. Alternatively an 'intubating' laryngeal mask can be used with blind advancement of the tracheal tube.

The use of a tracheostomy under local anaesthesia, and the use of intubation under deep inhalational anaesthesia should be considered. Expired CO_2 should always be used to confirm successful intubation.

Failed intubation

Morbidity and cases of mortality occur following difficulty with intubation, not usually because of a failure to intubate but a failure to stop trying to intubate and attend to the resuscitation of the patient. Anaesthetic practice used to allow for the return of spontaneous respiration as muscle relaxants became metabolized and then deepening anaesthesia using a spontaneously breathing technique. Even in the case of an emergency Caesarean section for fetal distress, however, modern teaching tends to favour a positive wake-up approach. In the case of a failed intubation the patient should be maintained in the same position with cricoid pressure applied, and manual ventilation given with 100% O_2 until breathing recommences. Further help and an alternative technique of anaesthesia may then be employed. The disaster is not failing to intubate, but failure to intubate and failure to ventilate and oxygenate. Under these circumstances a laryngeal mask or an oesophageal/tracheal Combitube may allow oxygenation. If this fails then cricothyroid puncture with jet ventilation is indicated.

Further reading

Charters P, O'Sullivan E. The 'dedicated airway': a review of the concept and an update of current practice. *Anaesthesia*, 1999; **54:** 778–786.

Crosby ET *et al.* The unanticipated difficult airway with recommendations for management. *Canadian Journal of Anaesthesia*, 1998; **45:** 757–776.

Practice Guidelines for Management of the Difficult Airway. *Anesthesiology*, 1993; **78:** 597–602. Algorithm at http://www.asahq.org/practice/homepage.html

Related topics of interest

Inherited conditions (p. 136); Intubation – awake (p. 138); Laryngectomy (p. 144); Obstetrics – delivery (p. 178); Tracheostomy (p. 266)

LARYNGECTOMY

Two thousand people develop laryngeal cancer in England and Wales each year. The vast majority are smokers or ex-smokers. Laryngectomy is reserved for those with invasive tumours or if radiotherapy has failed to control the disease. It is mutilating but potentially life saving. Laryngectomy is performed on its own, or with a block dissection of the neck, or as part of a pharyngolaryngectomy. Consideration of the psychological aspects of the operation must be made.

Problems

- Elderly and cachectic patients.
- Shared airway with poor access.
- Abnormal airway anatomy – difficult intubation.
- Smoking related CVS and respiratory disease.
- Potentially large intraoperative blood loss.
- Carotid sinus stimulation with bradycardia and hypotension.
- Air embolism or pneumothorax may occur.

Anaesthetic management

1. Assessment and premedication. Partial airway obstruction may occur with stridor if there is a reduction in airway diameter of at least 50%. This usually means an acute reduction down to 4 mm or less, but in chronic obstruction the diameter may be less. If radiotherapy has been performed, scarring of the tissues may further complicate intubation. The surgeon will have performed indirect laryngoscopy or fibreoptic nasendoscopy and the record of this should be examined, and the CT scans reviewed. Investigations appropriate to the patient's age and other pathologies must be performed. Lung function tests, arterial blood gases and flow volume loops are often indicated. Premedication should include an antisialagogue and sedation only given if there is no suspicion of airway obstruction.

2. Conduct of anaesthesia. Monitoring should include capnography and oximetry. Direct arterial blood pressure monitoring may be indicated. It should be used whenever large blood loss, hypotension or repeated blood gases are anticipated. The CVP may be measured using a long line from the brachial or femoral veins. The method of induction will depend on the degree of airway obstruction. Preoxygenation should always be performed. If respiratory obstruction is severe, a tracheostomy under local anaesthesia may be indicated. Where complete airway obstruction is considered less likely on induction, a gaseous induction may be performed, with the plan to proceed to an emergency tracheostomy if airway control is lost prior to intubation. Difficult intubation aids should be immediately available including a range of smaller tracheal tubes.

If not contraindicated, a hypotensive technique may be required to minimize blood loss and to improve the surgical field. During neck dissection the cuff of the tracheal tube may be damaged. Prior to tracheal transection, the patient is preoxygenated and the pharynx suctioned. The tracheal tube is then withdrawn to allow the distal trachea to be intubated. A sterile catheter mount is used to reconnect the patient to the breathing system. The patient's chest is auscultated to check that endobronchial intubation has not occurred. A fine bore nasogastric feeding tube should be passed at the beginning to facilitate early postoperative enteral feeding.

3. Postoperatively. This major surgery in relatively poor candidates often necessitates ITU or high dependency care for 24 hours. The usual tracheostomy care must be given (see Tracheostomy). Attention to analgesia must be given as the patient may not be able to indicate that they are in pain. Stomal bleeding may occur. The difficulties in patient communication should not be underestimated and early referral for speech therapy is needed. Recurrent tumours or second primary tumours in the airway may occur.

Further reading

Gleeson M, Jani P. Longterm care of patients who have had a laryngectomy. *British Medical Journal*, 1994; **308:** 1452–1453.
Mason RA, Fielder CP. The obstructed airway in head and neck surgery. *Anaesthesia*, 1999; **54:** 625–628.

Related topics of interest

Airway surgery (p. 12); Elderly patients (p. 107); Hypotensive anaesthesia (p. 133); Intubation – awake (p. 138); Intubation – difficult (p. 141); Sleep apnoea (p. 237); Tracheostomy (p. 266)

LASER SURGERY

Laser is an acronym for light amplification of the stimulated emission of radiation. Laser light is monochromatic (of a single wavelength), coherent (all waves are in phase in both time and space) and parallel. It thus appears as a non-divergent pencil beam of light. Laser light is produced when a potential difference is applied across a tube containing the laser medium. Lasers are used medically as scalpels and electrocoagulators. The effect that a particular laser beam has on body tissues depends upon its wavelength and its power density (energy delivered per unit cross-sectional area, usually W/cm^2). Lasers are named from the substance that emits the light. The three lasers commonly used in medicine are CO_2, Nd-Yag (neodymium-yttrium aluminium garnet) and argon.

Carbon dioxide laser

Light wavelength = 10 600 nm (far infra-red).

Light energy is strongly absorbed by all tissues. CO_2 lasers penetrate to a depth of only 200 μm of tissue. Cellular water boils causing cells to burst. There is minimal heating of adjacent cells and little oedema is formed. This laser permits precise surgical cutting and achieves coagulation and sealing at the same time. It is widely used in laser surgery of the larynx.

Nd-Yag laser

Light wavelength = 1060 nm (near infra-red).

This light can be transmitted down fibreoptics and may thus be applied more directly to the lesion. It is absorbed principally by darkly pigmented tissue and is used for photocoagulation of gastro-intestinal bleeding lesions as well as bronchial carcinomata.

Argon laser

Light wavelength = ~500 nm (blue/green visible).

Argon lasers are used in the treatment of lesions such as port wine stains and for retinal work in ophthalmology.

The principal concern to anaesthetists regarding the medical use of lasers is that of laser surgery to the upper airway.

Problems

1. Risk of explosion and fire in the airway following ignition of anaesthetic gases by the laser.
2. Risk of fire in the airway following ignition of the tracheal tube by the laser.
3. Hazard to the patient and operating department personnel from misdirected or reflected laser beam.

Anaesthetic management

1. *Assessment and premedication.* Patients presenting for laser surgery to the airway may be children with papillomata or adults with supraglottic, laryngeal, or upper tracheal tumours that require debulking. Evaluation of the patient must include an assessment of the degree of airway obstruction, adequacy of ventilation, and feasibility of intubation as well as an understanding of the results of pre-operative endoscopic examination of the airway. Preoperative administration of an antisialagogue is recommended. Sedative and respiratory depressant agents should be avoided in those with respiratory impairment.

2. *Conduct of anaesthesia.* As usual, monitoring of the patient should be commenced prior to induction. Pulse oximetry is essential and capnography is recommended.

A technique of anaesthesia is chosen with due consideration to surgical requirements. During laser resection the patient must not move. Coughing or swallowing at an inappropriate moment could lead to damage of normal tissues or ignition of inflammable materials by the laser. The choice lies between per-oral intubation and ventilation, per-oral/nasal jet ventilation, tracheostomy and ventilation, or transtracheal jet ventilation. Methods of jet ventilation require an intravenous technique of anaesthesia to ensure unconsciousness.

3. *Tracheal tubes.* If an anaesthetic technique is chosen which involves the use of a tracheal tube or catheter it must be shielded from the laser. All plastics and rubbers are heated by a CO_2 laser at a rate of approximately 5000°C per second. This rapidly leads to the destruction of the tube leaving an O_2 rich atmosphere open to ignition by the laser. The tracheal tube itself may ignite producing not only thermal injury but also toxic substances which may then be inhaled by the patient. The patient is unlikely to survive such a catastrophe. A specific laser-proof tracheal tube should thus be used. A flexible stainless steel tracheal tube with two cuffs has been designed. The second cuff permits maintenance of the seal should the proximal cuff be ruptured by the laser. The cuffs of tracheal tubes used during laser surgery should be filled with saline and not air. This will more readily permit detection of a burst cuff and allow absorption of laser energy by the saline. A tracheal tube with a foam filled cuff is also manufactured for use in laser surgery.

4. *Gas mixtures.* Oxygen, and to an even greater extent, N_2O, both support combustion. Ignition of inspired gas will thus readily lead to an airway fire. Flammable anaesthetic agents are absolutely contra-indicated in laser surgery. Restricting the inspired O_2 concentration to less than 40% and carrying it in helium reduces the risk of fire. Further safety is achieved by using the laser in repeated bursts for up to 10 seconds rather than as a constant source.

5. *Theatre safety.* A formal safety programme should be operated. Personnel should be properly trained in the use of the equipment and regular servicing carried out to ensure its correct function. Notices restricting admission should be posted on the doors to the theatre in which the laser is being used. Personnel should wear protective glasses to prevent eye damage from a deflected laser beam. Thermal damage to the patient is avoided by the generous use of swabs soaked in saline. In laser surgery to the airway the surgeon places saline soaked swabs distal to the lesion to absorb stray laser energy.

6.   *Management of a fire.* In the event of a fire in the airway the following measures should be taken.

- Stop ventilation.
- Disconnect O_2 source and douse with water if the fire persists.
- Remove the burned tracheal tube.
- Re-intubate and ventilate.
- Assess the extent of thermal injury by bronchoscopy and by effect on pulmonary gas exchange. Plan further management accordingly.
- Commence steroid therapy.
- Provide antibiotic and ventilatory support as indicated.

Further reading

Jones GW. Anaesthesia for laser surgery in the airway. *Royal College of Anaesthetists Newsletter*, 1999; **49:** 247–249.
Rampil IJ. Anesthetic considerations for laser surgery. *Anesthesia and Analgesia*, 1994; **74:** 424–435.

Related topics of interest

Airway surgery (p. 12); Intubation – awake (p. 138); Intubation – difficult (p. 141); Laryngectomy (p. 144); Sleep apnoea (p. 237)

LIVER – THE EFFECTS OF ANAESTHESIA

Liver function is vital for detoxification, metabolism (carbohydrates, vitamins and proteins), immunological and haematological processes. Hepatic blood flow (HBF) is approximately 1.5 l/min. The liver receives 25% of the cardiac output, 30% of which is delivered via the hepatic artery (SaO_2 98%) and the remaining 70% via the portal vein (SaO_2 70%). Portal perfusion pressure is low (8 mmHg in afferent vessels and 2 mmHg in the efferents). Small changes in perfusion pressure will produce large alterations in blood flow. Hepatic blood flow is affected by cardiac output, BP and CVP. Autonomic, metabolic and hormonal factors may also alter the hepatic arterial or portal venous perfusion pressures.

The effects of anaesthesia

Decreased hepatic blood flow risks hepatic hypoxia and cellular damage. Although liver O_2 consumption falls during anaesthesia, the 25% fall in HBF (and therefore O_2 delivery) is greater. This occurs in regional and general anaesthesia. IPPV increases hepatic venous pressure and further exacerbates the fall in hepatic perfusion whilst hypercarbia raises splanchnic vascular resistance. Hypocarbia should be avoided as it decreases cardiac output. Abdominal surgery may also reduce HBF either by mechanical obstruction or the pathological processes related to the surgery (e.g. malignancy or obstructive jaundice). Hepatotoxic and enzyme inducing agents (e.g. barbiturates) may also cause liver damage.

Abnormal LFTs will almost inevitably be made worse by anaesthesia. Anaesthesia is, however, only one of a number of hepatic insults which may result in deteriorating liver function. Other causes include sepsis, trauma, blood transfusion, hepatic infection, intravenous feeding or the administration of hepatotoxic drugs. Perioperative fasting will deplete glycogen stores and with the metabolic response to surgery produce a state of protein and fat catabolism. Approximately 100 cases of fatal liver damage following enflurane have been reported, and 10 cases following isoflurane. Although metabolized less than halothane (enflurane 2% and isoflurane 0.2%), they have a common metabolic pathway involving cytochrome P450 2E1.

Halothane hepatitis

Halothane was introduced in 1956 with few initial reports of hepatitis. Postoperative jaundice is relatively common and the diagnosis of halothane hepatitis used to be one of exclusion. However, recent immunological advances have led to a sensitive and specific test. The National Halothane Study in the USA investigated 250 000 halothane anaesthetics (out of a total of 800 000) and found an incidence of fulminant hepatic failure of 1:35 000 with a high mortality.

Children appear to be more resistant and the diagnosis of halothane hepatitis in children is controversial. The incidence in children has been estimated at 1:82 000.

Obese middle-aged women having repeat frequent halothane exposures, particularly with a history of mild pyrexia or jaundice following anaesthesia are most at risk. Halothane hepatitis may, however, occur following a single exposure. A history of unexplained pyrexia or jaundice following halothane is a contraindication to its future use. A national database of fulminant hepatic failure patients is kept at St Mary's Hospital, London. Advice can be obtained regarding investigation of suspected cases.

Possible mechanisms of halothane hepatitis

Mild increases in aminotransferase enzymes are seen in 20% of patients after halothane exposure, whereas hepatic necrosis is uncommon. They may have different aetiological mechanisms.

1.   Hepatotoxic metabolites.   Halothane is 20% metabolized. Trifluoroacetic acid is produced. If the hepatitis is related to direct hepatotoxicity caused by a normal halothane metabolite then damage should be dose related. All those exposed should be affected to some degree and it would be easily reproducible in animal models. None of these criteria are met. A genetic susceptibility to halothane metabolites may exist.

2.   Hepatic hypoxia.   Hypoxia causes the usual oxidative metabolism to switch to a reductive pathway with a free radical hepatotoxic product.

3.   Immunological.   This is mediated by immune sensitization in susceptible individuals to trifluoroacetylated liver protein neoantigens. These result from oxidative halothane metabolism by cytochrome P450 2E1. An immune mediated response against hepatocytes then occurs on subsequent halothane exposure. Anti-trifluoroacetyl antibodies are found in 70% of patients with halothane-induced hepatitis and they can be tested for, although they do not correlate with the severity of damage or outcome. Exposure to one volatile agent may sensitize the immune system and exposure to a different volatile agent then causes a major immunological reaction with hepatic necrosis. This is called cross sensitization.

Further reading

Kharasch ED, Hankins D, Mautz D, Thummel KE. Identification of the enzyme responsible for oxidative halothane metabolism: implications for prevention of halothane hepatitis. *Lancet*, 1996; **347**: 1367–1371.

Kharasch ED, Hankins DC, Cox K. Clinical isoflurane metabolism by cytochrome P450 2E1. *Anesthesiology*, 1999; **90**: 766–771.

Related topics of interest

Liver disease and anaesthesia (p. 151); Sequelae of anaesthesia (p. 232); Stress response to surgery (p. 248)

LIVER DISEASE AND ANAESTHESIA

Surgery may be related to liver disease or be for unrelated pathology. Liver disease has many aetiologies and, as the liver has many functions, it can affect anaesthesia in a number of ways. Patients with liver failure represent a high risk group for anaesthesia. A classification system (modified from Child's) to assess risk in liver failure uses five criteria: ascites, encephalopathy, bilirubin, albumin, and prothrombin time.

Problems

1. **Pharmacokinetics.**
   - Distribution. Decreased plasma albumin leads to decreased protein binding which results in increased free drug concentration and an increased drug effect (e.g. thiopental). As the unbound proportion of drug is increased it is able to redistribute, hence the volume of distribution of protein bound drugs increases, e.g. pancuronium.
   - Detoxification. Reduced hepatocellular function results in decreased hepatic clearance of drugs, e.g. benzodiazepines, and opioids.
   - Elimination. Patients with abnormal liver function often have decreased biliary excretion.

2. **Ascites.** This indicates severe liver failure. Outcome is improved with diuretics (or a peritoneovenous shunt). Ascites raises intra-abdominal pressure and thus causes a fall in the FRC.

3. **Coagulopathy.** There is decreased production of vitamin K dependent factors (II, VII, IX and X), non-vitamin K dependent factors (V, XI, XII, XIII) and fibrinogen. Thrombocytopenia (due to associated hypersplenism) and altered platelet function also occur.

4. **Renal.** There is a risk of the hepatorenal syndrome (characterized by a very low urinary sodium) and acute tubular necrosis (sodium in the urine). Marked sodium and water retention (associated with a low serum sodium if water is retained over and above sodium retention) and an increased plasma volume with increased extracellular fluid also occur.

5. **CVS.** High cardiac output (up to 14 l/min) and reduced peripheral resistance occur in chronic severe hepatic disease.

6. **Respiratory system involvement** is characterized by a decreased PaO_2 due to intrapulmonary shunts, V/Q mismatch and pleural effusions.

7. **Metabolic changes** include a risk of hypoglycaemia and sodium retention. Dextrose solution is the most suitable intravenous fluid (but risks water intoxication). A metabolic alkalosis of unclear origin is often found.

8. **Neurology.** Encephalopathy is related to hepatic failure. Treatment with lactulose to trap gut ammonia and bowel sterilization with neomycin has been advocated.

9. Drug therapy. Corticosteroids are given for some liver disorders and their effects should be considered.

Anaesthetic management

Assessment and premedication

The patient with liver failure must be fully assessed and their condition optimized by a hepatologist prior to anaesthesia. It may take several days or weeks to optimize the preoperative state (especially nutrition). Minimum investigations include FBC, clotting, U+E, LFTs, blood sugar, ECG, CXR, arterial gases, and hepatitis B and C status. Premedication must take into account altered pharmacokinetics and should be light, avoiding opioids. Vitamin K and mannitol may be needed preoperatively.

Conduct of anaesthesia

Monitoring will include CVP, capnography (to assist in the maintenance of normocarbia), an arterial line (pressure and gases), urinary output via a catheter, temperature, a peripheral nerve stimulator (metabolism of relaxants may be abnormal) and PAOP if severe haemodynamic or myocardial abnormalities are present.

1. Regional anaesthesia. If possible, this may offer the best option. Hypotension should be avoided as this adds to the usual peroperative fall in hepatic blood flow.

2. General anaesthesia. Drugs which are mainly hepatically excreted and have an increased volume of distribution (e.g. pancuronium) should be avoided. The reduced protein binding of thiopental lowers the dose required. Although thiopental is metabolized by the liver, it is redistribution that causes reawakening and this is less affected by hepatic failure. Enzyme induction (e.g. alcohol) may raise the liver's capacity to metabolize barbiturates.

A small dose of opioid (but not if the patient is encephalopathic), atracurium, thiopental and isoflurane represents an acceptable choice of agents. Drugs should be titrated to effect due to the variable pharmacokinetics.

An increased FiO_2 and careful fluid balance are required. As ascitic fluid is in dynamic equilibrium with plasma, its rapid removal may precipitate a marked fall in the intravascular volume. The aim is to preserve splanchnic perfusion. Perioperative mannitol should be given to maintain urine output and glucose 5% as fluid replacement (avoid lactate and sodium containing solutions). The patient is kept warm.

Postoperatively

ITU support may be required. Accurate fluid balance and urine output monitoring remain vital in the recovery period. Analgesia is titrated to effect by experienced personnel. Patients with liver failure are at great risk of infection and prophylactic antibiotics should be considered.

Further reading

Gimson AES. Fulminant and late onset hepatic failure. *British Journal of Anaesthesia*, 1996; **77**: 90–98.
Hayes PC. Liver disease and drug disposition. *British Journal of Anaesthesia*, 1992; **68**: 459–461.

Related topics of interest

Adrenocortical disease (p. 1); Liver – the effects of anaesthesia (p. 149); Renal disease (p. 217)

MINIMALLY INVASIVE SURGERY

Following minimally invasive surgery reduced long-term morbidity, cost, pain and duration of hospital stay have encouraged its widespread use. Minimally invasive surgery continues to expand, with cardiac, renal, and axillary surgery being developed. Surgery may be prolonged and may require conversion to an open operation.

Problems

1. ***Patient position.*** Trendelenburg is necessary for pelvic laparoscopy and is associated with a 15–20% fall in FRC and an increased risk of regurgitation. Lithotomy may be required. Head up positioning (reverse Trendelenburg) is used for upper abdominal surgery.

2. ***Insufflation.*** Intra-abdominal insufflation of CO_2 up to a pressure of 15 mmHg causes diaphragmatic splinting and decreased compliance, with an increased risk of regurgitation and impairment of venous return. Pneumothorax is possible, especially if the pleuro-peritoneal canals are patent. Pneumomediastinum, pneumopericardium, pneumoscrotum and surgical emphysema can also occur. Embolism of the insufflation gas may occur and acidosis, dysrhythmias and hypotension may follow CO_2 absorption. There is a 30% increase in the CO_2 to be removed, and the minute ventilation should be increased.

3. ***Instrumentation.*** Endoscopes are usually between 2 and 10 mm in diameter and inadvertent damage may occur. Cervical or peritoneal stimulation may cause vagally mediated bradycardia or asystole.

4. ***The environment.*** Haemorrhage may not be immediately obvious, theatre lighting is often dimmed, and lasers may be used.

Specific procedures

1. ***Pelvic laparoscopy.*** This is used predominantly for gynaecological procedures, but general surgical operations such as hernia repair are increasingly performed. A laryngeal mask airway, with spontaneous or assisted ventilation can be used for short procedures, but this is controversial due to the risk of regurgitation, and a 50% reduction in pulmonary compliance.

2. ***Abdominal laparoscopy.*** Laparoscopic cholecystectomy requires the insertion of four intra-abdominal cannulae. It shortens hospital stay, decreases the incidence of postoperative complications and allows an earlier return to work. Approximately 3% have to be converted to open operation. It is suggested that an end tidal CO_2 of 4 kPa prior to the insufflation of CO_2 will prevent hypercarbia occurring perioperatively. Perioperative hypotension is common. Other procedures include fundoplication, appendicectomy, vagotomy and colorectal and splenic surgery.

3. Thoracic laparoscopy. This may be performed for diagnosis, or for lobectomy, sympathectomy or cervical dissection of the oesophagus. A capnothorax is produced, and a lung permitted to deflate by using a double lumen tracheal tube. Overinflation risks a tension pneumo-thorax and a pneumothorax can develop on the contralateral side. Hypotension is common. A chest drain may be needed postoperatively.

Anaesthetic management

1. Assessment and premedication. Preoperative investigation and preparation is as for any anaesthesia and surgery. Shorter laparoscopic procedures may be performed as day cases. Consider H_2 antagonists, gastric prokinetic agents (e.g. metoclopramide), and anxiolytic premedicants.

2. Conduct of anaesthesia. Capnography, oximetry and ventilatory pressure monitoring will allow detection of endobronchial intubation, pneumothorax, surgical emphysema and CO_2 embolism. Pelvic laparoscopy can be performed under local anaesthesia, but the pneumoperitoneum may be very uncomfortable. Halothane is not used as it increases arrhythmias in the presence of hypercarbia. Head down tilt should be limited to 30°. Prophylaxis against bradycardia with atropine or glycopyrrolate should be considered.

3. Postoperatively. Local anaesthesia is given to the wounds and internal structures and further analgesia provided by NSAIDs or opioids. The incidence and severity of shoulder tip pain may be reduced by removing as much intra-abdominal gas as possible at the end of the procedure. A temporary percutaneous gas drain may be inserted to help with this.

Further reading

Alexander JI. Pain after laparoscopy. *British Journal of Anaesthesia*, 1997; **79:** 369–378.
Plummer S, Hartley M, Vaughan RS. Anaesthesia for telescopic procedures in the thorax. *British Journal of Anaesthesia*, 1998; **80:** 223–234.

Related topics of interest

Air embolism (p. 9); Day surgery (p. 80); Positioning (p. 207); Thoracic anaesthesia (p. 257)

MRI

Atoms with a net electrical charge will become aligned parallel to a strong static magnetic field. If a second, high frequency pulsating magnetic force is applied at 90 degrees to the first, these same atoms will deflect causing a release of high frequency energy. This is used to create the image. Sensitive atoms are hydrogen, carbon, sodium, fluoride and phosphorus. Magnetism is measured in tesla. One tesla (T) is equal to 10 000 Gauss and the earth's magnetism is 0.5–2.0 Gauss. Modern MRI magnets are approximately 1.5 T. Such powerful magnetic fields require cryogenic magnets which usually function in liquid helium at 4°K. There is no ionizing radiation and there appears to be no oncological or genotoxic effect. MRI scanning is used for neurological, cardiac, orthopaedic and research investigations. It is particularly for soft tissue investigation.

Problems

1. *Ferromagnetic objects* are attracted to the magnet and distort the image.

2. *Environment.* An enclosed and noisy (up to 95 dB) space with limited patient access as the whole body magnet is 2 m long with a diameter of 60 cm. Horseshoe shaped magnets allow better access, but are slower.

3. *Radiofrequencies* from monitoring distort the image.

4. *Interference* with monitoring by the changing magnetic field.

Indications for general anaesthesia

1. *Airway protection.* For unconscious patients.

2. *Movement.* Young children, anxious or confused adults. Scanning may take 1 hour and the patient must stay still. Children over 8 are often able to cope without anaesthesia.

3. *Claustrophobia.*

Anaesthetic management

1. *Assessment and premedication.* Contraindications to MRI scanning are sought. These include patients with pace-makers, automatic implantable defibrillators, cerebral aneurysm clips and metal foreign bodies (particularly intraocular). Prosthetic implants and valves, cochlea implants and IUCDs may be safe (as they are either non-ferromagnetic or very well attached) but will degrade the image, as may make-up and tattoos that can contain metals. Specific considerations depend on the indication for scanning e.g. neuroanaesthetic. Familiarization with the MRI suite should include knowledge of the outer limits of ferromagnetic attraction (usually the 50 Gauss line), the method of radiofrequency shielding for the magnet, and the anaesthetic equipment and monitoring. An anxiolytic premedicant may be required. For infants <6 months old, 'feed and sleep' or oral sedation may be attempted with general anaesthesia only if these techniques fail.

2. Conduct of anaesthesia. Induction should occur outside the magnetic field with appropriate monitoring. A tracheal tube or laryngeal mask airway may be used and the patient ventilated or allowed to breath spontaneously. Maintenance of anaesthesia may be intravenous or gaseous. An intravenous cannula is sited where it is easily accessible. Gadolinium is often given as an intravenous contrast media. The patient is transferred to the MRI on a trolley that can enter the magnetic field. If the anaesthetic machine and monitoring are ferromagnetic they must stay outside the 50 Gauss line and the radio-frequency field (usually a modified wall). Long tubes and wires are required for gases, infusion pumps and monitoring. Machines and monitoring devices are available that are MRI compatible and can be placed close to the magnet. Care should be taken that any infusion pumps used are accurate in a magnetic field and are attached to non-magnetic poles.

Monitoring causes specific problems:

(a) ECG. Conventional leads and electrodes cause image degradation and the changing magnetic field can induce currents in the leads causing ECG spike artefacts (interpreted as QRS complexes) and skin burns. Large T waves may be produced by induced currents from the transverse aorta. Better quality ECG monitoring can be obtained by using carbon fibres, electronic filters, keeping monitoring outside the shield, removing loops of wires and keeping electrodes close together. Telemetry may also be used.

(b) Pulse oximetry. Image degradation and induced currents can produce false readings. Optical fibre cables overcome this problem. The probe should be placed as far as possible from the scanning site.

(c) Non invasive blood pressure. Provided non-metallic connectors and long tubes are used, this does not produce problems.

(d) Capnography and inspiratory gas composition. Non-magnetic side-stream gas analysis can safely be used but the long tubing produces an increased lag time.

If possible two anaesthetists should be present, one outside and one inside the magnetic field.

3. Postoperatively. The patient is removed from the magnetic field to wake up. Full monitoring and resuscitation facilities should be immediately available.

Further reading

Groh J, Ney L. Anaesthesia for magnetic resonance imaging. *Current Opinion in Anaesthesiology*, 1997; **10:** 303–308.

Hatch DJ, Sury MRJ. Sedation of children by non-anaesthetists. *British Journal of Anaesthesia*, 2000; **84:** 713–714.

Peden CJ, Menon DK *et al.* Magnetic resonance for anaesthetists. Parts 1 and 2. *Anaesthesia*, 1992; **47:** 240–255 and 1992; **47:** 508–517.

Related topics of interest

Head injury (p. 124); Neuroanaesthesia (p. 167); Neurological disease (p. 170)

MYASTHENIA GRAVIS

Myasthenia gravis (MG) is an autoimmune disease. The majority of patients (~90%) have anti-bodies to the nicotinic acetylcholine receptors in the post-synaptic membrane of the neuromuscular junction, although the correlation between absolute antibody levels and disease severity is weak. Muscarinic acetylcholine receptors, and thus the autonomic nervous system, are spared. Thymus disease is associated with MG; 75% of patients have histological evidence of an abnormality (e.g. germinal centre hyperplasia) whilst 10% have a benign thymoma. Other autoimmune disorders are associated with MG (e.g. thyroid disease, pernicious anaemia) as are certain HLA subgroups. The prevalence of MG is around 5 per 100 000 population with young women being affected most commonly (peak onset 20–30 years of age). Men over the age of 50 are the next most commonly affected, though most patients with a thymoma associated with MG fall in this group.

Neonatal myasthenia is rare and is seen in infants of myasthenic mothers. It presents at birth and results from the passage of anti-acetylcholine receptor antibodies across the placenta. Congenital myasthenia is very rare and is not associated with antibodies to the acetylcholine receptor. Anaesthetists may be asked to care for myasthenics during surgery, especially for thymectomy, or in critical care when the patient is in crisis (myasthenic or cholinergic) or has developed respiratory failure.

Problems

1. Muscle weakness especially of the bulbar (aspiration risk) and respiratory muscles.

2. Abnormal response to muscle relaxants both depolarizing and non-depolarizing.

3. Complications of drug therapy difficulty interpreting response to muscle relaxants, immunosuppression.

Clinical features

The muscle weakness of MG is typically made worse by exertion and improved by rest. The characteristic distribution of affected muscles, in descending order, is extra-ocular, bulbar, cervical, proximal limb, distal limb and trunk. Thus patients frequently complain of ptosis, diplopia and dysphagia. Severe bulbar weakness leaves them at risk from frequent pulmonary aspiration.

The Eaton-Lambert syndrome, by contrast, is characterized by muscle weakness which improves on exertion and spares the ocular and bulbar muscles. It is a condition associated with small-cell carcinoma of the bronchus and sufferers, like myasthenics, are exquisitely sensitive to non-depolarizing muscle relaxants.

Investigations

1. Edrophonium test. The diagnosis of MG is established by administering an intravenous dose of the short-acting anticholinesterase edrophonium. Anti-cholinesterases increase the amount of acetylcholine available at the neuromuscular junction. An improvement in muscle function following edrophonium thus supports the diagnosis. Prior to administering the drug, intravenous access, continuous ECG monitoring, and full resuscitation facilities should be established. Patients weak due to cholinergic crisis may become apnoeic after edrophonium. A muscle group appropriate for the patient (i.e. where they are weak) is chosen for assessment. For those with respiratory weakness, forced vital capacity is measured. A test dose of 2 mg of edrophonium is administered intravenously, followed, in the absence of adverse effects, by 8 mg one minute later. Muscle function is assessed prior to, and one and ten minutes following, the administration of edrophonium.

2. *Electromyography.* A decremental response in the size of the compound motor action potential after repeated electrical stimulation of a motor nerve can confirm the diagnosis. This is true even in the majority of those with only ocular symptoms.

Treatment

1. *Anticholinesterases.* Pyridostigmine bromide 60 mg is given four times a day and increased until an optimal response is achieved. It may not be possible to abolish all weakness and increasing the dose in an attempt to do so may precipitate a cholinergic crisis.

2. *Anticholinergics.* May be required to control side effects of anticholinesterase administration such as salivation, colic and diarrhoea. They are not used as a matter of routine in all patients.

3. *Immunosuppression.* Corticosteroids may benefit those patients with pure ocular symptoms and those whose response to anticholinesterases is suboptimal. Their administration may be associated with an initial deterioration and improvement may take several weeks. Plasma potassium levels should be monitored to ensure that steroid-induced hypokalaemia (enhanced renal potassium loss) is not adding to muscle weakness. Azathioprine has been used in those with severe myasthenia unresponsive to other measures.

4. *Plasma exchange.* Some patients show a short-lived but dramatic improvement in weakness following plasma exchange. Maximum response is usually seen about a week after a series of five or so daily exchanges. Improvement lasts for around a month. It may be a useful technique for those is severe myasthenic crisis or to allow weaning from ventilation.

5. *Thymectomy.* Thymectomy results in clinical improvement in around 80% of all myasthenics. It produces a more rapid onset of remission and is associated with a lower mortality than medical therapy alone. Patients due to undergo thymectomy should have their respiratory function optimized preoperatively. Plasma exchange and steroids may help with this. The dose of pyridostigmine should be reduced as much as possible without compromising respiratory function. This is because thymectomy often leaves patients more sensitive to the effects of anticholinesterases and cholinergic crisis may ensue after surgery. Also, the intraoperative management of neuromuscular blockade is easier in the presence of a mildly myasthenic patient.

Anaesthetic management

Assessment of muscle function is essential and might include assessment of the patient's ability to sustain a head-lift off the pillow, generate a negative inspiratory pressure >25 cmH$_2$O, and arterial blood gas analysis to ensure an adequate minute ventilation. Almost all procedures will require tracheal intubation and assisted ventilation. An anaesthetic technique is usually chosen that will either reduce the dose of neuromuscular relaxants given or avoid their use altogether. If a non-depolarizing agent is required, atracurium or cis-atracurium in one-tenth to one quarter of the usual dose may be used with monitoring of the response. Neuromuscular function should be allowed to return spontaneously as the administration of reversal agents may cause confusion in the presence of continued weakness.

Myasthenic crisis

This is a severe life-threatening worsening of MG. It can progress rapidly to respiratory failure necessitating urgent tracheal intubation and respiratory support. Myasthenic crises can be precipitated by infection, pyrexia, surgical or emotional stress, and certain drugs. These drugs include aminoglycoside (e.g. gentamicin) and polymixin (e.g. neomycin) antibiotics, membrane-stabilizing antiarrythmics (e.g. quinidine, procainamide, lidocaine (lignocaine)), anticonvulsants (e.g. phenytoin), and antidepressants (e.g. lithium). If the patient's FVC falls below 10–15 ml/kg or they are unable to adequately expectorate secretions, they require intubation and respiratory support. Many then withdraw all anticholinesterase therapy and rest the patient, believing that the sensitivity of the motor end plate to acetylcholine will increase under such circumstances.

Subcutaneous heparin should be given for prophylaxis against thromboembolism.

Plasma exchange or immunosuppressive therapy may be required to wean the patient from mechanical ventilation.

The differential diagnosis of an acutely weak patient with MG includes cholinergic crisis.

Cholinergic crisis

A cholinergic crisis is caused by an excess of acetylcholine available at the neuromuscular junction and usually follows excessive administration of anticholinergics. It too may present with respiratory failure, bulbar palsy and virtually complete paralysis. It may be difficult to distinguish from a myasthenic crisis but often includes an excess of secretions, which may worsen the respiratory failure. Other symptoms more likely during a cholinergic crisis include abdominal pain, diarrhoea and blurred vision. The differential may be made be administering a small dose of intravenous edrophonium. Patients in myasthenic crisis should improve whereas those with a cholinergic crisis will get worse.

Further reading

Drachman DB. Myasthenia gravis. *New England Journal of Medicine*, 1994; **330:** 1797–1810.

Related topic of interest

Neurological disease (p. 170)

MYOTONIA

These hereditary diseases are characterized by delayed muscle relaxation following contraction. Myotonia congenita has little systemic involvement, a normal life expectancy and is very rare. Myotonic dystrophy is more common (prevalence 4 per 100000) and the discussion will be limited to this. It exhibits autosomal dominant inheritance with anticipation (i.e. increasing severity with successive generations). A mutation of chromosome 19 is found in 99% of families with males and females equally affected. Sufferers have characteristic facies with frontal balding, a smooth forehead, ptosis, cataracts and a 'lateral smile'. There is muscle wasting of the neck (especially of the sternomastoids), shoulders and quadriceps. Muscle tone and reflexes are reduced once wasting has developed and foot drop is common. Myotonia is precipitated by cold, exercise, shivering, hyperkalaemia, suxamethonium and neostigmine. The myotonia is due to abnormal closure of sodium and chloride channels in the muscle membrane following depolarization, leading to repetitive discharge and contraction. The disease is associated with a low IQ in 40%, gonadal atrophy, diabetes mellitus, dysphagia, constipation, respiratory muscle failure, cardiac conduction defects and cardiomyopathy. Patients usually present aged 20–40 years and die in their sixth decade from cardiac disease or bulbar muscle involvement. There is a progressive worsening of cardiac conduction with an increasing risk of tachyarrhythmia and sudden death.

Problems

1. Increased sensitivity to anaesthetic drugs e.g. propofol and thiopental.
2. Drug precipitation of myotonia e.g. suxamethonium and neostigmine.
3. Respiratory and cardiac involvement.

Anaesthetic management

1. Assessment and premedication. The clinical diagnosis is confirmed by EMG which shows myotonic discharges occurring spontaneously. Genetic testing is used as a screening test in affected families. Preoperative investigation should include an ECG and possibly a 24-hour tape, lung function tests (reduced maximum breathing capacity and expiratory reserve volume), and blood potassium. Cardiac pacing may be necessary.

Patients are sensitive to all depressant drugs so any such premedicant agents should be avoided. Quinine, procainamide or phenytoin may be used as symptomatic treatments for myotonia.

2. Conduct of anaesthesia. An ECG is essential and invasive CVS monitoring including a pulmonary artery catheter may be indicated. Body temperature and neuromuscular blockade should also be monitored.

Regional anaesthesia avoids the use of known precipitating agents but the myotonic reflex is not blocked as this is due to the intrinsic muscle disorder.

If a general anaesthetic is given, suxamethonium and neostigmine should be avoided as they can cause a generalized myotonic response. Atracurium, in very small doses due to an increased sensitivity, may be given with spontaneous recovery of neuromuscular function. Alternatively mivacurium is hydrolysed rapidly by plasma cholinesterase and reversal can also be avoided. Patients are very sensitive to opioids, barbiturates and volatile agents. As little as 1.5 mg/kg of thiopental may cause apnoea. The use of propofol in low doses has been reported as safe in myotonic dystrophy. Potassium worsens myotonia and should be avoided in intravenous fluids. Patients must be kept warm.

3. Postoperatively. Patients may require admission to ITU if they have CVS instability or have been slow to regain consciousness or normal neuromuscular function. Opioids should be carefully titrated to effect. Swallowing is often impaired and gastric emptying delayed. Asymptomatic aspiration is common and an early return to feeding should be avoided.

Further reading

Boyle R. Antenatal and preoperative genetic and clinical assessment in myotonic dystrophy. *Anaesthesia and Intensive Care*, 1999; **27**: 301–306.
Russell SH, Hirsch NP. Anaesthesia and myotonia. *British Journal of Anaesthesia*, 1994; **72**: 210–216.

Related topic of interest

Neurological disease (p. 170)

NEONATAL SURGERY

A neonate is a child in its first month after delivery. Congenital abnormalities are usually detected shortly after birth, and the neonate presented for emergency surgery. As well as small size there are marked anatomical and physiological differences from adults and older children. Neonates undergoing major surgery may require postoperative ventilation. Opioids and volatiles with muscle relaxation are therefore popular. However, tracheal tubes in neonates are more likely to migrate into the right main bronchus, kink or dislodge than in adults and postoperative ventilation should not be the automatic norm. If elective ventilation is not planned, high dose opioids must be avoided. Awake intubation has declined in popularity due to the delicate nature of the neonatal cerebral circulation and the risk of intracranial haemorrhage. Awake intubation is occasionally performed in the moribund or the actively vomiting. A neonate is heart rate dependent (to maintain BP) and has a tendency to large amounts of secretions. Anticholinergic agents are sometimes used as premedicants. The patient–monitor interface is a particular problem and it can be difficult to obtain continuous and reliable data. A neonate with one congenital abnormality has an increased incidence of other congenital malformations, particularly cardiac. Intra-uterine diagnosis and prenatal transfer of care to specialized centres is becoming more common.

Congenital diaphragmatic hernia

The incidence is 1:5000, with a male:female ratio of 2:1. Cardiovascular defects are found in 20%. The diagnosis is made either antenatally by ultrasound, or by CXR if poor respiratory function is noted. The hernia results from an embryological failure to close the pleuroperitoneal canals permitting herniation of abdominal contents into the thorax. This causes hypoplasia or agenesis of the lung. Eighty per cent are left sided through the foramen of Bochdalek. The severity of the hypoplastic lung affects outcome.

Problems

1. **Gastric dilatation** compressing the lungs. A nasogastric tube should be positioned.

2. **Gas exchange** is compromised requiring a high F_IO_2 and minute volume, while trying to minimize inspiratory pressure and PEEP. Following intubation 2–3 days of preoperative ITU stabilization are necessary. There is a risk of barotrauma. Pulmonary hypertension may occur and require treatment (nitric oxide).

3. **Nitrous oxide** is avoided as it causes bowel distension and will worsen pulmonary function.

4. **Postoperative ventilation** is required, particularly if the abdomen is closed in stages. Extracorporeal membrane oxygenation has been used to allow time for the hypoplastic lung to mature.

5. *Outcome.* There are three groups, the first having limited ventilatory disturbance do well. The second group have marginal gas exchange and have an improved outcome with ITU care. The last group have severe disease and do badly or die.

Inguinal hernia

These occur more commonly in premature low-birth-weight babies (13% of those born at less than 32 weeks gestation). They present for elective repair in fit and well babies, or having strangulated requiring emergency surgery, or in the ex-premature baby with other problems. Full term babies, older than one month may be suitable for elective daycase repair. A gaseous induction is usually performed and after venous access is obtained either a laryngeal mask or a tracheal tube placed. Opioids are used sparingly, and local anaesthetic infiltrated into the wound, and rectal paracetamol administered.

Problems

1. *Prematurity.* Due to opioid sensitivity and the risk of apnoea, general anaesthesia may best be avoided. A caudal or spinal may be given. The apnoea risk is increased if < 50 weeks gestational age, and if anaemic.

2. *Strangulated hernias.* Intravenous fluid resuscitation, a nasogastric tube and rapid sequence induction are required. A caudal may then be given, particularly to expremature babies to minimize the use of opioids.

3. *Postoperatively.* The neonate should be monitored with an oximeter and apnoea alarm for the first postoperative night. Caffeine has been shown to decrease the incidence of apnoea.

Intestinal obstruction

This can occur at several sites in the gastrointestinal tract, e.g. duodenal obstruction (1 in 25 000), jejunoileal atresia (1 in 5000), malrotation, volvulus, Hirchsprung's disease or imperforate anus. Upper gastrointestinal obstruction presents earlier and the neonate tends to be less unwell. Meconium ileus occurs in 20% of neonates with cystic fibrosis. Surgery may be required to evacuate the bowel.

Problems

1. Fluid and electrolyte balance.
2. A rapid sequence induction is required. Avoid nitrous oxide in lower obstructions where it is not possible to decompress the bowel.
3. Aspiration pneumonitis – if severe preoperative vomiting.
4. Bowel perforation and sepsis.
5. Respiratory embarrassment from bowel distension and diaphragmatic splinting.

Omphalocele and gastroschisis

Omphalocele is an embryological defect caused by failure of the abdominal viscera to return to the abdominal cavity (they are covered by a membrane). It has an incidence of 1 in 5000 live births. Gastroschisis has an incidence of 1 in 30000 and is caused by intra-uterine occlusion of the omphalomesenteric artery leading to an ischaemic deficit in the anterior abdominal wall (usually right-sided). The bowel lacks covering and the condition is not associated (unlike omphalocele) with other congenital abnormalities.

Problems

1. ***Fluid loss.*** heat loss and sepsis (particularly in gastroschisis). The lower body is placed in a plastic bag, and the neonate transferred for immediate surgery.

2. ***Bowel distension.*** A nasogastric tube is used and nitrous oxide avoided. A rapid sequence induction is indicated.

3. ***High intra-abdominal pressures.*** This occurs when the abdominal contents are resited and may cause a fall in cardiac output, decreased pulmonary compliance, bowel ischaemia, renal vein thrombosis, anuria and inferior vena caval compression. The bowel may be placed in a silastic sac and gradually 'wound' back into the abdominal cavity over 7–10 days. Dopamine can be used to increase mesenteric blood flow.

4. ***ITU care.*** Postoperative ventilation is usually required. Prolonged parenteral nutrition may be needed whilst the bowel recovers.

Necrotizing enterocolitis

The immature intestine has an impaired circulation resulting in stasis and proliferation of bacteria causing infection. There is a different incidence between neonatal ITUs. Intestinal distension with pooling of fluid and the risk of perforation leads to sepsis and acidosis with the potential for DIC. If conservative management with nasogastric suction, antibiotics and ITU support fails, bowel resection may be required. A laparotomy is indicated if gangrene or perforation is suspected. The terminal ileum, caecum and ascending colon are at particular risk.

Problems

1. Immaturity, commonly < 1500 g birth weight.
2. Sepsis.
3. Multisystem failure.
4. Fluid losses which may be very large.
5. A rapid sequence induction (if a tracheal tube is not *in situ*) is used. Avoid nitrous oxide, especially if an X-ray shows gas bubbles in the bowel wall and portal system.
6. Postoperative ventilation is essential. The mortality rate is about 50%.

Tracheoesophageal fistula

The incidence is 1:3500 with males equal to females, 50% have associated congenital abnormalities (VATER syndrome – Vertebral, Anal, Tracheal, oEsophageal, Radial or Renal). Six types exist, the commonest (85%) has a blind oesophageal pouch with a fistula between the distal oesophagus and the lower trachea (polyhydramnios may be noted in the obstetric history). Secretions may spill over through the fistula into the lungs. If a catheter cannot be passed down the oesophagus, a CXR (without contrast media) is taken to confirm the diagnosis. A suction catheter (Replogle tube) is left in the oesophageal pouch, the neonate nursed head up, and early repair performed if possible. If dehydration and aspiration pneumonia occur a gastrostomy can be performed and preoperative ITU care given. Intubation following an intravenous induction is performed. A right thoracotomy, with an extra-pleural approach is used. Postoperatively a nasogastric tube and a paraoesophageal drain are left *in situ* for one week, and parenteral nutrition given.

Problems

1. Tracheal tube positioning – distal to the fistula to seal it, but avoiding endo-bronchial intubation. The bevel on the tube is positioned anteriorly. The stomach is likely to become distended with gas, and the tracheal tube is repositioned during surgery to allow closure of the tracheal defect.

2. Surgical retraction may result in tracheal or bronchial obstruction. The SaO_2 is monitored and ventilation performed by hand to detect changes in pulmonary compliance. Postoperatively a chest drain may be needed, and ventilation should be avoided if possible to prevent stress on suture lines.

3. An oesophageal stricture may require regular dilation under anaesthesia later in life.

Further reading

Hughes D, Mather S, Wolf AR. A handbook of neonatal anaesthesia. London: Baillière Tindall, 1995.
Somri M *et al.* Postoperative outcome in high-risk infants undergoing herniorrhaphy: comparison between spinal and general anaesthesia. *Anaesthesia*, 1998; **53**: 762–766.

Related topics of interest

Paediatric anaesthesia – basic principles (p. 193); Paediatric anaesthesia – practical (p. 196); Pyloric stenosis (p. 215); Thoracic anaesthesia (p. 257)

NEUROANAESTHESIA

Anaesthesia for craniotomy is based on an understanding of techniques for controlling intra-cranial volume, and the effects of anaesthetic interventions.

Problems

1. Altered neurological function.
2. Effect of anaesthesia on cerebral function.
3. Positioning of the patient. The patient may be supine, prone, sitting, or in the park bench position. However, all neurosurgical procedures which include a craniotomy carry a high risk of air embolism.
4. Control of intracranial pressure (ICP).
5. Control of epilepsy.

Intracranial pressure

Normal ICP is 10–15 mmHg. An intracranial mass (tumour, oedema, or blood) will cause an increase in ICP. Initially, CSF moves from the cranium to the spinal sub-arachnoid space and there is little increase in volume. The brain is relatively non-compressible and this compensatory mechanism is soon exhausted. The intracranial contents then become non-compliant and any further volume increase results in large increases in ICP. Signs that a patient with raised ICP is decompensating include:

- Headache, restlessness, mental confusion, nausea and vomiting.
- Hypertension and bradycardia (the Cushing response).
- Hypotension, deep coma, periodic respiration, fixed and dilated pupils. Death from respiratory or cardiac arrest is the natural progression from this stage. The ultimate consequence of ever increasing ICP is brain herniation (coning).

Cerebral perfusion pressure (CPP)

The above changes are largely a result of the influence of ICP on cerebral blood flow (CBF). The prime determinant of CBF is CPP; this is equal to the mean arterial pressure (MAP) minus the sum of the ICP and CVP:

$$CPP = MAP - (ICP + CVP).$$

CVP at the jugular venous bulb is usually zero. Normal MAP is ~80 mmHg. Therefore,

$$CPP = 80 - (10 + 0)$$
$$CPP = 70 \text{ mmHg.}$$

The critical value for CPP is of the order of 30–40 mmHg. The brain, like other organs, shows autoregulation with respect to perfusion pressure over a range of MAP (~50–150 mmHg). Outside this range, or when autoregulation is lost, CBF is entirely pressure-dependent. Autoregulation is impaired under the following conditions.

- Hypotension.
- Hypertension.
- Profound hypoxia.
- Hypercarbia or hypocarbia.
- Cerebral ischaemia – including focal.
- Cerebral vasospasm e.g. following subarachnoid haemorrhage.
- Trauma.
- Seizure activity.
- In the presence of volatile anaesthetic agents.

Anaesthetic management

*1. **Assessment and premedication.*** The level of consciousness may be depressed, varying from mild confusion to deep coma. The airway may not be protected, and intubation may be required prior to surgery. The neurological status is assessed and recorded immediately prior to anaesthesia. Postoperatively, a rapid return to being alert and able to co-operate with a further neurological examination is essential. Anaesthetic techniques should accommodate these needs. Sedative premedication is avoided. Opioid premedication is contraindicated in those with raised ICP; respiratory depression will result in an increase in ICP secondary to an elevated $PaCO_2$. Anxiolytic or dissociative premedication is often prescribed. For example, an oral benzodiazepine with oral droperidol. The latter has the added advantage of antiemesis, important in the control of ICP postoperatively. Monitoring to detect air embolism (usually Doppler) should be instigated.

*2. **Conduct of anaesthesia.*** Invasive haemodynamic monitoring is used for many neurosurgical procedures including craniotomy. This is especially important in those undergoing cerebral vascular surgery in whom blood loss may be sudden and large. Urgent and profound hypotension may be required. Urine output and core temperature are monitored.

Anaesthesia is induced with thiopental or propofol. Methohexitone is not used (epileptiform changes on EEG), nor are ketamine or etomidate (increase ICP). Propofol is often used as a total intravenous anaesthetic by simple infusion or using a target controlled infusion. Enflurane is avoided during the maintenance of anaes-thesia as it also causes spike and wave changes on the EEG. Isoflurane appears to pro-duce the best flow-metabolism coupling at low CPP and is currently the volatile agent of choice for craniotomy. Nitrous oxide should not be used if there is reduced intracranial compliance or in situations with cerebral ischaemia.

The patient is paralysed and the trachea intubated as smoothly as possible to reduce surges in MAP (and thus ICP). It is essential that the patient does not cough, strain, or buck during the procedure as this will produce large increases in ICP or brain herniation. Neuromuscular blockade is thus continued throughout surgery (by bolus or infusion) and monitored with a peripheral nerve stimulator. Tracheal tube tapes and ties are placed with care to ensure obstruction of jugular venous return does not occur. The eyes are taped closed and padded. The use of PEEP is avoided as this, too, will increase CVP and therefore reduce CPP.

Arterial blood pressure should be close to preoperative levels to balance the risks of bleeding, and ischaemia from vasospasm and hypoperfusion. The use of mild hypothermia (32–35°C) is returning to fashion as neuroprotective effects have been demonstrated in animal models of cerebral ischaemia. Brain oxygenation can be monitored by 'global' methods such as jugular bulb oxygen saturation, but more local brain tissue oxygen monitoring probes are being developed.

Intracranial pressure may be controlled in a number of ways.

(a) Intravenous fluids. These are given in restricted amounts, sufficient to maintain haemodynamic stability. Crystalloid solutions containing glucose are avoided as hyperglycaemia worsens reperfusion injury following a period of cerebral hypoperfusion. This may be because the high glucose levels permit a greater build up of cerebral lactic acid during conditions of low flow. A balanced isotonic electrolyte solution is preferred.

(b) Diuretics. Loop diuretics (e.g. furosemide (frusemide) 0.3 mg/kg) or osmotic agents (e.g. mannitol 0.5–2 g/kg) may be given to reduce ICP. An intact blood–brain barrier is required for mannitol to exert its full effect and draw fluid from the interstitial space.

(c) CSF drainage. A spinal drain inserted prior to surgery will reduce CSF volume and thus ICP. The risks of brain herniation in those with a raised ICP must be considered.

(d) Hyperventilation to a $PaCO_2$ of ~3.0 kPa (end-tidal CO_2 = 3.5–4.0 kPa) causes cerebrovasoconstriction and thus a reduction in cerebral blood volume. There is little evidence that a $PaCO_2$ <3.0 kPa produces further benefit. It may in fact produce detrimental EEG changes. Even mild hyperventilation is now avoided in some centres with normocarbia being the aim.

3. *Postoperatively.* Attempts should be made to allow an immediate return of consciousness at the end of the operation, permitting full neurological assessment. Patients who remain obtunded should not be extubated if they are unable to protect their airway. Regular neurological observations should be recorded. Any neurological deterioration postoperatively should raise the suspicion of intracranial bleeding or swelling. In such an event a CT scan should be performed to exclude any treatable cause. Where post-operative raised intracranial pressure is anticipated an intra-cerebral pressure monitor may be inserted before completion of the operation.

Further reading

Matta B, Menon D, Turner J. *Textbook of neuroanaesthesia and critical care.* Greenwich Medical Media, 2000.

Owen-Reece H, Smith M, Elwell CE, Goldstone JC. Near infrared spectroscopy. *British Journal of Anaesthesia*, 1999; **82**: 418–426.

Spiekermann BF, Stone DJ, Bogdonoff DL, Yemen TA. Airway management in neuroanaesthesia. *Canadian Journal of Anaesthesia*, 1996; **43**: 820–834.

Related topics of interest

Air embolism (p. 9); Brain death and organ donation (p. 37); Epilepsy (p. 113); Head injury (p. 124); Neurological diseases (p. 170); Positioning (p. 207)

NEUROLOGICAL DISEASES

Multiple sclerosis

This chronic disease has an unpredictable episodic course. Classically it presents in patients aged 20–40, with a transient neurological deficit that develops over a few days and resolves over a few weeks. It has an equal sex incidence. Demyelination of white matter occurs in the brain and spinal cord leading to retrobulbar neuritis, and upper motor neuron and sensory deficits. Ocular, cerebellar and bladder dysfunction are also common. The disease may occur with mild infrequent episodes causing little interference with life, or may show a chronic progressive course leaving the sufferer severely handicapped. The aetiology is unclear, with environmental, genetic and immunological factors suspected. The incidence varies dramatically with geographical latitude. In the UK the prevalence is 50 per 100000. A minimum of two episodes is required for a clinical diagnosis. MRI, with gadolinium enhancement, demonstrates plaques of demyelination (proton dense) and has replaced CSF gamma-globulin and visual evoked responses as the best investigation. Symptoms may be exacerbated by stress, pyrexia, infection, trauma and exertion.

1. Problems
- Risk of exacerbation.
- Existing neurological deficits.
- Drug history, e.g. steroids, ACTH, azathioprine.

2. Anaesthetic management.
A careful assessment of the existing neurological deficit should be made. If deterioration occurs postoperatively then anaesthesia or surgery is likely to be blamed. This should be carefully discussed with the patient and his/her family. Any changes that occur should be carefully documented. Anticholinergic agents (which may increase temperature) should be avoided. There is no evidence that general anaesthesia has adverse effects on multiple sclerosis. In severe cases with muscle wasting it is best to avoid suxamethonium, although if laryngeal and pharyngeal muscles are involved a rapid sequence induction is indicated. Nondepolarizing relaxants have normal effects. The incidence of relapse following regional anaesthesia is no higher than would be expected by chance alone. Experimentally, there is an increased risk of local anaesthetic histotoxicity in plaques in the spinal cord and therefore spinal anaesthesia is contraindicated. There is, however, no clinical evidence to support this. Hyperthermia should be avoided as this may exacerbate the neurological deficit.

Motor neurone disease

A progressive degeneration in motor function occurs while sensory and higher functions remain normal. The incidence is 1 per 100000 and males are affected more commonly than females. A familial link is seen in 5% with an abnormality on chromosome 21. Aetiological theories include excess excitatory neurotransmitters (particularly glutamate), free radicals, abnormal growth factors and immunological causes. The diagnosis is made clinically and on EMG studies. There is currently no treatment of proven benefit. Three forms exist but any combination of symptoms and signs from these groups may occur together.

1. 'Progressive muscular atrophy' with lower motor symptoms initially occurring in the arms.
2. 'Amyotrophic lateral sclerosis' with upper motor symptoms initially occurring in the legs.
3. 'Progressive bulbar palsy' with lower motor symptoms affecting the brain stem. A pseudo-bulbar palsy results as lower not upper motor neurons are affected. Dysarthria and dysphagia are often the initial presentations.

1. Problems
- Increased sensitivity to non-depolarizing relaxants.
- Respiratory muscle involvement.
- Risk of aspiration if the brain stem is involved.

2. Anaesthetic management. The degree of respiratory muscle and brain stem involvement must be assessed. An appropriate premedication is then given. Suxamethonium should be avoided and nondepolarizing relaxants titrated to effect with a nerve stimulator. Controlled ventilation is often necessary. Regional anaesthesia may be performed but care must be taken to avoid further compromise of respiratory muscles. Postoperative ventilation in ITU is often required.

Guillain-Barré syndrome

This progressive (but reversible) polyneuropathy usually starts one week after an infective illness, often viral. Motor symptoms occur in the lower limb, although it can present with upper limb or cranial nerve involvement. The flaccid lower motor neuron paralysis, with loss of reflexes, progresses and can involve the respiratory muscles. Sensory symptoms are less severe. Diagnosis is clinical, but a high CSF protein is found (usually >3 g/l).

1. Anaesthetic management. Patients require meticulous nursing and physiotherapy. Daily vital capacity, FEV_1, and PEFR are performed to assess disease progression. Intensive care with ventilatory support may be needed if the vital capacity falls below one litre. Secondary infection, autonomic disturbance and DVTs all contribute to the 5% mortality rate. Management is supportive with specific therapy comprising either plasma exchange (plasmaphoresis) or immunoglobulin administration. Induction of anaesthesia may cause a marked worsening of the cardiovascular instability. There may be an exaggerated hypotensive response following the administration of intravenous induction agents. Serious arrhythmias are common especially after suxamethonium which should be avoided. Tracheostomy may be needed as the paralysis may take several weeks to improve. Psychological counselling is vital.

Further reading

Hambly PR, Martin B. Anaesthesia for chronic spinal cord lesions. *Anaesthesia*, 1998; **52**: 273–89.

Neurological diseases. In: Benumof JL, ed. *Anesthesia and Uncommon Diseases*, 4th edn. Philadelphia: WB Saunders, 1997.

Related topics of interest

OBESITY

In the USA the prevalence of morbid obesity is 10% and 4% in Europe, but this is increasing. The Body Mass Index (BMI) is the weight (kg) divided by the height squared (m^2). The normal range is 22–28 whilst obesity is defined as a BMI > 30 and morbid obesity >35. The ideal body weight in kilograms = height (cm) minus 100 for males or height (cm) minus 105 for females. The distribution of adiposity may be central – android (which is associated with more complications) or be to the buttocks (peripheral – gynaecoid). Obesity is caused by a higher calorific intake than required or by medical conditions such as diabetes mellitus, Cushing's syndrome, hypothyroidism, or the hypothalamic syndrome. It may occur with specific syndromes such as Prader–Willi or Lawrence–Moon–Biedl. Morbid obesity doubles the risk of premature death.

Problems

1. Respiratory. Oxygen consumption and CO_2 production are increased. The compliance and FRC are reduced resulting in inadequate gas exchange and hypoxaemia. This may lead to pulmonary vasoconstriction, pulmonary hypertension, right ventricular hypertrophy and failure. The expiratory reserve volume may be reduced and the closing capacity increased, adding to V/Q mismatch, especially when supine. Intrapulmonary shunt increases from 2–5% to 10–25% in the obese. The Pickwickian syndrome (loss of sensitivity to CO_2) occurs in up to 5%. Sleep apnoea and difficulty with intubation can occur.

2. CVS. Increased body mass is associated with an increase in the total blood volume and cardiac output (by increasing stroke volume). This causes cardiomegaly, LVH and predisposes to LVF. Hypertension, hyperlipidaemia, ischaemic heart disease, conduction defects, arrhythmias, CVAs, DVTs, polycythaemia and varicose veins are all more common in the obese. The diastolic blood pressure rises by 2 mmHg for every 10 kg of weight gained.

3. Gastrointestinal. Intra-abdominal pressure is increased and hiatus hernia is very common. Seventy five per cent of obese patients have a gastric residue of >25 ml with a pH <2.5. The risk of regurgitation and aspiration is high. Gallstones and fatty deposits in the liver are common, with a tendency for hepatic dysfunction.

4. Endocrine. Insulin resistance and type II diabetes mellitus occur secondary to the high calorific intake.

5. Pharmacological. The decreased total body water and lean body mass, together with increased body fat, alters the volume of distribution of many drugs. It is increased for fat soluble agents. Drug clearance may be altered by organ dysfunction. Sympathomimetic agents and methylxanthines may be used to treat obesity, but they can have significant interactions with anaesthetic agents.

6. Other. Psychological aspects of obesity.

Anaesthetic management

1. *Assessment and premedication.* The history and examination will identify any of the above problems. Investigation should include respiratory function tests, blood gases, a CXR and ECG, blood glucose and liver function tests. Consider premedication with H_2 antagonists or gastric prokinetic agents. Avoid sedatives and opioids if there is a history of respiratory problems or sleep apnoea.

2. *Conduct of anaesthesia.* Intravenous access may be difficult and necessitate a central line. It is essential to intubate and ventilate obese patients having a general anaesthesia. A rapid sequence induction or awake intubation should be performed and a difficult intubation expected. Opioids should be used sparingly. An FiO_2 of 0.5 should be used and PEEP added. Noninvasive blood pressure measurement may be unreliable, therefore direct measurement should be used for longer procedures. Capnography and pulse oximetry are used. The response to relaxants may be unpredictable and neuromuscular function should be monitored.

Active prophylaxis against DVT is taken. Two operating tables may be required if the patient weighs more than 130 kg and extra help needed to position the patient. Whenever possible the patient should be placed in the operative position prior to induction and the pressure points carefully padded. Two anaesthetists may be required.

Regional anaesthesia offers the potential to avoid the problems of a general anaesthetic but may be technically difficult. Patients may be unable to tolerate lying supine. The dose of agent for epidural or subarachnoid block is 80% of normal on a mg/kg basis. Blocks of unpredictable height and onset may occur. The CSF volume is reduced by approximately 20% in the morbidly obese.

3. *Postoperatively.* Extubate only when the patient is awake. Supplementary O_2 is required for longer than usual, and CPAP is often beneficial. High-dependency care may be needed and the patient should be extubated and nursed sitting up at a 45° angle and mobilized as early as possible. There is a higher incidence of chest infection, wound infection, DVT and pulmonary embolism in the obese. Analgesia is difficult; intramuscular absorption is variable and opioids risk respiratory depression. PCA may be the safest and most reliable means of delivering opioids. Where technically possible an epidural or regional block may be best.

Further reading

Adams JP, Murphy PG. Obesity in anaesthesia and intensive care. *British Journal of Anaesthesia*, 2000; **85:** 91–108.

Shenkman Z, Shir Y, Brodsky JB. Perioperative management of the obese patient. *British Journal of Anaesthesia*, 1993; **70:** 349–59.

Related topics of interest

OBSTETRICS – ANALGESIA

Jenny Tuckey

There is great variation in pain thresholds in labouring patients. During the first stage of labour, uterine pain afferents enter the cord at T10–L1. During the second stage, pain from other pelvic viscera is transmitted via sensory neurones from L5–S1. The pain caused by stretching of the perineum travels via S2–S4. Several methods of pain relief are available.

Methods of pain relief

1. ***Non-pharmacological*** means include the use of hypnosis, acupuncture homeopathic methods and transcutaneous electrical nerve stimulation (TENS). With TENS, a variable electrical stimulus passes through skin plates applied to the back on either side of the spine at T11–L1. Currents vary from 0–40 mA at a frequency of 40–150 Hz. Up to 25% mothers report good pain relief from TENS.

2. ***Entonox*** nitrous oxide 50:50) should be administered via a 2-stage reducing demand valve via a breathing filter. Analgesia takes 45 seconds to become effective. Inhalation must therefore commence concurrent with the start of each contraction. Entonox does not accumulate. It provides satisfactory relief for 30% of mothers.

3. ***Systemic opioids.*** The standard opioid in the UK is pethidine given by i.m. injection. Midwives may administer pethidine in doses and at intervals agreed locally, without a doctor's prescription. It causes maternal drowsiness, dissociation and marked nausea and vomiting. Fetal levels average 70% of maternal levels. It causes loss of beat to beat variability of the fetal heart rate in labour. Neonatal respiratory depression is greatest 3 hours after maternal i.m. injection. Pethidine affects feeding and depresses the neuro-behaviour of the neonate for up to 48 hours.

4. ***Invasive methods of pain relief*** include epidurals (by intermittent midwife top-up, continuous infusion or patient controlled epidural analgesia [PCEA]), or combined spinal epidural analgesia (CSE).

   Establishing an obstetric epidural should result in reliable pain relief for the labouring patient, achieving a sensory block of T10–S5. Advances have seen clinical practice progress from the use of intermittent boluses of concentrated local anaesthetic solutions, to infusions of low-concentration local anaesthetic solutions with or without opioids, and CSE blocks.

Epidurals

When an epidural is to be sited, informed maternal consent must be given and there should be no contraindications (see Obstetrics – delivery (p. 178) and Spinal and epidural anaesthesia (p. 241)). A sterile technique must be used. Following a test dose, the epidural is 'topped-up'. The blood pressure and sensory level are measured and recorded regularly. Once epidural analgesia has been established, electronic fetal heat rate recording is recommended. In the UK, 90% of consultant obstetric units offer a 24 h epidural service. The average epidural rate is 24%.

1. *Drugs.* In the UK the most commonly used local anaesthetic is bupivacaine. Newer regimens avoid the use of concentrated solutions at any time. Many advocate initial boluses of 15–20 ml 0.1% bupivacaine with 2 µg/ml fentanyl with the first 8–10 ml of the mixture acting as the test dose. Bupivacaine is a chiral drug. The L. form of the drug is less cardiotoxic and equally efficacious. Ropivacaine is a relatively new local anaesthetic. It is more selective for sensory (rather than motor) neurones than bupivacaine. The most commonly used epidural opioid in the UK in labouring patients is fentanyl.

2. *Test dose.* The purpose of the epidural test-dose is to demonstrate the accidentally misplaced catheter (intravenous or subarachnoid). In the labour ward setting, without routine ECG monitoring in the parturient, the purpose of the test dose is to exclude accidental subarachnoid placement. A suggested safe test dose (which avoids unnecessary motor block) is 8 mg bupivacaine (8 ml bupivacaine 0.1% bupivacaine with fentanyl 2 µg/ml). With subarachnoid injections, it is the dose and not the volume that is the most important determinant of the extent of the block.

3. *Method of drug administration.* Intermittent bolus may result in breakthrough pain if the top-up is delayed and hypotension may occur with the top-up. The cumulative dose of local anaesthetic is reduced with intermittent bolus versus continuous infusion. Reduced cumulative local anaesthetic dose is associated with reduced motor blockade.

Continuous infusions avoid troughs in pain relief. This results in more stable analgesia and cardiovascular status. With continuous infusion there is less handling of the epidural and fewer 'breaks in the system', reducing the risk of epidural infection.

Patient Controlled Epidural Analgesia (PCEA) allows individual titration of epidural drug delivery. PCEA minimizes periods of inadequate analgesia and periods of over-medication. There is a 35% cumulative hourly dose-sparing effect in contrast with a continuous epidural infusion. Opponents point out that it requires a complex delivery device and that parturients can receive boluses of local anaesthetic in the absence of a trained attendant. Meticulous monitoring of the sensory level is required.

4. *Adjuvant drugs.* Opioids and local anaesthetics produce synergistic mechanisms of analgesia. The site of action of the opioid is the spinal opioid receptor in the substantia gelatinosa; the site of action of the local anaesthetic is at the nerve axon. Addition of short-acting lipid-soluble opioids (e.g. fentanyl) has a local anaesthetic dose-sparing effect without analgesia being compromised. Incorporating opioid can ameliorate intractable back and rectal pain and enhance the quality of analgesia. There is improved maternal satisfaction with reduced motor block.

5. *Disadvantages of epidurals.* Complications include pruritis, urinary retention, nausea and vomiting, and dural tap. The management of a dural tap resulting in a dural puncture headache is to resite the epidural for a painfree delivery. Following delivery, encourage oral fluids (especially caffeine-containing), consider an epidural saline infusion (e.g. 1 l over 24 h), give simple oral analgesics and offer epidural 'blood patch' from 24 h. Immediate patch has a 75% failure rate. Bed rest is not therapeutic but gives symptomatic relief. Other complications are rare.

6. *Combined spinal epidural (CSE).* This technique combines the rapidity and reliability of a spinal anaesthetic (including sacral roots), with the flexibility of a continuous epidural to extend the duration and if necessary, the extent of the analgesia.

Proponents of the CSE technique suggest that the local anaesthetic-sparing effect, which results in reduced motor block, enables walking during labour. Risk of falls is a factor against widespread use. The theoretical advantages of ambulatory epidurals in terms of improved obstetric outcomes have not been substantiated in early clinical trials. However there is improved maternal satisfaction with reduced motor block. If parturients intend to walk, there must be clear guidelines including:

- No obstetric or anaesthetic contraindication for mobilization.
- Bromage score testing to demonstrate normal leg strength.
- Exclude orthostatic hypotension.
- Accompanying person must be suitably robust if the parturient should 'collapse'.
- Regular reassessment of motor and sensory block, and fitness to ambulate.

Further reading

Burnstein R, Buckland R, Pickett JA. A survey of epidural analgesia for labour in the United Kingdom. *Anaesthesia*, 1999; **54**: 634–640.
Collis RE, Davies DWL, Aveling W. Randomised comparison of combined spinal-epidural and standard epidural analgesia in labour. *Lancet*, 1995; **345**: 1413–1416.

Related topics of interest

Obstetrics – delivery (p. 178); Obstetrics – medical emergencies (p. 181); Spinal and epidural anaesthesia (p. 241)

OBSTETRICS – DELIVERY

Jenny Tuckey

In the UK the caesarean section rate is approximately 18–20%. In the report on Confidential Enquiries into maternal deaths in the UK (1994–1996), 0.8% of direct maternal deaths ($n = 1$) were due to anaesthesia. The death was associated with a combined spinal epidural block. The reduction in the death rate associated with anaesthesia is due to the general change in practice from general to regional anaesthesia.

Caesarean section (LSCS)

This may be elective, urgent or emergency. With urgent and emergency cases, there is often less time to achieve anaesthesia, and maternal or fetal physiology may be acutely deranged. Anaesthesia may be *regional* or *general*. Regional anaesthesia includes subarachnoid (spinal), epidural and combined spinal epidural (CSE) blocks.

1. Pre-operatively. Acid aspiration is a risk. Histamine (H_2) receptor blocker (e.g. ranitidine 150 mg p.o.) should be given regularly to high-risk labouring patients and 2 doses pre-operatively to elective cases. Ranitidine 50 mg may be given slowly intravenously to emergency cases when time precludes oral route. Metoclopramide increases lower oesophageal sphincter tone. A non-particulate antacid (e.g. 30 ml 0.3 M sodium citrate) should be given immediately pre-operatively.

2. Peroperatively. A skilled assistant must always be present. To prevent aorto-caval compression, the patient should be positioned either with a left lateral tilt or with a wedge beneath the right buttock. Prophylactic antibiotics reduce the incidence of puerperal infections. Thrombo-embolic events are the single greatest cause of maternal death. Calf compression devices should be used.

3. Postoperative analgesia should be multimodal. Where feasible it should involve 'spinal' opioids, non-steroidal anti-inflammatory drugs and paracetamol. For patients who have undergone general anaesthesia, ilio-inguinal/iliohypogastric nerve blocks and patient controlled analgesia may be useful. Heparin prophylaxis should be considered in all patients postoperatively. Sufficient time should have elapsed after administration of heparin before epidural catheter removal (e.g. 6 h).

Regional anaesthesia

Regional anaesthesia is the preferred technique providing maternal consent is obtained and there are no contraindications. It reduces the risk of failed intubation, aspiration of stomach contents and maternal awareness under general anaesthesia. Regional anaesthesia is relatively contraindicated in placenta accreta where there is the potential for severe haemorrhage.

Subarachnoid blocks are increasingly the technique of choice in patients with severe pre-eclampsia in place of epidurals providing they are not contraindicated by coagulopathy. The advantage is the improved quality of the block and, because of the smaller spinal needle and absence of epidural catheter, the reduced risk of epidural haematoma.

General anaesthesia

General anaesthesia is indicated where it is the maternal choice and in patients without existing regional block in certain urgent situations such as cord prolapse, severe sustained fetal bradycardia and significant antepartum haemorrhage.

Maternal hazards

1. Failed intubation. The incidence of failed intubation in obstetrics is between 1 in 250 and 1 in 300. During pregnancy, there is capillary engorgement of the nasopharynx and larynx. Total body water increases and generalized oedema may occur. Enlargement of the breasts may make insertion of the laryngoscope blade difficult.

The experience of general anaesthesia for LSCS is diminishing, especially amongst trainees. Displacement and distortion of the larynx by cricoid pressure may be exacerbated by left lateral tilt. The *failed intubation drill* should be well rehearsed. Most agree that the patient should be left supine with tilt to optimize the ability to maintain the airway and apply cricoid pressure. If there is difficulty maintaining the airway, some advocate a trial of release of cricoid pressure. The laryngeal mask airway is now an accepted part of most failed intubation algorithms. Where oxygenation still fails, the supine position is required for cricothyroidotomy.

2. Aspiration of gastric content. A rapid sequence induction should be used.

3. Awareness. To reduce the risk of awareness, a generous dose of induction agent is followed by overpressure to achieve an end-expired isoflurane of 1.2% prior to delivery. Following delivery, opioid and 70% nitrous oxide can be given. At this stage, if the uterus is not well contracted, the isoflurane may be reduced to achieve an end-expired concentration of 0.8%.

4. Hypertensive response to laryngoscopy may result in cerebral haemorrhage or acute left ventricular failure. Recommended treatments include alfentanil 15 mcg/kg, lidocaine (lignocaine) 1.5 mg/kg, esmolol 0.25–0.5 mg/kg and magnesium sulphate 4 g slowly (>5 minutes) if not already loaded with magnesium.

Fetal hazards

1. Asphyxia. Avoid aortocaval compression. In cases with fetal compromise, the FIO_2 should be 1.0 prior to delivery to optimize fetal oxygenation. Avoid maternal hyperventilation.

2. Effect of drugs on fetus. Unless induction-delivery time is unduly prolonged, insignificant amounts of induction agent or volatile agent cross the placenta. Avoid maternal opioids until after delivery of the fetus.

3. Uterine incision to delivery time should not exceed 90 seconds. If it is prolonged, it may result in fetal acidosis and low Apgar scores. This occurs as a result of uterine incision-induced changes in utero-placental blood flow.

Further reading

Husaini SW, Russell IF. Intrathecal diamorphine compared with morphine for postoperative analgesia after Caesarean section under spinal anaesthesia. *British Journal of Anaesthesia*, 1998; **81**: 135–139.

Department of Health, Welsh Office, Scottish Office Department of Health, Department of Health and Social Services, *Report on Confidential Enquiries into Maternal Deaths in the United Kingdom 1994–1996*. Northern Ireland. Norwich, HMSO, 1998, pp. 7–8, 92–102.

Related topics of interest

Audit – National (p. 30); DVT and PE (p. 101); Emergency anaesthesia (p. 109); Intubation – difficult (p. 141); Obstetrics – analgesia (p. 175); Obstetrics – medical emergencies (p. 181); Spinal and epidural anaesthesia (p. 241)

OBSTETRICS – MEDICAL EMERGENCIES

Jenny Tuckey

Pulmonary thromboembolism

There were 48 deaths due to thromboembolism reported to the Confidential Enquiry into Maternal Deaths (CEMD) during 1994–1996 (rate 21.8 per million pregnancies). Of the 48 deaths, 46 were due to PE and two to cerebral embolism secondary to DVT. Thromboembolism occurs in approximately 1 in 2000 pregnancies and is the single greatest cause of direct maternal deaths in the UK.

Eclampsia

Eclampsia is diagnosed if one or more grand mal convulsions (not related to other conditions) occurs in pre-eclampsia. The incidence (according to the British Eclampsia Survey Team, 1994), is 4.9 per 10 000 maternities. Two per cent of eclamptics die, whilst 35% suffer major complications. Eclampsia is more common in teenagers and in cases of multiple pregnancy.

HELLP syndrome

The HELLP syndrome is a form of severe pre-eclampsia and is associated with a maternal mortality of up to 24%. HELLP syndrome presents with malaise in 90%, epigastric pain (90%) and nausea and vomiting (50%). Physical signs include right upper quadrant tenderness (80%), weight gain and oedema. Blood pressure may be normal and proteinuria may be absent. Resolution of symptoms following delivery may be slow. These patients may develop multiple organ failure. Corticosteroids may normalize platelets and liver enzymes and hasten recovery.

Pregnancy-induced hypertension

There were 20 direct deaths due to pregnancy-induced hypertension reported to the CEMD during 1994–1996 (rate 9.1 per million pregnancies). Pre-eclampsia may be defined as 'gestational proteinuric hypertension developing during pregnancy or for the first time in labour'. It occurs in approximately 10% of pregnancies, most commonly between 33 and 37 weeks gestation. The only cure is delivery of the placenta. Pre-eclampsia generally resolves within 48–72 hours of delivery. The most common causes of death due to hypertensive diseases of pregnancy (CEMD 1994–1996) are ARDS, cerebral oedema, intracranial haemorrhage, pulmonary oedema and ruptured liver.

The American College of Obstetricians and Gynecologists use any one of the following to define severe pre-eclampsia: systolic blood pressure (BP) > 160 mmHg, diastolic BP > 110 mmHg, mean arterial pressure > 120 mmHg, proteinuria (5 g in 24 hours or +3/+4 on 'dipstick' testing), oliguria (< 500 ml in 24 hours), headache or cerebral disturbance, visual disturbance, epigastric pain or raised liver enzymes (transaminases), pulmonary oedema or cyanosis, HELLP (haemolysis, elevated liver enzymes, low platelets).

The prognosis in mild pre-eclampsia is good.

1. ***Management of pre-eclampsia.*** The general aims are to minimize vasospasm, improve perfusion of uterus, placenta and maternal vital organs, and assess fetal maturity.

- Antihypertensive agents are given if the diastolic blood pressure persistently exceeds 100 mmHg (e.g. labetolol, nifedipine or hydralazine).
- Regular assessment of proteinuria, urate, platelet count, and the fetus is required.
- If the pregnancy is < 34 weeks two doses of dexamethasone (12 mg) are given to aid maturation of the fetal lungs. Delivery is ideally delayed for 48 hours for maximal benefit.

Magnesium sulphate may be given as prophylaxis against convulsions. It is a central nervous system depressant, cerebral vasodilator and mild antihypertensive. It increases prostacyclin release by endothelial cells, increases uterine and renal perfusion, and decreases platelet aggregation. Conversely, its tocolytic effect may prolong labour and increase blood loss. A bolus dose of 4 g is given followed by an infusion of 1–3 g/h. Tendon reflexes, respiratory rate, SpO_2 and mental state should all be monitored. Therapeautic blood levels are 2.0–3.5 mmol/l. Heart block and respiratory paralysis occur at 7.5 mmol/l. Calcium gluconate antagonizes the actions of magnesium.

2. ***Fluids.*** In severe pre-eclampsia, CVP correlates poorly with left ventricular end diastolic pressure. If the CVP is zero, there is scope for a fluid challenge. Measurement of pulmonary artery occlusion pressure may be useful if there is evidence of pulmonary oedema, if blood products are required because of haemorrhage, or if there is prolonged oliguria.

Amniotic fluid embolism (AFE)

Between 1994 and 1996, there were 17 maternal deaths due to AFE (7.7 per million maternities). The incidence is 1 in 8000 to 1 in 80 000 live births. Mortality is as high as 86%, with 50% dying within the first hour. Amniotic fluid embolus can occur in early pregnancy, at the time of termination of pregnancy or amniocentesis, or following closed abdominal trauma. It can also occur during caesarean section or artificial rupture of the membranes, as well as during the more widely described oxytocic driven vigorous labour of an elderly multipara with a large baby.

1. ***Clinical features.*** Typically, there is a sudden onset of dyspnoea, cyanosis and hypotension out of proportion to blood loss, followed quickly by cardiorespiratory arrest. Up to 20% will have seizures and up to 40% will have DIC with bleeding from the vagina, surgical incisions, and intravenous cannula sites. Non-cardiogenic pulmonary oedema will follow in up to 70% of initial survivors.

Management of AFE is symptomatic and supportive.

Intracranial bleed

Between 1994 and 1996 there were 24 maternal deaths reported due to intracranial haemorrhage (14 subarachnoid haemorrhage and nine primary intracerebral).

Cardiac arrest in pregnancy

Hypoxia develops rapidly due to the reduced FRC and increased oxygen consumption of pregnancy. Early intubation is essential to prevent aspiration and because of the reduced pulmonary compliance. Caval compression should be avoided and chest compressions performed with a wedge beneath the victim's right hip, or the gravid uterus displaced manually. If spontaneous circulation is not restored rapidly the fetus should be delivered by immediate ceasarean section. Resuscitation should not be abandoned until after delivery of the fetus.

Local anaesthesia toxicity

Circumoral numbness, tinnitus, light-headedness, confusion and a sense of impending doom are typical complaints. Muscle twitching and grand mal convulsions may occur. All these symptoms and signs are exacerbated by acidosis and hypoxia. CNS symptoms usually occur before cardiovascular collapse.

Further reading

Department of Health, Welsh Office, Scottish Office, Department of Health and Social Services, Northern Ireland. *Report on Confidential Enquiries into Maternal Deaths in the United Kingdom 1994–1996.* Norwich; Her Majesty's Stationary Office, 1998.

Related topics of interest

Audit – national (p. 30); CPR (p. 75); DVT and PE (p. 101); Obstetrics – analgesia (p. 175); Obstetrics – delivery (p. 178)

OPHTHALMOLOGY
Richard Innes

Patients are often at extremes of age with coincidental illnesses including diabetes, cardio-respiratory disease and renal impairment. Some ocular abnormalities are manifestations of congenital disease, e.g. Downs syndrome. Anaesthesia aims to provide an immobile eye with low to normal intraocular pressure (IOP) avoiding spasm of extraocular muscles, coughing and vomiting.

Ocular physiology

1. IOP. A balance between production and drainage (via the canal of Schlemm) of aqueous and vitreous humour. Two thirds of aqueous is actively secreted dependent on carbonic anhydrase. Normal IOP is 16 ± 5 mmHg and is measured with a tono-meter. Factors affecting IOP are similar to ICP (coughing, straining, neck position). IOP increases with venous congestion, external pressure, choroidal blood volume and vitreous humour volume. Laryngoscopy via its pressor effect will also significantly elevate IOP. Choroidal blood flow is autoregulated over MAP 90–130 mmHg. Raised $PaCO_2$ will increase blood flow and hence IOP.

IOP is reduced pharmacologically by:

- Increasing aqueous drainage (miotics, e.g. pilocarpine).
- Reducing aqueous production (carbonic anhydrase inhibitors, e.g. acetazolamide).
- Both (beta blockers, e.g. timolol).
- All inhalation and induction agents (except ketamine due to CVS effect).
- Muscle relaxants (except suxamethonium).

2. Oculocardiac reflex. This manifests itself as sinus bradycardia and occurs with traction on extraocular muscles, pain or raised IOP. The afferent pathway is via the ciliary ganglion to the ophthalmic division of the trigeminal nerve through the Gasserian ganglion to the sensory nucleus in the fourth ventricle. Treatment involves release of eye traction, intravenous atropine or glycopyrrolate. Prophylactic treatment is controversial.

Anaesthesia

General anaesthesia is usually required in children however in adults most surgery is now performed using regional techniques. Premedication should aim to allay anxiety, prevent nausea and vomiting and avoid raising IOP.

1. Regional anaesthesia. Peri-operative monitoring should be employed. A mixture of lidocaine (lignocaine) and bupivacaine with hyaluronidase and epinephrine (adrenaline) may be used to achieve rapid response, long duration and good spread. Tetracaine (amethocaine) eye drops are applied to the conjunctiva to facilitate painless injection. The aim is to achieve an anaesthetized, akinetic and hypotonic eye.

Retrobulbar block penetrates the muscle cone and is performed with the patient looking straight ahead. A 25 gauge needle is passed backwards from the lower, outer angle of the orbit until the eye moves. Up to 4 ml of local anaesthetic solution is then injected slowly. Orbicularis oris also needs blocking with 3 ml of solution injected directly below the posterior portion of the zygoma.

Peribulbar block is safer as the needle remains outside the muscle cone. A 25 gauge needle is passed posteriorly from a point between the lateral and medial two thirds of the lower orbital margin. Up to 5 ml of local anaesthetic solution are injected slowly at a depth of 25 mm. A second injection passes posteriorly for 25 mm beside the medial canthus again injecting up to 5 ml. This block requires spread of solution to all compartments of the eye which is facilitated by compression of the eye for about 10 minutes postinjection with a pressure device.

Complications are more frequent with a retrobulbar block and include globe perforation, optic nerve damage, retrobulbar haematoma, subarachnoid or i.v. injection. Rare but serious complications have led to the concept of non-akinetic regional anaesthetic techniques for cataract extraction. These include:

- Sub-tenons block.
- Topical corneoconjunctival anaesthesia.
- Subconjunctival injection of local anaesthetics.

These techniques whilst safer and less invasive require good doctor:patient co-operation as the eye will not be akinetic.

2. General anaesthesia.   Secure control of the airway is required using a tracheal tube or a laryngeal mask. The latter leads to smaller increases in IOP and significantly reduced post-operative coughing and sore throat. Thus the LMA and in particular the reinforced LMA have found widespread acceptance for ophthalmic surgery using spontaneous ventilation or IPPV. Stable IOP is sought and capnography is recommended aiming for normocarbia. If IOP rises perioperatively despite adequate depth of anaesthesia, analgesia and hypocarbia, mannitol (0.5 g/kg) or acetazolamide (500 mg) may be administered. Intraocular air or sulphur hexafluoride are used in certain retinal procedures. Nitrous oxide may then raise IOP and should be discontinued 15 min before their introduction. Emergency surgery may require suxamethonium with its attendant risk of a temporary rise in IOP. Theoretically therefore, suxamethonium is contraindicated in penetrating eye injuries. Strategies to avoid or attenuate these risks include:

- High dose non-depolarizing muscle relaxants (providing it is anticipated tracheal intubation will be uneventful).
- Pretreatment with lignocaine, clonidine or an opioid to reduce pressor response. However the anaesthetic technique chosen should balance the risk of pulmonary aspiration or difficult intubation with the risk of vitreous extrusion and possible loss of sight if IOP rises. In this respect suxamethonium is not proven to adversely effect outcome.

Following general anaesthesia smooth emergence avoiding coughing and straining is required and deep extubation should be considered. The use of an LMA will avoid many of these problems. Postoperative pain is usually minimal and opioids should generally be avoided. The patient is nursed operated eye uppermost with head-up tilt and an antiemetic given as required.

Further reading

Hamilton RC. Techniques of orbital regional anaesthesia. *British Journal of Anaesthesia*, 1995; **75**: 88–92.

Johnson RW, Forrest FC. *Local and general anaesthesia for ophthalmic surgery*. London, Butterworth Heinemann, 1994.

Related topic of interest

Elderly patients (p. 107)

ORGAN TRANSPLANTATION

Anaesthesia may have profound influences on the ultimate outcome following transplantation of organs. This may stem from management of the organ donor in the intensive care, management of the patient during organ harvesting, anaesthesia for a living donor, or anaesthetic management of the organ recipient. Cardiovascular instability is common in the brain dead patient and donors frequently require administration of vaso-active agents. Fluid balance may be erratic especially if neurogenic diabetes insipidus occurs. Poorly functioning transplanted organs in the immediate postoperative period may require specific interventions involving anaesthetists.

Patients who have undergone organ transplantation may require anaesthesia for subsequent operative procedures.

Problems

1. Care of the organ donor.

2. Care of the organ recipient.   Patients are by definition usually in poor health often with limited cardiovascular reserve.

3. Concomitant drug therapy.   Especially immunosuppressives. Cyclosporin A is a cyclic compound comprising 11 amino acids. It inhibits T-lymphocyte activation. Other commonly used immunosuppressives include azathioprine and steroids.

Renal transplantation

Chronic cardiovascular disease is especially common in kidney transplant recipients. Hypertension is present in most patients with end stage renal disease (ESRD). Diabetes, left ventricular hypertrophy and chronic fluid retention are also common features. Pericarditis and pericardial effusions may be found especially in patients with raised blood urea. Respiratory compromise may result from fluid overload. Pleural effusions and basal atelectasis are common complications of CAPD. Hepatitis and CMV infections are more common in chronic dialysis patients.

1. Anaesthetic management.   Patients should be dialysed preferably the day before transplantation. This will optimize fluid and electrolyte balance whilst avoiding large fluid shifts and hypokalaemia associated with dialysis immediately before surgery.

Both regional and general anaesthesia have been used for renal transplantation. The former carries the risk of neurological complications from a potential epidural haematoma in patients who may have residual heparinization (from recent dialysis) or a tendency to be coagulopathic. Fluid overload is also a concern with regional techniques. General anaesthesia is thus preferred in many centres. A rapid sequence induction is recommended as many ESRD patients have delayed gastric emptying. Modern short-acting drugs rely little on the kidney for their elimination and consideration of the avoidance of certain agents (e.g. gallamine) because of prolonged action is now of historic interest only.

Delayed graft function after transplantation is most commonly due to acute tubular necrosis. Close attention to perioperative hydration is thus of paramount importance. Monitoring the CVP is considered to be mandatory by many. Administration of mannitol and/or furosemide (frusemide) has also been shown to improve graft survival.

Liver transplantation

Child's classification of risk associated with surgery and liver disease (an assessment of hepatic synthetic and excretory function) is of little help in assessing risk and survival from hepatic transplantation. Rather, the state of the patient's general health, surgical technique, intraoperative blood loss, and the quality of the donor organ have a greater bearing on outcome.

The majority of patients presenting for liver transplantation have a hyperdynamic circulation with a low systemic vascular resistance and high cardiac output. At particular risk are those with co-existing ischaemic heart disease, especially when associated with alcoholic liver disease (possible cardiomyopathy, increased risk of dysryhthmias).

Pulmonary disease and liver failure are intimately linked. Patients with advanced liver disease are almost all hypoxaemic. In most this is as a result of a restrictive pattern from ascites, pleural effusions or atelectasis. In a few a true hepatopulmonary syndrome exists which results from intrapulmonary vascular dilatations. These vascular anomalies are commonly associated with pulmonary hypertension and manifest as an increase in ventilation/perfusion mismatching. Pulmonary hypertension, especially if unresponsive (e.g. to nitrates, epoprostenol, or nitric oxide), is associated with a poor outcome following liver transplantation.

1. Anaesthetic management. The main considerations are to anticipate major intraoperative blood loss, disorders of coagulation, hypothermia (especially if an extracorporeal circulation is employed), abnormalities of electrolyte balance (in particular hypocalcaemia and hypomagnesaemia), and citrate toxicity from massive transfusion of citrated blood. Following removal of the diseased organ there is a brief an-hepatic phase prior to transplantation of the donor organ. This is frequently achieved by clamping the inferior vena cava above and below the liver. This produces a marked fall in cardiac output (~50%) that is best managed with volume loading and inotropic infusions. In patients unable to tolerate these haemodynamic disturbances a femoral/portal vein bypass circuit may be used though it appears to be associated with greater reperfusion injury after completion of the an-hepatic phase. Piggy-backing the transplanted organ on top of the native liver (via an anastomosis to the hepatic vein) avoids the need for caval clamping and its associated haemodynamic changes.

Postoperatively gut function recovers quickly and enteral nutrition should be commenced within the first 24 hours. Excessive catabolism is not a feature.

Heart transplantation

All patients selected for heart transplantation have, by definition, end stage cardiac disease not amenable to medical or surgical treatment and with an expected survival rate of <10% at 1 year. The two leading causes for this state are ischaemic heart disease and cardiomyopathy.

A thorough assessment of the potential recipient is essential. It should include cardiac catheterization and angiographic evaluation of cardiac function. The pulmonary vascular resistance should be calculated and if elevated the response to vasodilators such as nitrates assessed. Contraindications to heart transplantation include: fixed high pulmonary vascular resistance, severe obstructive pulmonary disease, malignancy, active infection, and severe end organ dysfunction (e.g. renal failure).

1. Anaesthetic management. The endstage cardiac disease in transplant recipients results in a low cardiac output and slow circulation time. Drug distribution is thus likely to be quite different from that in patients with a normal heart and a delayed onset of drug action should be expected. Induction of anaesthesia may be achieved with opioids alone (e.g. fentanyl) or with the addition of small doses of agents such as thiopental (1–2 mg/kg), or ketamine. Some centres use etomidate. Opioid-induced bradycardia is common in these patients and the resulting fall in cardiac output may be dramatic. Pancuronium remains a popular choice of muscle relaxant as its associated tachycardia helps offset any opioid-induced bradycardia. An adequate and sometimes very high filling pressure is required to maintain a cardiac output in the presence of poor ventricular function. Monitoring of the CVP is usually performed with avoidance of right jugular vein cannulation. This vessel is the preferred access point for post-transplantation endomyocardial biopsies.

A transplanted heart is denervated so temporary atrioventricular pacing wires are usually inserted and ino/chronotropic drugs given by infusion to maintain an adequate heart rate and cardiac output.

Infection remains a major source of morbidity and mortality in any transplant recipient so strict asepsis is essential for any invasive procedure.

Lung transplantation

Lung transplantation may be performed as part of a combined heart–lung transplantation, as a single lung transplantation, or as bilateral lung transplantation. The chief problem limiting the success of the operation was for many years ischaemic dehiscence of the bronchus, followed by chronic organ rejection and infections. Surgical techniques have improved and an adequate bronchial blood supply and healing is now the norm. Indications for lung transplantation (with or without heart) include pulmonary fibrosis, emphysema, cystic fibrosis, Eisenmenger's complex, primary pulmonary hypertension and obliterating bronchiolitis. Potential recipients should have end stage heart or lung disease. Some consider poor right or left ventricular function to be a contraindication to lung transplantation and all attempt to get the patient either steroid-free or on very low doses prior to transplantation. Steroid therapy is detrimental to healing of the new bronchial anastomosis. The advantage of single lung transplantation is that the procedure is performed without cardiopulmonary bypass.

1. Anaesthetic management. Sedatives should be used with care in patients with end-stage pulmonary disease. Cardiovascular collapse may follow the abrupt abolition of sympathetic tone so induction of anaesthesia should be slow. The transition from spontaneous ventilation to positive pressure ventilation may be accompanied by similar haemodynamic instability. Patients not undergoing cardiopulmonary bypass may benefit from a thoracic epidural.

During the operation episodes of severe hypoxia and pulmonary hypertension should be anticipated. Occlusion of the pulmonary artery may result in right ventricular failure. Systemic vasodilators such as nitrates may be required. If hypotension is a problem inhaled nitric oxide is an alternative. After declamping of the pulmonary artery a large part of the cardiac output may be diverted through the transplanted lung resulting in pulmonary oedema. Positive end expiratory pressure ventilation and diuretic therapy will help alleviate this.

Postoperative pulmonary oedema may be a result of volume overload, ventricular failure, reperfusion injury (and capillary leak) or acute rejection. The transplanted lung is denervated so there is loss of the cough reflex. Good quality analgesia is essential to ensure early extubation and vigorous chest physiotherapy.

Further reading

Booij LHDJ. Anaesthesia and organ transplantation. *Current Anaesthesia and Critical Care*, 1999; **10:** 285–350.

Klinck JR, Lindop MJ. *Anaesthesia and intensive care for organ transplantation.* London: Chapman & Hall, 1998.

Related topics of interest

Brain death and organ donation (p. 37); Cardiac assessment (p. 55); Liver disease and anaesthesia (p. 151); Renal disease (p. 217)

ORTHOPAEDICS

Orthopaedic surgery has two distinct branches: acute trauma and elective surgery. (For trauma surgery see Emergency anaesthesia and Anaesthesia for spinal injury.) Elective orthopaedic patients tend to be at the extremes of age, they may have multisystem disease and the procedures performed can have special hazards. Patient positioning, prophylactic antibiotics, laminar flow theatres, prolonged procedures, hypothermia and postoperative pain are problems common to many orthopaedic operations.

Prosthetic surgery

Predominantly older patients with osteoarthritis or rheumatoid arthritis (q.v.) present for knee or hip replacement. Hypotensive anaesthesia may be required as this improves the cement/bone bond. Blood loss with total hip replacement may be large. Regional techniques are frequently performed, with or without the addition of sedation or a light general anaesthetic (GA). Postoperative epidural infusions may be used for analgesia. If methylmethacrylate cement enters the circulation, it causes vasodilation and mast cell degradation with histamine release leading to hypotension, hypoxaemia and potentially, cardiac arrest. This is minimized by using a cement gun (rather than placing it by hand), using a high pressure saline wash prior to cementing and by using a vent to avoid high pressure (up to 600 mmHg) within the bone. Cement, fat or surgical debris forced into the circulation, resulting in pulmonary microemboli, are responsible for the cardiovascular and respiratory changes seen. Patients should be fluid preloaded prior to cementing and vasopressors may be needed. Falls in SaO_2 and end tidal CO_2 may be seen. Patients undergoing joint replacement are at high risk of DVT.

Scoliosis surgery

Scoliosis is usually congenital or idiopathic but muscle diseases may be associated. Restrictive pulmonary defects may result in abnormal gas exchange leading to pulmonary hypertension with right ventricular hypertrophy or failure. Careful preoperative assessment must be made. Surgery to correct, or prevent further progression of kyphoscoliotic deformities should stop further respiratory and CVS impairment. Positioning, blood loss, the need for hypotension and the risk of pneumothorax are particular problems. Harrington rods are inserted posteriorly, although anterior approaches requiring one lung anaesthesia may be needed. Spinal cord function is monitored using somatosensory evoked potentials (dorsal cord) or a 'wake up test' once the spine is straightened (ventral cord assessment). Relaxation is reversed and anaesthesia lightened until the patient moves their feet to command. A benzodiazepine is given immediately and anaesthesia deepened to permit completion of the operation. Recall following the test is unusual.

Limb tourniquets

Tourniquets are contraindicated in peripheral arterial disease, crush injuries and sickle cell disease. The limb is exsanguinated by compression (e.g. with an Esmarch bandage) or elevation for 4 minutes prior to inflation to 100 mmHg above the systolic blood pressure. Maximum inflation times, which should be documented, are 1 hour for the arm and 2 hours for the leg. Even with a fully functioning regional block, considerable discomfort from the tourniquet may be seen. Problems include skin and soft tissue damage, nerve palsies, ischaemic contracture, pulmonary embolism and severe hypotension on release. Sudden reperfusion of the ischaemic and acidotic limb can result in a severe systemic acidosis with cardiac arrest. Bilateral tourniquets should be deflated with at least a 5-minute interval between them.

Fat embolism

Fat embolism occurs in 2% of femoral fractures and after 0.1% of hip and knee replacements. It is much more common after multiple trauma (up to 90%). Fatty marrow is released, embolized and causes lung damage. A triad of respiratory compromise, cerebral dysfunction and petaechial haemorrhages is described. Cardiovascular, respiratory and nervous system signs are similar to those with air embolism (q.v.). Fat emboli may also be seen in the urine, sputum and retinal blood vessels. It may be complicated by secondary infection, acute lung injury, DIC and multiorgan failure. Supportive treatment is needed and fixation of any fractures is performed. Steroids, heparin and dextran have all been advocated.

Further reading

Borghi B, Zimpfer M, Blaicher AM (editors). 2nd European Congress of Orthopaedic and Trauma Anaesthesia. *Anaesthesia*, 1998; **53** Supplement 2: 1–80.
Loach A. *Orthopaedic Anaesthesia*, 2nd edn. Edward Arnold, Kent, 1994.

Related topics of interest

Air embolism (p. 9); DVT and PE (p. 101); Emergency anaesthesia (p. 109); Hypotensive anaesthesia (p. 133); Pain relief – acute (p. 199); Rheumatoid arthritis (p. 220); Spinal and epidural anaesthesia (p. 241); Spinal injury (p. 245)

PAEDIATRIC ANAESTHESIA – basic principles

Respiratory system

By comparison with adults, infants have the following characteristics.

A large head, short neck, and a large tongue. They have narrow nasal passages and are obligate nasal breathers. Infants have a high anterior larynx which is narrowest at the level of the cricoid (C3/4). The epiglottis is U shaped and angled at 45°. The carina is wider and is at the level of T2 (T4 adult). The main bronchi arise at equal angles.

At birth there are 21–22 generations of airway, 23 by age three. At birth there are 10% of the adult number of alveoli.

The chest wall is compliant and the FRC low. Airway closure occurs in the neonate at the end of expiration. Closing volume is greater than FRC up to the age of five years. There is an increased V/Q mismatch.

The tidal volume is relatively fixed due to horizontal ribs, weak intercostal muscles and a large abdomen. The alveolar minute ventilation is increased by increasing respiratory rate and not tidal volume. The respiratory rate of a neonate is ~32 breaths per minute. Between the ages of 1 and 13 years it may be estimated by $(24-[age/2])/min$. The respiratory cycle is sinusoidal with no expiratory pause.

Oxygen consumption is relatively high (3 ml/k/min adult, 6 ml/kg/min neonate). Both the PaO_2 and the $PaCO_2$ are low at birth.

Cardiovascular system

At birth there is a marked fall in pulmonary vascular resistance. Air-filled alveoli offer mechanical support to the vessels and the pulmonary vascular tone falls as alveolar O_2 tension rises. The increased flow of blood to the left atrium elevates left atrial pressure and the atrial septum closes the foramen ovale. Cessation of flow through the placenta (a large low-resistance vascular bed) results in an increase in the SVR. This, coupled with the fall in PVR, reverses the flow of blood through the ductus arteriosus (i.e. left to right). The resultant local increase in PaO_2 causes the muscular wall of the DA to constrict and functional (but not permanent) closure occurs. Neonates tend to revert to transitional circulation following hypoxia or acidosis due to a labile pulmonary vascular resistance.

Blood volume at birth is ~85 ml/kg. Transfusion should be started if >10% of the blood volume is lost. The haemoglobin at birth is ~18 g/dl, falling to ~10 g/dl by 3 months.

Children have a high pulse rate and a low BP (approximately 110 beats/min and 95/55 at 2 years). Sinus arrhythmia is common, all other irregular rhythms are abnormal. They have a large percentage of non-contractile cardiac mass (60% versus 30% in adults). Cardiac output is increased by increasing the heart rate and not the stroke volume. There is right axis deviation due to a thick right ventricular wall in the neonate but ventricular thickness is equal by 6 months of age and then becomes greater on the left.

Nervous system

Myelination is incomplete during the first year of life. At birth there is no reaction to pin prick, by 2 weeks it is diffuse and at 3 months there is withdrawal. The MAC of halothane is increased from the adult level of 0.75% to 0.87% in neonates and 1.20% in the infant. This may be due to CNS immaturity, but neonates also have high levels of endorphins and encephalins (three to four times that of adults).

Narcotics readily depress the ventilatory response to CO_2. Intramuscular codeine (1 mg/kg) provides safe analgesia. Control of ventilation is altered with an increased incidence of periodic breathing and sleep apnoea.

The sympathetic response to bleeding is reduced.

The neuromuscular junction is immature for the first 4 weeks of life and thus there is sensitivity to non-depolarizing relaxants.

Renal system

Extracellular fluid volume is increased at birth. It is 40% of total body water rather than 30% in the adult. The volume of distribution of many drugs is also increased, e.g. suxamethonium.

Renal function is not fully matured, but may be 80% mature by one month. Neonates are unable to handle large fluid or sodium loads. Fluid requirements are low in the first week of life, rising to 4 ml/kg/h if under 10 kg. Daily requirements may be calculated from the following formula.

Weight	Rate
Up to 10 kg	100 ml/kg/day
10 to 20 kg	1000 ml + 50[wt (kg) – 10]ml/kg/day.
20 to 30 kg	1500 ml + 20[wt (kg) – 20]ml/kg/day.

Electrolyte requirements are sodium 2–3 mmol/kg/day and potassium 1–2 mmol/kg/day.

Temperature

Infants have a high surface area:body weight ratio. The head represents a large proportion of the body surface and children therefore lose heat readily if the head is exposed. They have immature responses to hypothermia (unable to shiver and poor vasoconstriction). They produce heat in brown fat which increases O_2 requirement.

Term infants cope with small temperature changes but the preterm or sick infant should be placed in a thermoneutral environment. The critical temperature is that below which the naked subject is unable to maintain body temperature. The critical temperature for an adult is 6°C, whilst for a term infant it is 23°C.

Glucose homeostasis

Infants younger than 1 year may become seriously hypoglycaemic during preoperative fasting and postoperatively if recommencement of feeding is delayed. Healthy children aged 1–5 years are able to maintain normal glucose homeostasis after 8 hours of fasting.

Further reading

Aun CST, Panesar NS. Paediatric glucose homeostasis during anaesthesia. *British Journal of Anaesthesia*, 1990; **64:** 413–418.

Hatch DJ, Fletcher M. Anaesthesia and the ventilatory system in infants and young children. *British Journal of Anaesthesia*, 1992; **68:** 398–410.

Related topics of interest

Neonatal surgery (p. 164); Paediatric anaesthesia – practical (p. 196); Temperature – hypothermia (p. 255)

PAEDIATRIC ANAESTHESIA – Practical

Safe paediatric anaesthesia relies upon careful preoperative assessment of the child and meticulous planning of perioperative care.

Problems

1. Size. Different equipment is required, e.g. a paediatric breathing system is necessary for a child < 20 kg. Such equipment may appear unfamiliar to an occasional paediatric anaesthetist.

2. Metabolic. The higher metabolic rate and immature respiratory physiology of a child make desaturation and hypoxia occur more rapidly.

3. Homeostatic mechanisms are less able to tolerate change (e.g. temperature and glucose).

Assessment of an infant will include meeting the parents. They may feel helpless and fear the loss of their child. An explanation of the planned perioperative management should be given and inviting parents to accompany the child during induction considered. Children as young as five years have been shown to fear death as well as pain and parental separation at the time of surgery.

Premedication

Pre-anaesthetic medication with atropine in children less than 1 year will dry oropharyngeal secretions and reduce the incidence of bradyarrhythmia. Sedative or analgesic agents may be prescribed for the older child. A variety of routes of administration may be considered including oral, i.m., i.v., sublingual, intranasal, and rectal. Topical anaesthetic agents may prevent the pain of cannula insertion. An occlusive dressing should be applied to topical anaesthesia creams as rapid absorption across mucous membranes (e.g. from licking) may result in methaemaglobinaemia. Tetracaine (amethocaine) gel is more rapid in onset and has less potential for side-effects.

Fasting

The residual volume of gastric juice is no greater, and may even be less, if children are allowed clear fluids to within 2 hours of anaesthesia than after a longer fast. Milk takes longer to empty from the stomach and it is recommended that milk feeds be stopped 3 hours prior to induction.

Parental presence

Having parents present at the time of induction of anaesthesia may relieve the stress of separation, reduce postoperative behavioural problems, and reduce the need for premedication. Disadvantages include the logistics of getting parents in and out of the operating environment, the unpredictability of both the child and parent in response to the latter being present at induction, and increased stress for the anaesthetist. Parental characteristics associated with a reduced benefit to the child are mothers of only children and parents who are health-care workers.

Induction

Drug doses, including those used for resuscitation, should be calculated before commencing anaesthesia. The child's blood volume should be estimated and the 10% loss allowable before transfusion noted. The choice of induction lies between intravenous or gaseous, but adequate vascular access must be established before the airway is instrumentated or surgery starts.

Awake intubation is only of use in the neonate with special indications, e.g. tracheo-oesophageal fistula.

Combined general anaesthetic and regional/local infiltration techniques reduce the need for perioperative opioids. Non-opioid analgesics such as paracetamol or diclofenac (suppositories = 1–2 mg/kg/day in divided doses for children over 1 year) should also be considered.

Tracheal intubation

Tracheal tube size up to 1 year is as follows.

- Tracheal tube size (mm) after 1 year = age/4 + 4.0.
- Length of tracheal tube (cm) = age/2 + 12.
- Weight at birth (term infant) = 3–4 kg.
- Weight 1–10 years = $2 \times$ (age + 4) (kg).

Peroperative care and monitoring

Monitoring of breath and heart sounds is achieved with the use of a precordial or oesophageal stethoscope. Core temperature should also be monitored. Rapid respiratory rates and small tidal volumes require expired gas to be sampled from close to the tracheal tube and the use of short sampling lines.

An uncuffed tracheal tube which allows a small audible leak is used in prepubertal children. Meticulous attention to the fixing of the tube and its connections is essential. Movement of the tracheal tube or breathing system may result in trauma to the airway, kinking of the tube or inadvertent bronchial intubation.

Children over 20 kg in weight have no special breathing system requirements. In younger children, especially infants and neonates, a system of low internal resistance and deadspace must be used. The Jackson-Rees modification of Ayre's T-piece is one such system, being valveless and of low resistance. For positive pressure ventilation the fresh gas flow requirements are 200 ml/kg with a minimum flow of 3 l/min. For spontaneous ventilation a fresh gas flow of three times the minute ventilation should be used. The minute ventilation is ~100 ml/kg + 1 litre. Disadvantages of this system include difficulty in scavenging and the use of cold unhumidified fresh gas.

Measures to conserve temperature and humidity should be taken. The temperature of the operating room is increased and active measures (e.g. forced warm air blankets) used. It is especially important to keep the head covered. Small babies may be anaesthetized under a radiant heat source. The child may be placed on a thermostatically controlled hot water mattress. Surgical fluids such as those used for skin preparation and cavity washout should be warmed. Intravenous fluids should also be warmed. A heat and moisture exchange device may be inserted in the breathing system but this will increase deadspace.

Careful measurement of fluid balance includes accurately weighing bloodstained swabs. Swabs are changed and weighed frequently as drying and evaporation will rapidly lead to a significant underestimation of losses. Infusion of intravenous fluid should account for the preoperative fluid status, including fasting as well as peroperative losses and postoperative requirements. Crystalloid solutions with low salt concentrations are used for infants as the immature kidney cannot tolerate large solute loads.

Following the completion of anaesthesia supplementary O_2 is given until the child is fully awake and able to return to its parents on the ward. Oral feeding should recommence as soon as possible.

Postoperative nausea and vomiting

This remains a significant problem and is associated with the type of surgery (incidence of over 80% in strabismus surgery), as well as the use of certain anaesthetic drugs. Opioids, especially morphine, in particular increase the incidence of postoperative nausea and vomiting. Perioperative analgesic techniques that reduce or obviate the need for opioid administration should be used. The use of local anaesthetic nerve blocks is especially beneficial in children.

Further reading

Bösenberg AT. Recent developments in paediatric regional anaesthesia. *Current Opinion in Anaesthesiology*, 1996; **9**: 233–238.
Hatch DJ, Hunter JM, eds. The paediatric patient. *British Journal of Anaesthesia*, 1999; **88**: 1–197.

Related topics of interest

Neonatal surgery (p. 164); Paediatric anaesthesia – basic principles (p. 193); Pain relief – acute (p. 199); Preoperative preparation (p. 209); Temperature – hypothermia (p. 255)

PAIN RELIEF – ACUTE

Acute pain relief in the postoperative patient is not an isolated intervention but part of a package of perioperative care. Effective pain management is frequently not achieved. A survey of just over 5000 patients who had recently been discharged from hospital included the following recollections from the patient's perspective. Pain was present all or most of the time in 33% of patients, pain was severe or moderate in 87%, pain was worse than expected in 17%, 42% of responders had had to ask for drugs and in 41% the drugs did not arrive immediately. These findings are true despite the availability of effective drugs and effective methods for administering them. The introduction of clear-cut guidelines or recommendations and the development of organizational structures such as acute pain services are probably the most efficient ways to ensure that the management of acute pain improves to acceptable standards.

Problems
- Insufficient education (of clinical staff and patients).
- Lack of interest by the medical professions, especially surgeons.
- Fear of side-effects.
- Huge interindividual variation in analgesic needs between patients.
- Difficulty in reliably assessing pain.
- Insufficient organisational structures to monitor and improve treatment.

Pain assessment
It is difficult to make an objective measure of a subjective experience. Tools of assessment include adjective, numeric, behavioural and physiological parameters.

1.   Adjective scale.   None, mild, moderate, severe, intolerable.

2.   Visual Analogue Scale (VAS).   Pain is indicated on a 10 cm scale continuum or expressed as a numeric value from 0 to 10.

3.   Happy and sad faces.   A qualitative scale for paediatric patients.

4.   Observer scale.   For non-communicative or intubated patients. This scores a series of behavioural and physiological parameters including vital signs, non-vocal communication, facial expression, posture and agitation.

Pain assessment must be continuous and should include the response to an intervention and subsequent adjustments in therapy.

Managing acute pain
Successful management of acute pain depends upon appropriate planning of perioperative care as well as education of the patient. Non-pharmacological methods of managing pain include attention to nursing issues such as limb positioning and pressure area care, physiotherapy (both passive and active) and psychological support of the patient.

Pharmacological pain management

1. Non-steroidal anti-inflammatories (NSAIDs).

(a) *Paracetamol.* Paracetamol is an analgesic and antipyretic. It inhibits central and peripheral prostaglandin synthesis. It is a poor anti-inflammatory. It has few irritant side-effects and is renally excreted following hepatic conjugation. Paracetamol has a ceiling effect and is used for mild pain. It is administered orally (or NGT) or rectally. A parenteral form is available in some countries. It should be given regularly if it is to have an opioid sparing effect.

(b) *Other NSAIDs.* These non-opioids are reversible inhibitors of cyclo-oxygenase, reducing levels of prostaglandin, prostacyclin and thromboxane A_2 pain mediators. They have both a central and peripheral role in blocking the prostaglandin mediated lowering of pain receptor thresholds. Salicylates are non-reversible inhibitors of prostaglandins. They are useful for the management of mild to moderate pain. They can be used in combination with opioids and regional analgesic techniques.

2. Opioid analgesics.

Opioids are those analgesics with morphine-like actions. They may be opiates; derivatives of the opium poppy *Papaver somniferum* (morphine and codeine) or synthetic analogues (pethidine, fentanyl, methadone). They are agonists at opioid receptors in the central and peripheral nervous systems.

Opioid receptors are subclassed as mu, kappa and delta. Opioid analgesics are primarily mu receptor agonists. They produce both excitatory and inhibitory phenomena including: analgesia, respiratory depression, euphoria, bradycardia, pruritis, meiosis, nausea and vomiting (via the chemoreceptor trigger zone) and inhibition of gut motility.

In equianalgesic doses and in most patients, the incidence of side effects is similar regardless of the opioid used.

In general, dosage varies inversely with age (not size). There is, however, a ten-fold variation in dose requirements between individuals of the same age. The initial dose should be based on patient age and subsequent doses titrated to suit the individual with respect to renal and hepatic function and cardiorespiratory function.

Equianalgesic doses

Opioid i.m./i.v.(mg)		oral (mg)	$t\frac{1}{2}b$ (elimination half life; h)
Morphine	10	30–60	2–3
Pethidine	100	400	3–4
Fentanyl	0.1	N/A	3–4
Codeine	130	200	3–4
Oxycodone	15	10–20	2–3
Diamorphine	5	60	0.5 (rapidly hydrolysed to morphine)
Methadone	10	20	15–40

Epidural analgesia (see spinal/epidural anaesthesia, p. 241)

The combination of epidural opioids and local anaesthetic agents can provide better pain control with fewer side-effects than epidural or systemic opioids alone. Intraoperative and postoperative epidural analgesia reduces thromboembolic complications, is associated with a better recovery of gastrointestinal function, probably preserves immune function, and reduces cardiovascular complications. It inhibits endocrine metabolic stress from surgery and may help shorten the time of rehabilitation, hospital stay, and return to work. Epidural analgesia may reduce the incidence and severity of chronic pain syndromes.

Patient controlled analgesia (PCA)

The premise behind any PCA technique, administered by whatever route, is that for each individual there is a minimum effective analgesic concentration (MEAC). This varies with changes in the level of pain perceived (usually decreasing over time) and appears to be largely independent of pharmacokinetic variables. For any given individual it is inversely related to the level of endogenous opioids. Therefore, if a patient has a low level of endogenous opioids, they are likely to need a higher plasma level of exogenous opioids to obtain their MEAC. There is no means of predicting this in an individual and thus the planning of conventional intramuscular dosage regimens is unlikely to provide safe and adequate analgesia. Experimentally, patients use PCA to maintain a relatively constant drug level around their individual MEAC level.

1. *Drug choice.* Virtually all opioids have been tried in a variety of PCA techniques. There is no clear best agent. In a well-controlled study of intravenous PCA neither patients nor observers could distinguish between morphine, pethidine or fentanyl.

2. *Drug dose.* The correct dose will allow the patient to appreciate the analgesic effect of each dose. Too small a dose will decrease this feedback effect and will result in multiple requests for further analgesia (prevented by the lockout time) and loss of confidence in the technique. Too large a dose will result in toxicity. There is an optimal dose range for each agent.

3. *Loading dose.* Achieving adequate analgesia before handing over control to the patient is important. Loading infusions can be used.

4. *Lockout interval.* This safety feature prevents over-administration by too frequent dosages. It denies the patient a subsequent dose for a fixed time following a successful request for a dose of analgesic. It should be greater than the length of time taken for the maximal analgesic effects of a dose to be perceived.

5. *Background infusion.* A constant rate background infusion can assist in providing constant drug levels. It aims to decrease the number of demands the patient needs to make and helps prevent 'breakthrough pain' when the patient sleeps and fails to make regular demands. However, there is no evidence to show that background infusions improve the quality of analgesia. More drug is used to provide the same degree of analgesia. Background infusions thus increase the risk of side-effects with no gain in analgesia. Most centres no longer use background infusions in adults.

6. *Routes of administration.* PCA can be administered transdermally, orally, sublingually, intranasally, via the epidural space, and, most commonly, intravenously.

Acute pain service

The introduction of PCA and epidural analgesia on postoperative wards does not guarantee efficient and safe pain control. Only after organizational changes (e.g. establishing an acute pain nurse) do significant improvements in pain relief and reduction in side-effects occur.

An acute pain service (APS) should develop from a multidisciplinary background. One of its principal roles is to educate staff (rather then deliver the acute pain care). It should develop guidelines both for the administration of analgesia and for the monitoring of the recipient. It should offer patient information (usually written) and ensure that new techniques are introduced in a controlled manner. Finally, it should audit the efficacy of its efforts.

Further reading

Alexander-Williams JM, Rowbotham DJ. Novel routes of opioid administration *British Journal of Anaesthesia*, 1998; **81**: 3–7.

Zenz, M. Pain therapy. *Current Opinion in Anesthesiology*, 1997; **10**: 367–368.

Related topics of interest

Obstetrics – analgesia (p. 175); Spinal and epidural anaesthesia (p. 241); Vomiting (p. 279)

PHAEOCHROMOCYTOMA

This is a tumour of chromaffin cells usually within the adrenal medulla. Ninety per cent are benign, 10% are extra-adrenal and it may be familial (occasionally it is bilateral). Phaeochromocytomata may secrete epinephrine (adrenaline), norepinephrine (noradrenaline) or dopamine. The most common extra-adrenal site is the organ of Zuckerkandl (found at the aortic bifurcation). Phaeochromocytoma is associated with neurofibromatosis, medullary thyroid carcinoma, and multiple endocrine adenomata.

It usually presents with paroxysmal or persistent hypertension, sweating, palpitations, headache, postural hypotension, anxiety and nausea. It may be an unexpected finding during laparotomy for abdominal pain of unknown aetiology. Epinephrine (adrenaline) is predominately secreted in a 'crisis'.

Diagnosis is confirmed by finding raised plasma/urinary catecholamines, raised urinary vanilyl mandelic acid or with a CT scan. Selective venous sampling or ^{99}Tc scanning may be used in order to isolate the site of the tumour.

Problems

1. Uncontrolled hypertension.
2. Potential for cardiac dysfunction from long standing disease (e.g. left ventricular hypertrophy).
3. Marked changes in arterial pressure, myocardial excitability, and arrhythmias following induction of anaesthesia, laryngoscopy, intubation and during surgical manipulation of the tumour.

Assessment

Consider decreasing catecholamine synthesis with alpha methyltyrosine. The BP is controlled pre-operatively using α-blockade, which causes peripheral vasodilatation. Phentolamine is a short-acting α-blocker while phenoxybenzamine is longer acting; it binds irreversibly to α-receptors. Prazosin produces $α_1$-blockade with less tachycardia. Doxazosin has been used in some series with a reduction in the need for concomitant β-blockade except in those with predominantly norepinephrine (noradrenaline) secreting tumours.

Patients, especially those presenting in an emergency state, usually have a low intravascular volume. A regimen of vasodilators and fluids should be given with pre-operative CVP monitoring. Premedicant agents which increase BP (e.g. atropine) are avoided. An anxiolytic/sedative premedicant is usually given.

Peroperative management

Direct arterial blood pressure and CVP measurement are used. Muscle relaxants which cause histamine release and halothane (which sensitizes the myocardium to catecholamines) are avoided.

The blood pressure is controlled as above or with sodium nitroprusside.

Alternatively, esmolol, an ultra-short-acting β-blocker may be used to control intraoperative tachycardia or hypertension.

If the diagnosis becomes apparent for the first time during laparotomy, stop any further surgery or manipulation of the tumour until the circulating volume is fully restored and the BP controlled.

The BP may fall markedly following removal of the tumour (a low blood volume and persistent α-blockade) and an α-agonist (norepinephrine (noradrenaline)) may be required.

Phaeochromocytomata may also be removed laparoscopically.

Postoperative care

ITU/HDU care with invasive haemodynamic monitoring for the first 24 hours is recommended. Hypoglycaemia, adrenal failure, and left ventricular dysfunction may occur. However, hypertension may persist for up to 4 days.

Further reading

Hull CJ. Phaeochromocytoma. Diagnosis, preoperative preparation and anaesthetic management. *British Journal of Anaesthesia*, 1986; **58:** 1453–1468.

Prys-Roberts C. Phaeochromocytoma – recent progress in its management. *British Journal of Anaesthesia*, 2000; **85:** 44–57.

Related topics of interest

Cardiac assessment (p. 55); Hypertension (p. 131).

PORPHYRIA

Porphyrias are metabolic disorders of porphyrin metabolism. They are uncommon diseases which may have a fatal outcome following exposure to certain anaesthetic agents. Four common forms exist. Acute intermittent porphyria (AIP), variegate porphyria (VP), porphyria cutanea tarda and congenital porphyria. Only AIP and VP occur with any frequency and both provide potential anaesthetic problems. Acute attacks present with acute abdominal pain (intra-abdominal autonomic neuropathy), nausea and vomiting, confusion, psychosis, seizures, motor neuropathy and labile hypertension associated with tachycardia and sweating. Diagnosis in the latent phase is made in AIP by finding aminolaevulinic acid (ALA) in the urine and in VP by the presence of faecal porphyrins. Management of an acute attack includes analgesia (pethidine), carbohydrate loading (2000 kcal/day), β-blockade, fluids and haematin solutions to suppress ALA synthetase activity.

AIP is caused by a deficiency of uroporphyrinogen-1-synthetase and is most commonly found in Scandinavia. VP occurs more commonly in South Africa (caucasians 1 in 15000) and is due to deficiency of protoporphyrinogen oxidase. Both enzymes are involved in the production of haemoproteins and their deficiencies show autosomal dominant inheritance. The symptoms and signs of porphyria follow the build up of the precursors ALA and porphobilinogen and may result from their stimulation of presynaptic GABA receptors. Acute attacks may be precipitated by stress, pyrexia, menstruation or dieting.

Problems
1. Drug precipitation of attacks.
2. Management of acute attacks.

Anaesthetic management

1. _Assessment and premedication._ The diagnosis is already likely to have been made, with affected families being traced and tested. Establish that anaesthesia is absolutely necessary. Urinary porphyrins are only present during an acute attack. An anxiolytic premedicant, e.g. temazepam, is recommended to reduce stress.

2. _Conduct of anaesthetic._ A search for the latest recommendations for drug safety should be made. The British National Formulary (BNF) includes such data in Section 9.8.2. There is not total agreement between authorities e.g. the BNF lists lidocaine (lignocaine), prilocaine and halothane as unsafe, whereas the _BJA_ 2000;**85**:151 states that these agents should be used. These differences are due to the poor quality of the evidence from clinical and laboratory studies. Regional anaesthesia minimizes the exposure to potential precipitating drugs. Bupivacaine is safe and should be used as the agent of choice.

For general anaesthesia the following are thought to be safe:

- Analgesics: pethidine, morphine, fentanyl, salicylic acid, paracetamol.
- Induction agents: midazolam, propofol.
- Volatile agents: ether, N_2O, halothane, isoflurane.
- Relaxants: suxamethonium, curare, vecuronium.

- Psychotropics: chlorpromazine, droperidol.
- Anticholinesterases: neostigmine.
- Anticholinergics: atropine.
- Cardiovascular agents: adrenaline, phentolamine, β-agonists and -blockers, ephedrine.

A total intravenous anaesthetic using propofol should be considered. The following drugs are listed as definitely unsafe: barbiturates, etomidate and pentazocine. The following should be used with extreme caution only: NSAIDs, phenacetin, chlordiazepoxide, nitrazepam, hydralazine, nifedipine and phenoxybenzamine.

3. Postoperatively. Adequate analgesia must be provided as pain may precipitate an acute attack. Patients should be monitored for any signs of increased porphyrinogenesis, with the urine being tested with Ehrlich's aldehyde reagent for porphobilinogen. If an acute episode occurs the patient should be transferred to the ITU for further management.

Further reading

Ashley EM. Anaesthesia for porphyria. *British Journal of Hospital Medicine*, 1996; **56:** 37–42.
James MFM, Hift RJ. Porphyrias. *British Journal of Anaesthesia*, 2000; **85:** 143–53.

Related topics of interest

Evidence-based medicine (p. 118); Inherited conditions (p. 136)

POSITIONING

The position that an anaesthetized patient is placed in may expose him/her to potential injury and may affect physiological function. Optimal peroperative position improves patient safety and decreases the chance of litigation for which there is joint responsibility with the surgeon. Where possible, positioning of the patient prior to induction will help avoid these problems. When the surgical position cannot be adopted prior to anaesthesia, as 'normal' a position as possible should be achieved and protective padding used for vulnerable areas. The length of time spent in an 'abnormal' position will influence the likelihood of problems. Positioning is used to facilitate procedures, e.g. intubation, the spread of spinal anaesthesia, surgical access, and to influence physiological function. For the patient and staff, the transport of unconscious patients may be hazardous.

Patient injury

1. ***Pressure necrosis.*** Pressure points (e.g. the occiput, sacrum, buttocks, elbows and heels) must be protected in all unconscious patients. Contact with theatre apparatus such as supports, lithotomy poles, and anaesthetic masks may also create areas of necrosis. Patients at particular risk include the severely debilitated, the elderly, and those with connective tissue disorders or neurological deficits.

2. ***Nerve injury.*** Many nerves can be damaged perioperatively. The supra orbital and facial nerves are superficial, and at risk of injury. In the upper limb, the brachial plexus, radial and ulnar nerves may be affected by stretching or external pressure. Meralgia paraesthetica occurs if the lateral cutaneous nerve of the thigh is compressed. Lithotomy can damage the obturator and femoral nerves, the saphenous nerve (against a support), or the common peroneal nerve as it passes around the head of the fibula.

3. ***Tendon and joint injury.*** These result from pressure or an 'abnormal' position, e.g. neck pain following poor cervical spine positioning. Neuromuscular blockade can alter lumbar musculature and result in backache.

Systems

1. ***CVS.*** Anaesthesia affects cardiac output and vascular tone. If the legs are lowered, venous pooling may occur. In the sitting position cerebral hypoperfusion is possible, e.g. the dental chair or during certain neurosurgical procedures. Compression leggings or anti-shock trousers are used to prevent venous pooling and hypotension in prolonged sitting cases. Reverse Trendelenburg may be used as part of a hypotensive anaesthetic technique. Low venous pressure with 'open veins' predisposes to air embolism (q.v.).

Aortocaval compression can occur in the supine position with a gravid uterus, large intra-abdominal tumours or with morbid obesity. A left lateral tilt should be used. Venous stasis predisposes to DVT (q.v.). Obstruction of venous drainage will increase surgical bleeding.

2. *Respiratory system.* The supine position impairs lung function in those over 45 years. The FRC falls by 30% and the closing volume encroaches into the tidal volume. With IPPV in the lateral position ventilation is greater in the upper lung in comparison with spontaneous ventilation where the lower lung receives more. This increases ventilation:perfusion mismatch. Obstruction of abdominal excursion during inspiration decreases compliance and impairs ventilation. This occurs in the prone and Trendelenburg positions. Access to the airway is impaired and the tracheal tube may kink when prone.

3. *Gastrointestinal tract.* The sitting position provides the best protection against regurgitation although a lateral head-down position allows fluids to move with gravity away from the airway. Trendelenburg or external pressure on the abdomen may cause respiratory embarrassment and increase intragastric pressure. A high intra-abdominal pressure causes distension of epidural veins affecting spinal surgery or epidural catheter insertion.

4. *Central nervous system.* Trendelenburg impairs venous drainage and raises ICP. Sitting may decrease cerebral perfusion.

5. *Eyes.* Corneal abrasions may occur. Direct pressure, and a low BP, can result in central retinal artery ischaemia and blindness.

Further reading

Martin JT. *Positioning in Anesthesia and Surgery*, 3rd edn. Philadelphia, WB Saunders, 1997.
Porter JM, Pidgeon C, Cunningham AJ. The sitting position in neurosurgery: a critical appraisal. *British Journal of Anaesthesia*, 1999; **82:** 117–128.

Related topics of interest

Air embolism (p. 9); Critical incidents (p. 78); DVT and PE (p. 101); Neuroanaesthesia (p. 167); Sequelae of anaesthesia (p. 232)

PREOPERATIVE PREPARATION

Objectives of a preoperative visit

- To meet the patient.
- To discover the past and present medical history.
- To examine the patient.
- To review investigation results, and arrange for any others that are required.
- To plan the anaesthetic technique.
- To provide information for the patient and relatives about the anaesthetic, post-operative care and pain relief.
- To ask the patient to stop smoking preoperatively.
- To ensure appropriate postoperative facilities are available.
- To prescribe preoperative medication, if appropriate.

Investigations

These need to be tailored to each patient and operation. They must be justifiable to prevent 'blanket' investigations. Hospitals often have local guidelines for commonly used investigations. Studies have shown that there is no virtue in routine screening with many investigations, even in the elderly. History and examination miss few management altering conditions. Therefore investigations performed should:

- Potentially alter management.
- Find a condition whose risk can be decreased.
- Be sensitive and specific (and cost effective?).

Cardiovascular system

See Cardiac assessment – page 55.

Respiratory system

Respiratory function tests (RFTs) are used for patients short of breath at rest, asthmatics, chronic obstructive pulmonary disease (COPD), and prior to thoracic surgery. RFTs along with exercise tolerance, other systems disorder and blood gas analysis help assess operative risk. The most commonly used are the peak flow and the FEV_1/FVC (using a spirometer).

Patient co-operation with the tests is important as they are 'effort dependent'. A normal FEV_1/FVC ratio is greater than 70%. Low values with a normal ratio (restrictive pattern) are seen with lung fibrosis, effusion and sarcoidosis. Low values with a low ratio (obstructive pattern) are seen with COPD and asthma.

Less commonly used tests include flow volume loops, carbon monoxide transfer and helium dilution.

Haematology

1. FBC. For patients with clinical signs of anaemia, bleeding disorders, receiving chemotherapy, or when large blood loss is expected. Common abnormalities include:

- Low haemoglobin, low MCV and low MCH (microcytic/hypochromic). Seen in iron deficiency, thalassaemia, and sideroblastic anaemia.
- Low haemoglobin, high MCV and high MCH (macrocytic/hyperchromic). Seen in megaloblastic anaemia, chronic liver disease, alcohol abuse, hypothyroidism, or haemolytic anaemias.
- Low haemoglobin, normal MCV and normal MCH (normocytic/normo-chromic). Seen in chronic renal failure, chronic infections, malignancy, connective tissue diseases, or chronic gut diseases.
- High haemoglobin may be primary in polycythaemia rubra vera or secondary to hypoxic lung disease (including smoking) right-to-left shunt, high altitude, renal or hepatic disease, or cerebral tumours.

'Stress polycythaemia' has an unknown cause.

2. Sickledex test. See Sickle cell disease, page 235.

3. Blood crossmatching. Either a 'group and save' or a crossmatch should be arranged depending on the preoperative haemoglobin, and the degree and rapidity of expected blood loss. Many hospitals have guidelines for the amount of blood to order for various procedures.

4. Coagulation. Patients with a history of bleeding disorder, those taking or recently stopped anticoagulants, liver disease, or prior to cardiac or major vascular surgery.

Biochemistry

1. Urea and electrolytes. Recommended for all patients over 70, and those with any potential abnormality, e.g. diuretic therapy, renal disease, diarrhoea or vomiting.

2. Blood sugar. Diabetics and any patient with a cause for secondary diabetes.

3. Liver function tests. Patients with liver disease, alcohol abuse, altered nutritional status or on drugs that affect hepatic function.

4. Urine testing. Performed on all patients.

Radiology

1. CXR. For patients with a significant history of cardiorespiratory disease (acute or chronic), suspected lung carcinoma or metastases, prior to cardiothoracic surgery, and patients whose ethnic background makes tuberculosis more likely. Old age is not an indication for a CXR. A lateral should be requested if doubt exists as to a lesion's position.

2. Thoracic inlet views. For retrosternal expansion of a goitre that may cause tracheal compression.

3. Cervical spine. Lateral flexion/extension views in patients with rheumatoid arthritis looking for greater than 5 mm between the anterior arch of C1 and the odontoid peg in flexion.

Miscellaneous

- Pseudocholinesterase levels and genetic typing (suxamethonium apnoea).
- Caffeine/halothane tests – see Temperature – hyperthermia.
- Muscle biopsy/EMG studies (muscle disorder).
- Urine and stool porphyrins – see Porphyrias.
- HIV/hepatitis B.

Starvation

Convention states that 6 hours after the last ingestion of food and 4 hours after fluids, the stomach will be empty. However, in some situations this is not long enough, e.g. old age, pain, analgesic administration and pregnancy. Conversely, in otherwise fit patients, clear fluids up to 3 hours preoperatively will make the patient more comfortable, will decrease gastric volume and acidity and reduce the risk of hypoglycaemia.

Consent

Informed written consent should be sought before every operative procedure, with consent for anaesthesia being verbal. A preinduction check of the operation intended and the patient's identity should be made. Separate consent forms are used for minors, sterilizations, Jehovah Witnesses and for procedures on the mentally ill. In an emergency, the written informed consent of the next of kin should be sought. If not available an explanation of the situation should be written in the notes. Specific consent should be obtained if rectal drugs are to be administered, particularly to children.

Children

Special attention should be paid to the psychological aspects of paediatric preparation. Children less than one year old do not recognize parental separation. Older children do, and consideration should be given to allowing a parent to accompany the child to the anaesthetizing location. Pre-admission visits to hospital, information packs, videos of a hospital stay and role play with the nursing staff, all help to overcome a child's fears.

Children may suffer 3–8 upper respiratory tract infections per year but repetitive cancellation of surgery should be avoided. However, those with a temperature, productive cough or evidence of a lower respiratory tract infection should be postponed.

Premedication

Aims of premedication.

1. Amnesia. Certain benzodiazepines, e.g. lorazepam, may produce both antegrade and retrograde amnesia. This may be of benefit to an especially frightened patient but its occurrence is unpredictable.

2. Anxiolysis. A preoperative visit from the anaesthetist may be a more effective anxiolytic than simply administering preoperative medication. Neurotic and introverted patients tend to have higher anxiety scores preoperatively.

3. *Antacid.* Decreasing the gastric residual volume to less than 25 ml and its pH to > 2.5 is a frequently quoted aim. H_2 antagonists in combination with an antacid immediately prior to the induction of anaesthesia will raise gastric pH. Cimetidine inhibits the metabolism of benzodiazepines. Oral administration of clear fluids up to 3 hours before surgery decreases the gastric residual volume and acidity.

4. *Antiemetic.* They may have other actions which must be considered.

5. *Analgesia.* Pre-emptive analgesia is the administration of analgesic drugs before the onset of pain. It is suggested that this might decrease the dose of analgesic given, but this is controversial. Unless the patient has pain preoperatively it may be best given intravenously as the patient is anaesthetized.

6. *Antisialagogue.* This was the most important requirement of a premedicant when ether was used. Today, it may be desirable prior to ketamine anaesthesia, oral surgical procedures or fibreoptic intubation/bronchoscopy. However, it is unpleasant for the patient and risks inspissation of bronchial secretions and other adverse anticholinergic effects.

7. *Autonomic actions.* β-blockade will help attenuate the hypertensive response to laryngoscopy and intubation. Intravenous vagolytic agents may offer the most reliable protection from vagal responses such as the oculocardiac reflex.

8. *Allergy prophylaxis.* Atopic patients or those with known hypersensitivities may be treated with H_1 antagonists for 24 hours preoperatively and with H_2 antagonists as a single dose 1–2 hours prior to the induction of anaesthesia.

9. *Continuation of specific therapy.* Most regular medication should not be discontinued simply because an anaesthetic is to be given. Examples include steroids, antihypertensives, bronchodilators, and antibiotic therapy. Such agents may therefore be administered as part of the preoperative medication.

10. *Addition of specific therapy.* Prophylaxis against infection or DVT may be required preoperatively. Additional steroids are given to all patients who have received steroids in the preceding year.

Further reading

Seeking patients' consent: the ethical considerations. 1999. General Medical Council. at http://www.gmc-uk.org
Postgraduate educational issue. The Paediatric Patient. *British Journal of Anaesthesia*, 1999; **83:** 1–168.

Related topics of interest

Adrenocortical disease (p. 1); Anaemia (p. 18); Drugs of abuse (p. 97); Emergency anaesthesia (p. 109); Governance (p. 121); Porphyria (p. 205); Sequelae of anaesthesia (p. 232); Sickle cell disease (p. 235); Smoking – tobacco (p. 239); Temperature – hyperthermia (p. 251)

PULMONARY OEDEMA

Pulmonary oedema is the extravascular accumulation of fluid within the lung. There is a 'usual' leakage of fluid through the capillary endothelium, with the lymphatics returning it to the intravascular space (500 ml per day). Once fluid accumulates in the interstitial space it causes interstitial oedema. From here it can pass across the alveolar epithelium to enter the alveoli. It is a common clinical problem with a number of differing aetiologies. The Starling equation (describing the balance of hydrostatic and osmotic pressures) is fundamental to their understanding. Successful treatment will depend on diagnosing the cause correctly.

Symptoms and signs

Shortness of breath, orthopnoea, tachypnoea, paroxysmal nocturnal dyspnoea and a cough productive of blood-tinged frothy fluid may all indicate pulmonary oedema. Fine inspiratory crackles may be heard on auscultation of the chest and in the ventilated patient the inflation pressure may be elevated as pulmonary compliance is reduced. Gas exchange is impaired. The CXR may show upper lobe blood diversion, Kerley B lines, diffuse shadowing around the hilar (bats wing) and pleural effusions.

Aetiology

1. Raised pulmonary capillary pressure (PCP), i.e. cardiogenic with an increase in left sided preload, e.g. mitral stenosis or left ventricular failure. The pulmonary artery occlusion pressure (PAOP) usually reflects the PCP which is normally ~10 mmHg. Oedema tends to occur when this is raised to above 25 mmHg.

2. Decreased oncotic pressure makes the formation of pulmonary oedema more likely. It can therefore occur with hypoalbuminaemia (liver disease, protein loss and severe catabolism).

3. Capillary permeability can be increased in ARDS, sepsis, DIC, fat embolism, aspiration of gastric contents or the inhalation of toxins. Over-inflation of the lungs, bleomycin, heroin and cyclosporin may also cause endothelial damage and oedema.

4. Obstruction of lymphatic drainage, e.g. by malignancy. Increased superior vena caval pressure may also impair the lymphatic return. Any clinical therapies that raise this CVP may aggravate pulmonary oedema.

5. Rapid lung expansion resulting in a negative pressure in the interstitial tissues can lead to the development of pulmonary oedema. This can occur when a pneumothorax is rapidly drained or upper airway obstruction is relieved.

6. Neurogenic pulmonary oedema occurs when there is sympathetic overactivity following an acute brain injury. Rapid alteration in haemodynamic pressures are probably responsible.

7. Re-establishment of pulmonary perfusion after a period of hypoperfusion results in increased interstitial fluid and oedema.

8. High altitude with severe exercise leading to hypoxic pulmonary vasoconstriction and oedema. Acetazolamide is given prophylactically and nifedipine as treatment.

Management

The most likely aetiology must be determined so that the underlying physiological abnormality may be understood. Treatment of pulmonary oedema depends on optimizing pulmonary capillary pressure, normalizing plasma oncotic pressure, removing stimuli that increase capillary permeability and ensuring lymphatic drainage. The crystalloid versus colloid controversy has the above factors at its roots. Oxygen should be given by CPAP or IPPV. Diamorphine, diuretics and nitrates may also be required. Multiple aetiologies such as fluid overload, damaged lung lymphatics and endothelial damage combine following pneumonectomy (particularly right sided), to cause severe often fatal (> 50%) pulmonary oedema in approximately 3% of patients.

Further reading

Lang SA *et al.* Pulmonary oedema associated with airway obstruction. *Canadian Journal of Anaesthesia*, 1990; **37**: 210–218.

Slinger P. Post-pneumonectomy pulmonary edema: is anesthesia to blame? *Current Opinion in Anesthesiology*, 1999; **12**: 49–54.

Related topics of interest

ARDS/ALI (p. 24); Burns (p. 44); Drowning (p. 95); Sepsis and SIRS (p. 229); Ventilation (p. 276)

PYLORIC STENOSIS

This is the commonest neonatal surgical problem presenting to district hospitals in the UK. It has an incidence of ~1:350 live births. Approximately 80% of affected infants are male and ~50% are the first born child. It has a peak age of presentation between 3 and 6 weeks. The stenosis is caused by a gross thickening of the circular muscle of the pylorus of unknown aetiology. The typical presenting symptoms are of weight loss and projectile vomiting after feeds. Signs include those of dehydration, visible gastric peristalsis, and a palpable tumour in the epigastrium. Ultrasound can be used to confirm the diagnosis.

Problems
- Dehydration.
- Metabolic imbalance.
- Risk of aspiration.

Metabolic changes
Vomiting produces a loss of gastric hydrogen and chloride ions resulting in a metabolic hypochloraemic alkalosis. The initial response of the kidney is to conserve potassium and hydrogen and to excrete an alkaline urine. As dehydration continues, however, the kidney begins to conserve sodium and chloride (and therefore water) and to excrete hydrogen and potassium ions, thus exacerbating the alkalosis. The compensatory response to these metabolic changes is hypoventilation.

Anaesthetic management
1. Assessment and premedication. Pyloromyotomy should not be performed as an emergency. Rehydration and correction of metabolic imbalance must occur preoperatively. Normovolaemia is restored with 0.9% sodium chloride solution. In severe cases and those presenting late, additional potassium may also be required. A nasogastric tube is passed and stomach washouts with saline are performed every 4 hours. There is frequently a secondary gastritis and the gastric aspirate may be offensive. Before surgery is undertaken, the gastric residue should be clear and odourless. Laboratory investigation should confirm adequate resuscitation and indicate concentrations within the following plasma electrolyte limits: sodium >135 mmol/l, chloride >90 mmol/l, and bicarbonate >24 mmol/l and <30 mmol/l. Alternatively a urinary chloride >20 mmol/l suggests that adequate volume and electrolyte correction have occurred. Premedication with intramuscular atropine is usual.

2. Conduct of anaesthetic. Intravenous access is necessary preoperatively for resuscitation. The nasogastric tube should be aspirated and left on free drainage. Infants with pyloric stenosis are too old and too large for an awake intubation. Rapid sequence intravenous induction with cricoid pressure is the technique of choice for induction, with gaseous induction becoming less popular. Muscle relaxation is necessary and it is essential that the infant does not cough during surgical splitting of the muscle. The aim of surgery is to dissect down to but not through the pyloric mucosa. Breaching the mucosa is associated with increased postoperative morbidity. Intermittent suxamethonium or short-acting non-depolarizing agents such as mivacurium or atracurium may be used according to the speed of the surgeon. Anaesthesia is maintained with a volatile agent such as isoflurane or sevoflurane.

At the completion of the operation the nasogastric tube should again be aspirated and the baby turned on their side and muscle relaxation reversed if appropriate. Extubation should be performed awake and with full recovery of airway reflexes.

3. ***Postoperatively.*** Opioid analgesics are rarely required and postoperative analgesia may be provided by infiltration of the wound with a local anaesthetic agent and oral or rectal paracetamol. Feeding usually recommences within a few hours, although this may need to be delayed due to impaired gastric motility.

Further reading

Bissonnette B, Sullivan PJ. Pyloric stenosis. *Canadian Journal of Anaesthetics*, 1991; **35**: 668–676.
MacDonald NJ, Fitzpatrick GJ, Moore KP, Wren WS, Keenan M. Anaesthesia for congenital hypertrophic pyloric stenosis. A review of 350 patients. *British Journal of Anaesthesia*, 1987; **59**: 672–677.

Related topics of interest

Neonatal surgery (p. 164); Paediatric anaesthesia – basic principles (p. 193); Paediatric anaesthesia – practical (p. 196)

RENAL DISEASE

Patients with preoperative renal dysfunction are more likely to develop postoperative renal failure, particularly after cardiac or aortic surgery. The aetiology of the renal dysfunction is important in assessing the severity of the impairment, and careful evaluation allows a management strategy to be formulated. Associated medical problems (e.g. hypertension, diabetes mellitus, and rheumatoid arthritis) must be considered.

Problems

1. The effect of renal failure on drug handling. Renal failure has both pharmaco-kinetic and pharmacodynamic effects. Protein bound drugs have increased free fractions due to acidosis and hypoalbuminaemia. Lipid insoluble drugs are predominantly eliminated by the kidney whilst the hepatic metabolites of many lipid soluble drugs are excreted renally. Uraemia causes denaturation of protein and change of structure or binding site configuration and may thus affect drug action.

2. Fluid and electrolyte balance. Patients may be hypervolaemic with oedema and hypertension or recently dialysed with dehydration and limited cardiovascular reserve. Metabolic acidosis is usually present and compensated for by a respiratory alkalosis. Serum potassium may vary, although most patients are hyperkalaemic. It may rise further with acidosis, suxamethonium, catabolic stress (surgery, trauma, sepsis) and potassium sparing diuretics. Hyper-magnesaemia as a result of inadequate dialysis may increase sensitivity to relaxants. Hypocalcaemia induces secondary and tertiary hyperparathyroidism leading to bone resorption, osteoporosis, osteomalacia and fractures.

3. Medical conditions associated with uraemia. These include: hypertension leading to arrhythmias, cardiomegaly and failure; pericarditis and effusion, atherosclerosis and ischaemic heart disease; pulmonary oedema, atelectasis, pneumonia and ARDS. Immunosuppression occurs and may be related to poor nutrition and anaemia. Poor wound healing and an increased risk of bedsores result. Peptic ulceration, an elevated gastrin level, hiccups, and nausea and vomiting are more common and increase the risk of aspiration.

4. Anaemia. The anaemia associated with renal failure is usually normochromic, normocytic and secondary to decreased erythropoietin secretion. Multiple transfusions increase the risk of transfusion acquired infection, e.g. hepatitis. Uraemic coagulopathy with a prolonged bleeding time but a normal prothrombin time, partial thromboplastin time, thrombin time and platelet count increases the risk of cerebral, pericardial and surgical haemorrhage. It is improved with dialysis, cryoprecipitate and DDAVP (desmopressin).

Anaesthetic management

1. *Assessment and premedication.* Preoperative assessment should include reference to the above complications and the timing of dialysis. The site of any shunts or fistulae should be noted. The optimal timing for surgery is 24 hours following haemodialysis when the fluid volume is normal. Peritoneal dialysis can be continued until surgery. Blood transfusion, if required, is best performed during dialysis and may improve graft survival in patients for transplantation. An abnormal bleeding time should be corrected with DDAVP. Hypertension and hyperkalaemia should be corrected.

2. *Conduct of anaesthesia.* Spinal and epidural anaesthesia should not be undertaken in the presence of clotting abnormalities or following recent haemodialysis. Other regional techniques may be considered, e.g. brachial plexus block for vascular access procedures. Lactate containing intravenous solutions are avoided. Careful patient positioning ensures pressure points and shunt sites are protected. No intravenous lines should be placed in limbs with vascular shunts. Care must be exercised to prevent fluid overload and CVP monitoring is often required. Neuromuscular blockade is monitored. A urinary catheter should be passed and a urine output of greater than 0.5 ml/kg/h should be ensured. A rapid sequence induction is preferred as there is an increased risk of aspiration. Preoxygenation should be routine in view of the anaemia. Suxamethonium may have prolonged action due to reduced pseudocholinesterase levels and in non-dialysed hyper-kalaemic patients may cause arrhythmias or asystole. Thiopental appears safe, although care must be taken to avoid hypotension. Mivacurium, atracurium or vecuronium are the relaxants of choice as they do not accumulate. Anaesthesia may be maintained with N_2O, O_2 (50%) and a volatile agent. Enflurane should be avoided as its metabolism produces nephrotoxic fluoride ions. Sevoflurane also causes an increase in fluoride ions but to a lesser extent. Renal ischaemia initially affects the outer medulla, causing acute tubular necrosis, and this must be avoided. Renal perfusion may be improved by dopamine or dopexamine. Hypotension should initially be treated with volume expansion as vasopressors may reduce renal perfusion. If an inotrope is necessary, dopexamine has the advantage of increasing cardiac output without vasoconstricting the peripheral circulation. Ephedrine is the second choice as its chronotropic effect and increased cardiac output may negate the renal vasoconstrictive effect.

3. *Postoperatively.* Patients should be observed for signs of fluid overload, dehydration and residual neuromuscular blockade. Dialysis dependent patients are best observed on a renal unit where dialysis is readily available in the event of pulmonary oedema or hyperkalaemia.

Following transplantation, renal dopamine (1–5 μg/kg/min) may improve graft function. Hourly urine output determination is used as a basis for intravenous fluid replacement. Mannitol or furosemide (frusemide) may be given when oliguria or anuria occurs as a result of prolonged ischaemic times (>2 hours). They should be used only after an adequate renal perfusion pressure has been established. Analgesia for patients with renal failure may be achieved with titrated opioids. Non-steroidal anti-inflammatory drugs are avoided. Drugs with predominately renal excretion or active metabolites (e.g. morphine) should be titrated carefully to effect.

Further reading

Cranshaw J, Holland D. Anaesthesia for patients with renal impairment. *British Journal of Hospital Medicine*, 1996; **55:** 171–175.

Pollard BJ. Neuromuscular blocking drugs and renal failure. *British Journal of Anaesthesia*, 1992; **68:** 545–547.

Related topics of interest

Anaemia (p. 18); Diabetes (p. 89); Hypertension (p. 131); Organ transplantation (p. 187); Pulmonary oedema (p. 213); Rheumatoid arthritis (p. 220); Sepsis and SIRS (p. 229)

RHEUMATOID ARTHRITIS

This systemic connective tissue disease most commonly presents in the fourth decade with an insidious onset, although an acute onset can occur. A genetic link with HLA DR4 resulting in an abnormal immune response has been found. It affects 3% of women and 1% of men. Rheumatoid factor (IgM) is found in 70%. The classical pattern is of a symmetrical arthropathy involving the interphalangeal joints, the metacarpophalangeal joints, the wrists, and feet. Any joint may be involved. The cervical spine is of particular anaesthetic importance. Laxity of the atlanto-axial joint ligaments with erosion of the odontoid peg may result in subluxation during flexion, with the possibility of cord compression. Twenty-five per cent of rheumatoid arthritis sufferers have cervical instability but only 7% have clinical signs. The lower cervical vertebrae may be fused leading to fixed flexion. Cricoarytenoid involvement may cause hoarseness, stridor and airway obstruction. Involvement of the temporomandibular joint may limit mouth opening. Juvenile chronic arthritis (Still's disease) may present with a systemic illness including lymphadenopathy, a rash and pyrexia. It progresses to either polyarthritis or pauci-articular disease (less than 5 joints affected). It is a different disease from rheumatoid arthritis.

Systemic effects

1. Respiratory. Diffuse infiltration with fibrosis or localized rheumatoid nodules. Pleural effusions occur. Caplan's syndrome occurs very rarely in coal miners.

2. Haematological. Normochromic normocytic anaemia plus anaemia from chronic blood loss (NSAIDs). Felty's syndrome with hypersplenism.

3. Cardiovascular. Asymptomatic pericarditis is relatively common but tamponade occurs rarely. Conduction defects and valvular lesions can occur. Vasculitis with Raynaud's syndrome and nailfold infarcts may also involve cranial, coronary and mesenteric vessels.

4. Neurological. Peripheral neuropathy, mononeuritis multiplex and carpal tunnel syndrome.

5. Renal impairment from amyloidosis, or nephritis usually drug related.

6. Ocular. Sjögren's syndrome, scleritis and uveitis.

Drug effects

1. NSAIDs. Gastric erosions, renal impairment.

2. Gold. Nephrotic syndrome, bone marrow suppression.

3. Penicillamine. Nephropathy and thrombocytopenia.

4. Immunosuppressives. For example steroids, azathioprine, methotrexate or cyclosporin.

5. Methotrexate. Pneumonitis and liver toxicity.

6. Steroids. Osteoporosis, Cushing's syndrome, thin skin, purpura etc.

Problems

- Cervical subluxation.
- Systemic manifestations.
- Drugs used to treat rheumatoid arthritis.

Anaesthetic management

1. Assessment and premedication. Rheumatoid arthritics must be fully assessed to exclude the above problems. Investigations should be tailored to the clinical findings. As a minimum an FBC, U+E, CXR and cervical spine views (flexed and extended) should be performed. Neck movement and mouth opening should be assessed. A lateral cervical X-ray with a gap of more than 3 mm between the odontoid peg and the posterior arch of the axis is diagnostic of subluxation.

2. Conduct of anaesthesia. Monitoring should be appropriate to the surgery and the systemic involvement of the rheumatoid arthritis. Regional anaesthesia should be considered but may be difficult to perform in view of deformed anatomy. A difficult intubation must be anticipated and fibreoptic intubation considered. Patients with cervical involvement should demonstrate their normal range of movement immediately before induction. A protective collar should then be worn. An LMA may avoid the necessity to intubate. Abnormal protein binding may alter drug-free fractions. Positioning on the operating table must be performed with particular care.

3. Postoperatively. HDU may be required to provide analgesia, pressure area care and physiotherapy. Regional analgesic techniques may be used.

Further reading

MacKenzie CR, Sharrock NE. Perioperative medical considerations in patients with rheumatoid arthritis. *Rheum Dis Clin North Am*, 1998; **24:** 1–17.
Skues MA, Welchew EA. Anaesthesia and rheumatoid arthritis. *Anaesthesia*, 1993; **48:** 989–997.

Related topics of interest

Intubation – difficult (p. 141); Orthopaedics (p. 191); Positioning (p. 207)

SCORING SYSTEMS

Scoring systems are used in an attempt to predict outcome, improve planning and evaluate care. For a scoring system to be of use it must be able to yield valid, consistent and reproducible results. The validity and reliability of the scoring system must itself be rigorously tested and subjected to peer review.

1. *Anaesthesia.*
- Goldman index.
- Mallampatti score (see Intubation – difficult p. 141).
- Cormack and Lehane (see Intubation – difficult p. 141).

2. *Intensive care.*
- Apache II and III.
- Therapeutic intervention scoring system (TISS).

3. *Trauma.*
- Revised trauma score (RTS).
- Injury severity score (ISS).
- Paediatric trauma score (PTS).

4. *Neurological.*
- Glasgow Coma Score.

5. *Paediatric.*
- Apgar score.

Goldman risk index

1. **Aim.** To predict operative cardiovascular morbidity for non-cardiac surgery by weighting risk factors. Studies vary as to the accuracy of prediction, as hospital, patient and therapeutic variability will alter risk. More accurate risk determination requires knowledge of the results of the particular hospital.

2. **Risk factors.** S3 gallop, raised CVP, myocardial infarction within 6 months, premature ventricular beats (more than five per minute), atrial dysrhythmias, age >70 years, emergency operation, severe aortic stenosis, poor general condition, intraperitoneal or intrathoracic operation.

3. **Significance.** Each risk factor is scored and a total score derived. Scores of more than 26 suggest a high incidence of life-threatening complications of cardiac origin. In use the Goldman risk index has proven to be unreliable due to inter-hospital differences, changes in management, and the effect of the operation site and other diseases. Thus, whilst it guides the anaesthetist in likely signs equating to risk, an absolute risk value can only be determined by knowledge of results within that institution and for that anaesthetist and surgeon. For some years an alternative has been sought but as yet the Goldman risk index continues to inform risk assessment.

APACHE score (acute physiology and chronic health evaluation)

1. ***Aim.*** The primary objective is to measure case-mix and predict outcome for ITU patients as a group. It is not used to predict individual outcome or to influence the treatment that an individual receives. The pretreatment risk of death is scored according to the primary disease, the physiological reserve (age and chronic disease dependent), and the severity of the disease determined by derangements in acute physiological balance. The initial 33 physiological variables used to derive APACHE I were cut to 12 without losing predictive power in Apache II. The Apache II score is the sum of the patient's acute physiological score and the points awarded for chronological age, chronic health evaluation and whether admission followed emergency surgery. The primary diagnosis was found to have a great bearing on the outcome. A standardized mortality rate (SMR) is defined as the ratio between actual and predicted mortality and may reflect the quality of care.

2. ***Chronic health history.*** Chronic liver, cardiovascular, respiratory, renal, and immune conditions are scored.

3. ***Acute physiology score.*** This uses the worst value in the first 24 hours of admission of 12 variables including the Glasgow Coma Score.

4. ***Significance.*** Apache II assesses the quality of care rather than the use of resources. Its prediction of outcome applies to groups of patients rather than individuals and should not be taken to predict individual death. For predictive validity, the description of the disease is crucial. Apache III seeks to improve the scoring system by:
- The inclusion of six further variables.
- Chronic health, function and co-morbidity score as components of chronological age.
- Increased diagnostic categories from 42 to 230 to improve prediction.

Therapeutic intervention scoring system (TISS)

1. ***Aim.*** To score patient severity by analysis of their requirement for care. Each therapeutic intervention, e.g. ventilation, physiotherapy, or arterial blood pressure monitoring is scored from 1 to 4, and a total calculated.

2. ***Significance.*** It allows determination of the severity of illness, staff:patient ratio, and the resource usage to enable the planning of future needs. Variations in the use of therapies between units affect inter-unit comparisons.

Trauma score

1. ***Aim.*** To assess the status in triage and a quality assurance/outcome prediction. The score is based on five parameters.
- Respiratory rate per minute.
- Respiratory effort.
- Systolic blood pressure.
- Capillary refill.
- Glasgow Coma Score (q.v.).

2. *Significance.* A score of 12 or less suggests transfer to a trauma centre is indicated. Survival is closely related to the trauma score for blunt and penetrating injuries.

Revised trauma score (RTS)

Only the Glasgow Coma Score, the systolic blood pressure and the respiratory rate are recorded. Each parameter is coded and weighted and the sum forms the RTS, ranging in value from 0 to 7.8408. The higher the score the better the prognosis. The weighting for the GCS is greatest to allow for the identification of those with a severe head injury and little physiological change. The RTS has greater predictive reliability but is less suitable for triage.

Injury severity score

1. *Aim.* To score multiple injuries using the Abbreviated Injury Scale (AIS).

2. *Technique.* Every injury is assigned a score from 1 to 5 according to severity. Injuries are coded and classified into one of six regions; head and neck, face, thorax, abdomen and pelvic contents, extremities and pelvic girdle, and external or burns. The ISS is the sum of the squares of the highest AIS scores from three of the six body regions. Maximum score is 75 ($5 \times 5 \times 5$).

3. *Significance.* A validated scoring system with a significant correlation with mortality, morbidity and the length of hospital stay. It is used for all ages above 12 years.

Paediatric trauma score

1. *Aim.* Triage scoring for children as recommended by the ATLS (advanced trauma life support) system. It scores −1 to +2 according to the size of the child, quality of the airway, systolic blood pressure, state of consciousness, type of fractures, and extent of cutaneous injury.

2. *Significance.* A PTS of 8 or less correlates with an increased risk of morbidity and mortality and referral to a trauma centre is indicated.

Apgar score

1. *Aim.* Simple scoring system to assess neonatal wellbeing. Scores ranging from 0 to 2 are applied to heart rate, respiratory effort, muscle tone, reflex movement and colour.

2. *Significance.* A widely used scoring for neonatal condition at birth but uncertain as a prognostic index. Neurobehavioural scores may be more significant.

Glasgow coma score

1. *Aim.* To document the depth of coma by assessment of the best verbal, motor and eye responses to stimulation.

- Eye opening may be, spontaneous (4), to speech (3), to pain (2), absent (1).
- Best motor response is determined by: obeys commands (6), localizes to pain (5), withdraws to pain (4), abnormal flexion (3), extension (2), no response (1).

- Best verbal response: oriented (5), confused (4), inappropriate words (3), incomprehensible sounds (2), no verbal response (1).

2. Significance.   Scores range from 3 to 15. It is a useful index of depth of coma, has some prognostic significance and allows comparison between results at different centres. Scores of 8 or less indicate a requirement for ventilation. It lacks complete sensitivity as the same score can be achieved by different combinations.

Further reading

Knaus WA, Draper EA, Wagner DP, Zimmerman JE. APACHE II: A severity of disease classification system. *Critical Care Medicine*, 1985; **13:** 818–29.

Steele A, Bocconi GA, Oggioni R, Tulli F. Scoring systems in intensive care. *Current Anaesthesia and Critical Care*, 1998; **9:** 8–15.

Related topics of interest

Audit – national (p. 30); Head injury (p. 124)

SEDATION

Sedation of the surgical patient may be required when anaesthesia is provided by local or regional anaesthetic blocks. Even when dense local or regional anaesthesia has been achieved many patients experience anxiety, fear, or even panic at the thought of being awake during their procedure. As well as anxiolysis, amnesia may also be desirable to ensure patients do not have fear of returning for further procedures. Whilst much can be done to alleviate such feelings by a sympathetic approach from theatre staff, sedative agents may still be required. Anaesthetists may also be called upon to sedate nonoperative patients. Clinical research has shown that sedation by nonanaesthetists carries a higher risk of death than general anaesthesia.

Definitions

1. **Anxiolysis.** Awake but not anxious.

2. **Sedation.** Verbal communication maintained. Appropriate (though possibly slow) response to command.

3. **Deep sedation.** Eyes closed, may fall asleep if unstimulated, rousable, appropriate (though possibly slow) response to command.

4. **Sedoanalgesia.** Depressed conscious level achieved by use of combination of sedative and analgesic agents.

5. **Anaesthesia.** Loss of verbal communication, may respond to physical stimulation (e.g. pain) but not rousable.

Patient selection

Care should be taken when administering sedation to elderly patients (respiratory depression and hypotension occur more readily), uncooperative patients, those with sleep apnoea (airway obstruction occurs more easily in those supine and sedated). The administration of sedation outside the operating theatre should also be undertaken with caution.

Anaesthetic management

1. **Preoperative preparation.** All patients due to receive sedation should be fasted as per general anaesthesia guidelines. Loss of the protective airway reflexes may follow the administration of sedative drugs. Unsuccessful sedation may need to be converted to general anaesthesia. Emergency resuscitation equipment must be immediately available at the place at which patients receive sedation. Monitoring should be identical to that employed for a spontaneously breathing patient being administered general anaesthesia. As well as that the anaesthetist must remain in close contact with the patient to ensure an acceptable and appropriate level of sedation is maintained. Supplemental oxygen should be given to sedated patients. As with general anaesthesia, the patient's consent should be sought for the sedative technique and a written record of the drugs administered together with the patient's vital signs should be kept.

Drugs used for sedation

1. *Opioids.* Dependence occurs only in patients not in pain. All opioids exhibit great inter-patient variation. Morphine has a slow onset of action and is suitable for longer-term sedation but prolonged infusions result in accumulation of longer-acting metabolites, e.g. morphine 6-glucuronide. Fentanyl may appear to be shorter in duration but the elimination half-life (2–5 hours) is longer than morphine (1.5–4 hours). Alfentanil has a shorter half-life and may be used by infusion. Pethidine may be useful in patients with bronchospasm but norpethidine accumulation in renal dysfunction may lead to convulsions. Hepatic dysfunction prolongs its elimination. Phenoperidine may increase ICP, causes peripheral vasodilatation and occasionally profound cardiovascular depression. All opioids depress the cerebral response to CO_2 and decrease cough responses. All opioids decrease arterial pressure and pethidine has vagolytic effects. Hypovolaemia should be corrected and loading doses infused rather than given by bolus to reduce falls in arterial pressure associated with their use. All opioids delay gastric emptying and decrease intestinal motility.

2. *Benzodiazepines.* All induce sleep, anxiolysis and decrease muscle tone. Diazepam is unsuitable for infusion as its metabolite N-desmethyl diazepam has an elimination half-life of 96 hours. Unless formulated with soyabean extract, thrombophlebitis is a problem when administered peripherally. Midazolam has a rapid onset and shorter duration of action and no long-acting metabolites. It may cause cardiovascular depression. Benzodiazepines may fail to achieve sedation or prevent recall. Recovery may be prolonged after long term use. Flumazenil, a benzodiazepine antagonist may aid reversal of sedation but is not always successful. It has a short half-life and respiratory depression and resedation may occur.

3. *Intravenous anaesthetic agents.* Propofol by constant infusion has advantages over benzodiazepines in terms of ease of control and more rapid recovery. Ketamine has analgesic and bronchodilator properties. It may be useful in burns patients or for severe bronchospasm.

4. *Clormethiazole.* Sedative, anticonvulsant and antiemetic properties make it useful in the control of agitation and acute confusional states. The side-effects include an increase in upper airway secretions and thrombophlebitis. It is formulated as a 0.8% solution in 5% dextrose and may require large volumes resulting in hyponatraemia. Accumulation occurs after 48 hours, especially in cirrhotics and the elderly.

5. *Phenothiazines.* They have antipsychotic, sedative, antiemetic and antihistaminic activity. They also depress temperature regulation and prevent shivering. Chlorpromazine possesses α-adrenergic blocking activity, and cardiac depressant and antiarrhythmic actions. It may be useful in certain shock states and for psychotic reactions but has little place in general sedation.

6. *Inhalational agents.* Nitrous oxide is a useful agent for painful procedures but is toxic to the bone marrow. Sub-anaesthetic doses of inhalational anaesthetic agents have been used with success but require scavenging and low flow circle systems.

Patient-controlled sedation

There are many analogies between patient-controlled analgesia (PCA) and patient-controlled sedation (PCS). Patients having PCS use less drug than if it is administered by clinicians. There are thus fewer side-effects. Many patients benefit from the control of being in charge of their own level of sedation and therefore tolerate being less sedated. Syringe drivers designed for PCA have been adapted for PCS, usually by eliminating the lock out time. Drugs such as midazolam, fentanyl, and propofol have all been tried for PCS, either alone or in combination. Propofol alone remains the drug of choice at the current time.

Further reading

Hatch DJ, Sury MRJ. Sedation of children by non-anaesthetists. *British Journal of Anaesthesia*, 2000; **84:** 713–14.

Rudkin GE. Sedation. In: Millar JE, Rudkin GE, Hitchcock M (eds). *Practical anaesthesia and analgesia for day surgery*. BIOS, Oxford, UK, 1997.

Related topics of interest

Dental anaesthesia (p. 83); Pain relief – acute (p. 199)

SEPSIS AND SIRS

Jerry Nolan

The systemic inflammatory response syndrome, sepsis, shock and other related terms have been defined precisely by consensus:

- Infection is the inflammatory response to micro-organisms or the invasion of normally sterile host tissue by those organisms.
- Bacteraemia is the presence of viable bacteria in the blood.
- The systemic inflammatory response syndrome (SIRS) occurs in response to a variety of clinical insults. The response is manifested by two or more of the following conditions:
  (a) Temperature > 38°C or < 36°C
  (b) Heart rate > 90 beats/min
  (c) Respiratory rate > 20 breaths/min or $PaCO_2$ < 4.3 kPa
  (d) White blood count > 12 000 cells mm^{-3}, < 4000 cells mm^{-3}, or >10% immature (band) forms.
- Sepsis is the systemic response to infection as defined by the presence of two or more of the SIRS criteria (above).
- Severe sepsis is sepsis associated with organ dysfunction, hypoperfusion, or hypotension.
- Septic shock is sepsis-induced hypotension (systolic blood pressure < 90 mmHg or a reduction of > 40 mmHg from the baseline, or the need for vasopressors) despite adequate fluid resuscitation, along with the presence of perfusion abnormalities.
- Multiple organ dysfunction syndrome (MODS) is the presence of altered organ function in an acutely ill patient such that homeostasis cannot be maintained without intervention.

There are no universally agreed definitions of organ system failure largely because severity will be influenced strongly by treatment.

Pathophysiology of the inflammatory cascade

An initial insult (e.g. infection or trauma) triggers the production of proinflammatory cytokines (e.g. TNF, IL-1, and IL-8). These cytokines activate leukocytes and endothelium, and promote neutrophil-endothelial-cell adhesion and migration into tissues. The trapped leukocytes discharge a series of secondary inflammatory mediators, including other cytokines, prostaglandins and proteases. Ischaemia-reperfusion injury is also implicated in the inflammatory process. It generates toxic oxygen free radicals that cause cell membrane lipid peroxidation and increased membrane permeability. Depending on the severity of the initial insult and ischaemia-reperfusion injury, the inflammatory response will generate a SIRS and MODS. The arachidonic acid metabolites thromboxane A_2, prostacyclin, and prostaglandin E_2 contribute to the generation of fever, tachycardia, tachypnoea, and lactic acidosis. Anti-inflammatory mediators, such as IL-6 and IL-10, are also released and serve as negative feedback on the inflammatory process. They inhibit the generation of TNF, enhance the action of immunoglobulins, and inhibit T lymphocyte and macrophage function.

Tissue hypoxia

Some organs are particularly susceptible to ischaemia and hypoxia and may then form the trigger for multiple organ failure. Blood flow to the gut is not autoregulated for pressure; gut blood flow falls in response to reductions in cardiac output. Furthermore, plasma skimming of the blood in the gut mucosa results in a haematocrit of only 0.1, which reduces oxygen content substantially. Hepatic blood flow also has a limited capacity for autoregulation, thus the splanchnic organs are at particular risk from a systemic reduction in oxygen supply. Ischaemia-reperfusion injury increases gut permeability probably because of increased synthesis of nitric oxide by gut epithelium or vascular endothelium. The subsequent translocation of bacteria and endotoxin was thought to be a primary mechanism for the initiation of sepsis and multiple organ failure. However, there is little evidence that translocation causes systemic symptoms in humans. Instead, translocation is probably part of the normal physiological process of immune sampling by gut-associated lymphoid tissue (GALT).

Oxygen supply and demand

Severe sepsis and SIRS are associated with a marked increase in oxygen demand. Although systemic vascular resistance is low, hypovolaemia secondary to 'leaky' capillaries and relative myocardial depression may result in a global reduction in oxygen delivery. The activation of leukocytes and other cellular elements causes capillary obstruction, endothelial cell injury and microvascular shunting. Thus, even after fluid resuscitation and the institution of inotropic therapy, oxygen utilization may be significantly depressed. The persistent tissue hypoxia will be manifest as a lactic acidosis.

Gastric tonometry

The development of lactic acidosis is a global indicator of tissue hypoxia. Early warning of tissue ischaemia and hypoxia at a regional level may provide the opportunity for earlier intervention with the possibility of improving patient outcome. The precarious nature of gut mucosal blood flow makes this an appropriate organ to monitor for early evidence of global inadequate oxygen supply or utilization. Gastric tonometry is a method of monitoring the gastric mucosa for evidence of ischaemia. At equilibrium, the partial pressure of diffusible carbon dioxide in the lumen of the stomach is the same as that in the gastric endothelium. The gastric tonometer comprises a sampling tube with a distal semi-permeable silicone balloon. The balloon is filled with saline and after allowing 90 minutes for equilibration, the regional PCO_2 ($PrCO_2$) is measured in a blood gas analyser. The $PrCO_2$ is converted into an intramucosal pH (pHi) using a modified Henderson-Hasselbach equation. This calculation is based on the controversial assumption that tissue bicarbonate concentration is the same as that in arterial blood. A recent development of gastric tonometry, continuous air tonometry, is more convenient to use. Air is cycled through the balloon and the PCO_2 of the gas is measured. Calculation of the gastrointestinal-end-tidal 'PCO_2 gap' provides a convenient method of 'trending' the status of the gastric mucosa.

Treatment of SIRS and sepsis

1. General principles. The management of these inflammatory processes involves treating the cause and supporting vital organ function. Treatment of sepsis requires aggressive antimicrobial therapy and, where appropriate, surgical eradication of the focus of infection. Oxygen delivery is optimized through fluid resuscitation, supplemental oxygen and, if necessary, inotropes and mechanical ventilation. Enteral nutrition will increase gut blood flow and help to preserve gastric mucosal integrity. The maintenance of adequate mean arterial pressure and cardiac output will maximize renal blood flow. Dopamine or frusemide will help to maintain urine output but will not influence renal function per se. The onset of oliguric renal failure will require the institution of renal replacement therapy.

2. Goal directed therapy. In the past, the management of SIRS and sepsis has involved aggressively increasing oxygen delivery ($\dot{D}O_2$) (using fluid and inotropes) and oxygen consumption ($\dot{V}O_2$) until certain empirically derived goals were achieved. Earlier evidence had suggested that this strategy would reduce mortality. More recent evidence indicates that this approach either makes no difference or increases mortality. It is possible that global indices are not the best goals to aim for and, in theory, splanchnic focused resuscitation may be better. Whilst pHi appears to be a good predictor of outcome, efforts to use it as a target for goal-directed therapy have so far been unsuccessful. Thus, gastric tonometry remains largely a research tool. The commonest approach to resuscitation is to ensure normovolaemia and, using moderate inotropic support, increase cardiac output with the goal of minimizing the base deficit and/or serum lactate.

3. Specific therapies for septic shock. Considerable resource has been invested into developing a specific therapy for septic shock. Various therapies have been used in an effort to neutralize circulating endotoxin, TNF or IL-1. None of these studies have demonstrated significant beneficial effect. These disappointing results are a reflection of the complexity of the inflammatory cascade; individual cytokines are likely to have both protective and harmful effects. Clinical trials of nitric oxide synthase blockers have also produced disappointing results.

Further reading

Davies MG, Hagen PO. Systemic inflammatory response syndrome. *British Journal of Surgery*, 1997; **84:** 920–935.

Wheeler AP, Bernard GR. Treating patients with severe sepsis. *New England Journal of Medicine*, 1999; **340:** 207–214.

Related topics of interest

ARDS and ALI (p. 24); Scoring systems (p. 223)

SEQUELAE OF ANAESTHESIA

Richard Struthers

Anaesthesia and surgery have many effects on the patient. Some are inevitable consequences, but many are avoidable with knowledge and appropriate care. Air embolism, cardiac arrhythmias, DVT, hypotension, ischaemic heart disease, nerve injury and pressure necrosis are discussed in other topics (see Related topics of interest).

Airway

The patient remains the responsibility of the anaesthetist until they are fully recovered or that responsibility has been transferred to a competent person – commonly in a recovery ward or ITU. The recovering patient is at risk of the same respiratory and cardiovascular complications as at induction, but these often occur when the level of monitoring has reduced and there is a less skilled person attending them. Some units have now introduced a trained anaesthetist dedicated to the recovery room – both to increase the level of care for patients and to encourage research and training.

Atelectasis

Atelectasis occurs on induction of anaesthesia with collapse of lung in dependent areas causing ventilation–perfusion mismatch. While PEEP will maintain airways that are already open it will not re-expand collapsed airways. Atelectasis is reversible in normal patients by the maintenance of an airway pressure of 40 cm H_2O for 7–8 seconds. In patients with abnormal lungs this pressure may have to be maintained for much longer.

Cerebrovascular accident

1. Definition. Acute onset of focal neurological signs and symptoms lasting more than 24 hours and due to intracerebral infarction or haemorrhage.

2. Causes. Embolism from an extracerebral site, thrombosis or rupture of intracerebral vessel, and rarely hypotension, hyperviscosity, vasculitis and thrombophlebitis. Risk factors:

- atheromatous disease
- hypertension
- diabetes mellitus
- obesity
- cigarette smoking
- family history
- hyperlipidaemia
- atrial fibrillation.

3. Incidence. True incidence may be hard to judge as many patients with minor CVAs may be labelled as suffering from perioperative confusion. In the general surgical population the incidence is estimated as 0.2 to 0.7% in those with no history of cerebrovascular disease. This rises with age and the presence of risk factors.

In those with history of previous stroke the risk is 2.9% (i.e. 10 times). In carotid surgery the incidence is between 2 and 4%. Perioperative CVA has a mortality of 26% compared with 15% for a first stroke in the community.

4. Perioperative management. Cerebrovascular accidents often present 2 to 7 days postoperatively and are not correlated with perioperative events such as hypotension or dehydration.

5. Preoperatively. Treat hypertension and atrial fibrillation; consider anticoagulation and cardioversion. The treatment of asymptomatic carotid bruit is evolving but such patients might warrant vascular studies.

6. Intraoperatively. Maintain normal BP, and CO_2 to maintain autoregulation. Avoid excessive head rotation or extension.

7. Postoperatively. Maintain normal BP, keep well hydrated and consider anticoagulation if in AF.

Ophthalmic complications

Most cases of eye damage during anaesthesia are due to corneal abrasion. Anaesthesia may cause:

- failure of the eyelid to close (lagophthalmos).
- loss of blink reflex.
- central position of the pupil (loss of Bell's reflex – a protective reflex which causes the eyes to roll up when asleep).
- decrease in the production and quality of tears.

The incidence of corneal abrasion increases with operations lasting over 90 minutes, those on the head and neck and those where the patient is prone.

Taping the eyes and the use of aqueous gel or soft contact lenses reduces the risk of corneal abrasion. Paraffin based ointment increases morbidity – possibly by absorbing volatile agents that irritate the cornea.

Other cases of eye trauma include direct trauma or chemical irritation.

Pruritis

Itching has a diverse aetiology. Pruritis secondary to anaesthesia is commonly due to the administration of drugs or fluids.

1. Opioid drugs. Cause itching by an action on spinal opiate receptors especially the spinal nucleus of the trigeminal nerve leading to itching around the face. Increased incidence with epidural and intrathecal use and in obstetric patients. The itch may be treated with low dose naloxone, ondansetron and low dose propofol.

2. Histamine release. Secondary to drug administration. This may be short lived but will respond to antihistamine drugs.

3. Hydroxyethyl starch. Probably causes pruritis due to deposition of starch in the dermis. The incidence quoted ranges from 1% to 30% but is probably dose related. The itching lasts up to eight weeks and is unresponsive to antihistamines.

Shivering

Causes a large increase in oxygen consumption, problems with monitoring and patient discomfort. Its aetiology is poorly understood but its occurrence correlates poorly with axillary temperature. It may be due to differential recovery of spinal and higher centres. Shivering is related to the length of operation, epidurals, and the use of a volatile agent rather than TIVA. Shivering may be terminated by the use of pethidine or doxapram, although there is a 25% placebo response rate. Radiant warming is superior to the use of thermal blankets.

Sore throat

The rate of sore throat after operations depends on the technique used for airway control.

1. Tracheal tube. Intubation may cause epithelial loss, glottic oedema and haematoma and submucosal tears as well as recurrent laryngeal nerve palsy, and haematomata of the cord. Rate of sore throat ranges from 14–50%. This is more frequent with large tubes, high volume cuffs, high cuff pressure, and the use of local anaesthetic spray/gel or hydrocortisone gel. The use of suxamethonium does not lead to sore throat.

2. Laryngeal mask airway. This may cause pharyngeal trauma and there have been case reports of neuropraxia of the recurrent laryngeal and hypoglossal nerves, and epiglottic and arytenoid damage. Rate of sore throat reported as 6–34%. This is more frequent with pharyngeal trauma due to incorrect sizing and possibly trauma from the edge of a deflated cuff.

3. Face mask and oral airway. With warmed gases the rate of sore throat is reported as 15–22%. More if there is evidence of pharyngeal trauma – blood on the airway or on suction.

Most cases of sore throat are self-limiting and may be treated with simple analgesia. Vocal cord trauma usually resolves spontaneously but mucosal damage may rarely need microsurgical repair.

Further reading

McHardy F, Chung F. Postoperative sore throat: cause, prevention and treatment. *Anaesthesia*, 1999; **54:** 444–453.
White ET, Crosse M. The aetiology and prevention of perioperative corneal abrasions. *Anaesthesia*, 1998; **53:** 157–161.

Related topics of interest

Air embolism (p. 9); Anaesthetic records (p. 21); Cardiac arrhythmias (p. 50); Cardiac ischaemia (p. 58); Critical incidents (p. 78); DVT and PE (p. 101); Hypotensive anaesthesia (p. 133); Positioning (p. 207); Stress response to surgery (p. 248); Temperature – hypothermia (p. 255); Vascular surgery (p. 273)

SICKLE CELL DISEASE

A haemoglobinopathy with autosomal dominant inheritance found in Negroes and non-Negroes from around the Mediterranean and in parts of India. The β chain of haemoglobin A has valine substituted for glutamic acid in position 6. In the heterozygous form (sickle cell trait) some protection against falciparum malaria occurs. Ten per cent of Negroes in the UK have sickle cell trait. This is associated with a normal life expectancy, a Hb greater than 11 g/dl, no clinical signs or symptoms, and sickling only if the SaO_2 is less than 40%. There is, however, an increased risk of pulmonary infarcts. Co-dominant expression of the haemoglobin gene allows normal and abnormal haemoglobin to coexist. Haemoglobin S may be produced with mutant haemoglobins such as haemoglobin C (giving SC disease), and with β thalassaemia. In the homozygote (SS genotype), deoxygenated HbS becomes insoluble leading to red blood cells becoming rigid and sickle-shaped. This is more likely if hypoxia, acidosis, low temperature or cellular dehydration occur. Sickling is initially reversible, but when potassium and water are lost from the cell it becomes irreversible with haemoglobin polymerization. Sickled cells result in decreased microvascular blood flow (or occlusion) causing further local hypoxia, acidosis and thus more sickling. Local infarction causes the symptoms and signs of a sickle cell crisis. The acute chest syndrome (pleuritic pain, cough and fever), musculoskeletal complaints (bone pain, muscle tenderness, erythema), abdominal pain, splenic sequestration (acute anaemia and aplastic crisis), haematuria, priapism and cerebral vascular events (TIAs and strokes) may occur during a crisis. Chronic haemolytic anaemia, increased infection risk and specific organ damage such as 'autosplenectomy', gall stones, renal and pulmonary damage occur as the result of long-term sickling. Osteomyelitis and meningitis are more common and prophylactic antibiotics are often given. Homozygotes usually present in early childhood when HbF levels fall and HbS predominates. Survival beyond the fourth or fifth decade is rare.

Problems

- Chronic haemolytic anaemia.
- Prevention of an acute sickle cell crisis.
- Pre-existing organ damage.
- Surgical procedure (may be sickle related).
- Infection risk.

Anaesthetic management

*1. **Assessment and premedication.*** At risk patients should have a Sickledex test which detects HbS by causing sickling when the cells are exposed to sodium metabisulphite. It does not differentiate between the homozygote and the heterozygote and, if positive, formal electrophoresis must be performed. This will quantify the types and amounts of each haemoglobin. In the homozygote HbA concentrations >40% with a total Hb >10 g/dl but <12 g/dl should be achieved by exchange transfusion, but only in those undergoing elective procedures of intermediate or high risk. This optimizes oxygen delivery and blood viscosity. Patients are assessed for pre-existing organ damage and other pathologies consequent upon tissue infarction. The care of patients with haemoglobinopathies is increasingly being given in specialized centres and a haematological opinion must be sought. Sedation with the risk of hypoventilation and hypoxia should be avoided.

2. Conduct of anaesthesia. Normothermia, good hydration and oxygenation prevent the development of a sickle crisis. Following preoxygenation, a high F_IO_2 is used. Hyperventilation (respiratory alkalosis) shifts the ODC to the left and oxygen is more readily bound to haemoglobin thus preventing sickling. Cardiac output is maintained to prevent microvascular sludging, vasoconstrictors are avoided. Monitoring includes pulse oximetry, temperature, urine output and the state of hydration. Regional anaesthesia may be used, with the benefits of postoperative analgesia. It can also be of help in the acute crisis to provide analgesia. Tourniquets are avoided and patients carefully positioned to prevent venous stasis.

3. Postoperatively. High dependency care is given to provide oxygen and analgesia whilst good hydration is maintained. Shivering is avoided as this increases oxygen consumption. Prophylactic antibiotics may need to be continued. If an acute crisis develops, pain control is particularly important as the pain is characteristically very severe and patients may have previous opioid exposure with tolerance.

Further reading

Davies SC, Oni L. Management of patients with sickle cell disease. *British Medical Journal*, 1997; **315:** 656–660.
Vijay V, Cavenagh JD, Yate P. The anaesthetist's role in acute sickle cell crisis. *British Journal of Anaesthesia*, 1998; **80:** 820–828.

Related topics of interest

Anaemia (p. 18); Blood (p. 32); Temperature – hyperthermia (p. 251); Temperature – hypothermia (p. 255)

SLEEP APNOEA

During sleep, intermittent and repeated obstruction of the upper airway occurs in 4% of middle-aged men, and 2% of women. This increases to approximately 30% in morbidly obese patients. Upper airway muscle tone is abnormally decreased during sleep, and there may be abnormal anatomy and central control of breathing. Symptoms include snoring and daytime sleepiness, with an increased incidence of cardiopulmonary disease caused by chronic hypoxia and hypercarbia. Patients may also present having been involved in a road traffic accident after falling asleep at the wheel. Sedative premedicants, anaesthetic agents and opioids can therefore precipitate upper airway obstruction with further impairment of gas exchange.

Surgical treatments in adults include laser-assisted uvulopalatoplasty under local, uvulopalatopharyngeal surgery, operations on the tongue, and ultimately tracheostomy or weight reduction surgery. The aim is to increase the calibre of the upper airway, or to bypass it altogether.

In children, hypertrophy of the adenoids and tonsils can lead to chronic upper airway obstruction, pulmonary hypertension and right ventricular hypertrophy which can cause right heart failure. Symptoms include failure to thrive, hyperactivity, nightmares, enuresis and morning headaches. It is equally common in boys and girls, and obesity is rare. With superimposed infection or sedation, complete upper airway obstruction can occur. Treatment is by adenotonsillectomy which has a high success rate.

Problems

- Surgery to the upper airway.
- Airway obstruction.
- Abnormal control of breathing.
- Obesity.
- Incidental surgery.

Anaesthetic management

1. ***Assessment and premedication.*** History and examination may reveal obesity and the symptoms and signs of sleep apnoea. Whether surgery is performed to treat sleep apnoea or for an incidental indication great care is required. Patients can be receiving long-term nocturnal nasal CPAP. Haemogloblin levels may be elevated, with the ECG showing right heart strain. Cardiomegaly on a CXR may indicate the need for further cardiac investigation with echocardiography. Diagnostic sleep studies may have been performed, and the frequency and duration of apnoeic episodes with hypoxia, will indicate the severity of the disease. Sedative premedicants are avoided, but antisialogogues may be given.

2. ***Conduct of anaesthetic.*** All general anaesthetic agents can precipitate upper airway obstruction. After general anaesthesia there is a marked reduction in Rapid Eye Movement (REM) sleep on the first postoperative night, with a rebound in REM sleep on the 3rd night. REM sleep is associated with decreased muscle tone and therefore upper airway obstruction and sleep apnoea. Even topical local anaesthetic

to the oropharynx can cause obstruction as upper airway muscle tone is reduced. Nasal CPAP can be used throughout the perioperative period to prevent upper airway obstruction. Following preoxygenation, an intravenous or gaseous induction is performed. Muscle relaxation or deep inhalational anaesthesia will allow tracheal intubation which may be difficult. Intermittent positive pressure ventilation is used in cases with cardiac or pulmonary involvement.

3. Postoperatively. Following extubation, particular care must be taken to prevent upper airway obstruction, which can occur due to mechanical swelling related to the surgery or to tracheal intubation. Extubation should be performed awake. Nasal CPAP may be recommended following extubation, and severe cases should be nursed in a high dependency setting. This may be necessary for up to 3 days as there may be problems related to rebound REM sleep. Sedative analgesics should be used sparingly and their effects closely monitored.

Further reading

Boushra NN. Anaesthetic management of patients with sleep apnoea syndrome. *Canadian Journal of Anaesthesia*, 1996; **43:** 599–616.
Warwick JP *et al.* Obstructive sleep apnoea syndrome in children. *Anaesthesia*, 1998; **53:** 571–579.

Related topics of interest

Airway surgery (p. 12); Obesity (p. 173); Tracheostomy (p. 266)

SMOKING – TOBACCO

Dave Pogson

Smoking is a widespread addictive habit of clinical importance to the anaesthetist. The margin of safety of anaesthesia is reduced in smokers. Worldwide, the incidence of smoking is increasing. In the UK adolescent females are increasingly taking up the habit. The chronic deleterious effects of smoking mainly affect middle-aged adults, greatly increasing morbidity and mortality. Smokers commonly present for elective and emergency surgery. Complication risks are lessened the longer the period of abstinence. In emergency cases the benefits of a period of abstin-ence are lost and particular attention to the potential complications is required.

The effects of tobacco must also be considered in passive smokers, particularly children, who may have an increased risk of desaturation and postoperative respiratory complications.

The pharmacologically active ingredient of tobacco is nicotine. This increases HR, SVR and BP via adrenergic agonism. There is an increase in myocardial oxygen demand whereas coronary blood flow decreases. Several components of tobacco smoke are carcinogenic and adversely affect T-cell function.

Postoperative respiratory complications are 6–8 times more common than in non-smokers.

Problems

1. Airway complications are more common due to mucus hypersecretion and impaired clearance. There is small airway narrowing and sputum retention. Increased airway reflexes cause laryngospasm and bronchospasm.

2. Nicotine increases oxygen demand, blood pressure and catecholamine levels.

3. Carboxyhaemoglobinaemia up to 15% may occur, reducing oxygen delivery to tissues and shifting the oxyhaemoglobin dissociation curve to the left.

4. Thromboembolic events are more common due to increased platelet aggrega-tion and haematocrit.

5. Coexisting diseases are common, including obesity, alcoholism, COAD and CVS disease.

6. Surgical complications are more common due to tissue hypoxia and impaired wound healing.

Anaesthetic management

1. Assessment and premedication. A smoking history should be elicited and abstinence encouraged, even on the day of operation. Short-term abstinence mainly benefits the CVS as nicotine and COHb have short half-lives (1 hour and 4 hours). Ciliary activity takes 6 weeks to recover. Coexisting conditions must be assessed, including ECG findings and FBC for raised haemoglobin. Measuring COHb with a co-oximeter can assess compliance. Urinary cotinine can be assayed, but the long half-life of this nicotine metabolite prevents its use for short-term abstinence. Abstin-ence may precipitate anxiety, irritability, nausea and insomnia. Premedication may therefore include anxiolysis, bronchodilators, anticholinergics and prophylaxis against thromboembolism.

2. *Conduct of anaesthesia.* Preoxygenation is required; with increased inspired oxygen concentration throughout if carboxyhaemoglobinaemia is suspected. Gastric pH and emptying are unaffected in smokers. Intubation may produce an exaggerated pressor response, but allows bronchial toilet. Ventilation with neuromuscular blockade prevents coughing. Histamine-releasing drugs should be avoided if possible. Desflurane may cause a pronounced rise in heart rate and blood pressure in smokers. Tolerance to the effects of nicotine may attenuate the response to haemorrhage. If vasopressors are required they should be titrated carefully as nicotine may potentiate their effect. The response to opiates may be affected by liver enzyme induction. They should be titrated to effect. The use of regional anaesthesia may facilitate deep breathing postoperatively.

3. *Postoperatively.* Anxiety caused by abstinence may increase analgesic requirements. Humidified oxygen should be administered for 24 hours and deep breathing exercises encouraged. A productive cough may necessitate physiotherapy. The help of ward staff is needed to encourage the patient to abstain from smoking.

Further reading

Egan TD, Wong KC. Perioperative smoking cessation and anaesthesia: a review. *Journal of Clinical Anaesthesia,* 1992; **4:** 63–72.

Nel M, Morgan M. Smoking and anaesthesia revisited. *Anaesthesia,* 1996; **51:** 309–311.

Related topics of interest

DVT and PE (p. 101); Preoperative preparation (p. 209); Sequelae of anaesthesia (p. 232)

SPINAL AND EPIDURAL ANAESTHESIA

Spinal (subarachnoid) and epidural anaesthesia (neuroaxial anaesthesia) using local anaesthetics can produce profound analgesia, muscle relaxation, and a reduction in operative blood loss. Analgesia may also be provided by other agents (opioids, clonidine) injected into the cerebral spinal fluid (CSF) or epidural space. Neuroaxial anaesthesia is most effective when the site of injection is close to the affected dermatomes.

Spinal or epidural anaesthesia may be considered for any operation to the lower limbs, perineum or lower abdomen. There are certain circumstances where it is especially indicated either with or without general anaesthesia.

Indications

- Acute or chronic pulmonary disease.
- For the provision of profound analgesia for operations on the legs, perineum, or pelvis.
- To reduce the incidence of DVT and hypoxia during lower limb surgery especially for a fractured femoral neck. Neuroaxial anaesthesia does not, however, improve long-term perioperative mortality in this group of patients when compared with general anaesthesia.
- To obtund the stress response. The humoral response to the insult of surgery is reduced and the small bowel becomes shrunken, thus improving surgical access during laparotomy.
- Obstetric practice. Operative vaginal delivery, caesarean section, and manual removal of a retained placenta may all be performed under spinal or epidural anaesthesia.

Contraindications

1. Patient refusal.   In a properly prepared patient intravenous sedation may be used as an adjunct to neuroaxial anaesthesia in those who wish to be unaware of their surroundings.

2. Severe cardiovascular disease.   Spinal anaesthesia in particular is not a safe technique in those with cardiovascular disease such as fixed cardiac output states (e.g. valvular stenoses and obstructive cardiomyopathy; ischaemic heart disease; heart block; uncontrolled hypertension; or hypovolaemia). These patients have a cardiovascular system unlikely to tolerate abrupt alterations in haemodynamic physiology.

3. Abnormal coagulation   (including within 12 hours of a dose of heparin) and where there is the potential for severe blood loss (e.g. placenta accreta).

4. Local or systemic sepsis.

5. Raised intracranial pressure   (dural puncture risks coning and brain death).

6. Neurological disease e.g. multiple sclerosis (q.v.) is a relative contraindication as any postoperative neurological deterioration is likely to be blamed on the anaesthetic.

Drug actions

1. Local anaesthetic agents block sodium channels, preventing neural transmission. Higher concentrations are required to block motor nerves which have the thickest myelin sheath. Unmyelinated and lightly myelinated C and A delta pain and temperature fibres are blocked at low concentrations. Autonomic nerves are also blocked; vasodilatation and hypotension are thus side effects. Blockade at the level of the cardioaccelerator fibres (T1–T4) will cause bradycardia and further hypotension. Limiting the extent of the block to only those roots required and intravenous preloading will reduce the incidence of hypotension. Drugs such as atropine (if the patient is bradycardic), ephedrine (a combined α- and β-agonist), and methoxamine (a pure α-agonist), may be needed. Drugs such as bupivacaine are made hyperbaric in relation to CSF by the addition of glucose. Local anaesthetic agents are removed from the sub-arachnoid space by absorption into blood vessels. Rate of uptake is proportional to the agent's lipid solubility.

2. Opioids act at receptors in the dorsal horn to produce analgesia. Highly lipid soluble fentanyl will act near the site of absorption across the dura. The duration of action of 25 µg of intrathecal fentanyl is approximately 90 minutes. Less lipid soluble morphine may circulate in the CSF to the medulla and may cause respiratory depression.

Complications

1. Hypotension. This is the commonest complication and is usually due to blockade of the sympathetic outflow.

2. Headache following spinal anaesthesia may be due to dural stretching caused by the weight of the brain pulling down as a consequence of CSF loss. It is most common in young fit patients, especially in obstetric practice. The incidence of spinal headache may be reduced by the use of needles no larger than 25 gauge and those with a 'pencil point'. Post-spinal anaesthesia headache is managed with simple analgesics, a high fluid intake, and limited bed rest. Resistant headaches may require a blood patch. Accidental breaching of the dura with an epidural needle results in a larger hole; symptoms may consequently be more severe.

3. Itching. Intrathecal and epidural opioids result in a high incidence of widespread itching, especially in those not previously given an opioid. Nausea and vomiting are also common.

4. Other complications are rare but include spinal stroke, extradural haematoma, meningitis and extradural abscess, direct nerve damage, transverse myelitis and adhesive arachnoiditis.

Anaesthetic management

Close co-operation with the patient is essential in regional anaesthesia. An explanation of the insertion of the block should be given and the patient's consent to the procedure obtained. Anxious patients benefit from preoperative medication with agents such as benzodiazepines.

Full resuscitation facilities such as those found in a properly equipped anaesthetic room must be available prior to commencing neuraxial anaesthesia. Supplementary O_2 should be given and the O_2 saturation monitored. Intravenous access is established before the block is performed. Strict asepsis is essential.

The extent of the block is not solely related to the volume of agent used. It may be increased by the use of barbotage and changes in patient position with reference to the baricity of the agent. The total dose of agent administered is also important.

Patients with preoperative prostatism, a spinal block effective for a prolonged time, or those given large volumes of intravenous fluid may have difficulty passing urine in the immediate postoperative period. Those unable to pass urine should be examined for a full bladder and catheterized if necessary.

1. Management of an accidental dural tap. This may result in either a 'total spinal' or a postdural puncture headache. The management of a postdural puncture headache includes encouraging oral fluids (especially caffeine-containing), consider an epidural saline infusion (1 l over 24 h), give simple oral analgesics and offer epidural 'blood patch' from 24 h. Immediate patch has a 75% failure rate. Bed rest is not therapeutic but gives symptomatic relief.

2. Neuroaxial blockade and coagulation status. Bleeding within the vertebral canal may result in the formation of a haematoma which may compress the theca and result in irreversible neurological injury and paraplegia. Vertebral canal haematomata can occur spontaneously in those who have not received neuroaxial blockade. The question is do spinal and epidural techniques increase the incidence and if so in whom? Vertebral canal haematoma after neuroaxial blockade is extremely rare in the absence of abnormal coagulation or thromboembolic prophylaxis. The combination of neuroaxial blockade and thromboembolic prophylaxis appears safe provided that guidelines are followed. In Europe, for example, the recommended frequency of administration of low molecular weight heparin for thromboembolic prophylaxis is once daily. Permitting the maximum time interval between the administration of LMWH and the insertion of a spinal or epidural needle or the removal of an epidural catheter would seem prudent (12 h is frequently recommended).

Further reading

Checketts MR, Wildsmith JAW. Central nerve block and thromboprophylaxis – is there a problem? *Anaesthesia*, 1999; **82(2):** 164–167.

McCrae AF, Wildsmith JAW. Prevention and treatment of hypotension during central neural block. *British Journal of Anaesthesia*, 1993; **70:** 672–680.

Related topics of interest

Obstetrics – analgesia (p. 175); Pain relief – acute (p. 199); Sequelae of anaesthesia (p. 232); Urology (p. 271)

SPINAL INJURY

Patients are often transferred direct to a specialist unit. Resuscitation may be needed immediately after injury. Later, elective procedures are performed. Cord injury occurs in 1.5–3% of patients with major trauma, and must not be overlooked in head injuries or alcohol abuse. Traumatic cervical cord injuries are commonest in young men from road traffic accidents, falls and sporting injuries. At the time of injury there may be a massive sympathetic discharge with a parasympathetic response resulting in hypertension and myocardial, cerebrovascular or pulmonary impairment. This is followed by the acute post-transection period which transforms to the chronically injured state over several months. Low cervical and thoracolumbar lesions are the commonest lesions. Treatment aims to minimize secondary cord injury due to vasospasm, and biochemical changes resulting from the primary injury.

Problems

1. Airway. Impaired protective reflexes, poor clearance of secretions, gastric stasis, and hypoventilation often necessitate intubation following injury. Avoidance of further damage to the cord (particularly with neck flexion) is vital. Cervical in-line stabilization is provided by tongs or an assistant, whilst the rigid collar is removed. Anaesthesia is induced and laryngoscopy performed, with intubation aided by a gum elastic bougie. Cricoid pressure is used. The rigid collar is then replaced. Alternatives are blind nasal (not if there is a basal skull fracture), awake fibreoptic intubation or an intubating laryngeal mask.

2. Respiratory. Vital capacity, FRC, respiratory muscle power, and arterial oxygenation are decreased while residual volume and $PaCO_2$ is increased. Hypoventilation with failure to clear secretions results in a high acute mortality. Bronchopneumonia, neurogenic pulmonary oedema, pulmonary embolism, ARDS and sleep apnoea (Ondine's curse from damage in the C2–C4 region) may all occur. 'C3,4,5 keeps the diaphragm alive' via the phrenic nerve and with high cord transections diaphragmatic function may also be impaired.

3. Cardiovascular. Total sympathectomy whilst the parasympathetic system (vagus) remains intact results in hypotension, bradycardia, and arrhythmias (spinal shock) which may last a few days or up to 6 weeks. This needs active management to prevent cord ischaemia from extending the neurological impairment. In the chronic phase, autonomic dysreflexia results in severe hypertensive crises in 85% of those with lesions above T7. Headache, sweating and reflex bradycardia are seen. Ganglion blocking agents, α-antagonists, or direct vasodilators may be used. Volatile agents and regional anaesthetic techniques will also moderate this reflex. Impaired vasoconstriction increases the susceptibility to postural hypotension and the haemo-dynamic effects of IPPV. Preload is assessed with CVP or PAOP measurement.

4. Abdominal. Paralytic ileus increases the risk of regurgitation and aspiration. Gastric ulceration is common. Bladder and bowel atony may necessitate intermittent or permanent catheterization, and manual faecal evacuation. Recurrent urinary tract infections may impair renal function.

5. Muscles. These are initially flaccid, but in the chronically injured state spasms and contracture may develop.

6. Biochemical. Osteoporosis and hypercalcaemia may occur. Hyperkalaemia in response to suxamethonium may be life-threatening. It should not be administered after the first 48 hours until 9 months following the acute injury. Hypoventilation may result in respiratory acidosis while fluid loss from the stomach can cause a metabolic hypokalaemic alkalosis. Hyperglycaemia will cause ischaemic injury and should be prevented.

7. Temperature regulation. Sympathectomy results in an inability to vasoconstrict and hypothermia can occur.

8. Decubitus ulceration and infection are common in the quadriplegic or paraplegic patient. Such patients may present for plastic procedures. Great care of pressure areas must always be taken. There is an increased risk of thromboembolic disease.

Anaesthetic management

Assessment and premedication

1. Acute injury. Pain in the neck is an important indicator of an acute injury. A lateral cervical spine X-ray, odontoid and A–P views are taken. C7–T1 must be viewed as 20% of injuries involve this site. Anaesthesia may be required for the stabilization of the fracture site or for the management of associated injuries. Ventilation and oxygenation must be ensured, with intubation if necessary. 'Spinal shock' should be corrected with fluids and vasopressors, and ECG monitoring commenced. Spinal cord blood flow must be optimized to prevent secondary ischaemic injury. Methylprednisolone improves neurological outcome if given within 8 hours, with an initial dose of 30 mg/kg followed by an infusion for 24 hours. Mannitol to prevent oedema has been advocated. A nasogastric tube and urinary catheter should be inserted. Other injuries must be investigated and treated, while the spinal injury is assessed clinically and radiologically. CT or MRI may be indicated. Pressure area care must be instigated as soon as possible. The psychological effects of such an injury must never be forgotten.

2. Chronic injury. Stability of the fracture site and the possible complications of the injury must be assessed. Normochromic normocytic anaemia is common. Sedative premedication is avoided if respiratory function is impaired or a history of sleep apnoea obtained. Antisialogogues may be given.

Conduct of anaesthesia

Maintenance of gas exchange, blood pressure, biochemistry and temperature are imperative. Regional techniques are favoured as they decrease the incidence of autonomic dysreflexia. Cardiovascular support is often required whether a regional or general anaesthesia is performed, and invasive CVS monitoring may be needed. To prevent spinal reflexes, muscle relaxants are used if a general anaesthetic is given (cricoid pressure should always be used). Patient positioning is of particular importance. Spinal cord monitoring may be necessary in those with a vertebral column injury, but no neurological deficit.

Postoperatively

If necessary ventilation, CVS support and invasive monitoring should be continued postoperatively.

Further reading

Grundy D, Swain A. *ABC of spinal cord injury*. BMJ Publishing Group, 1993.

Hambly PR, Martin B. Anaesthesia for chronic spinal cord lesions. *Anaesthesia*, 1998; **53:** 273–289.

Petrozza PH. Anesthetic considerations for the patient with acute spinal cord injury. *Anesthesia and Analgesia*, 1998; **Mar** (Suppl): 85–90.

Related topics of interest

ARDS and ALI (p. 24); Emergency anaesthesia (p. 109); Orthopaedics (p. 191); Temperature – hyperthermia (p. 251); Temperature – hypothermia (p. 255)

STRESS RESPONSE TO SURGERY
Richard Struthers

Surgery is a form of trauma that causes marked neuroendocrine and inflammatory changes, which are referred to as 'the stress response to surgery'. These changes aim to ensure the survival of the organism while allowing wound healing and are triggered by a combination of afferent neuronal stimulation and cytokine release from traumatized tissue. While they have previously been considered separately there is considerable modulation of one response by the other.

The changes may be modified by the nature of the afferent stimuli from the injured area, starvation, dehydration, hypothermia, hypovolaemia, infection, immobilization, hypoxaemia, and emotional factors such as fear and apprehension.

The stress response can be divided into two phases – catabolic and anabolic. The catabolic or ebb phase may commence in the preoperative period if the patient is particularly anxious or is in pain but its full effects are seen shortly after the start of surgery. It may last for up to 5 days or longer if the trauma continues. It results in an increase in the production and delivery of fuel sources (glucose and free fatty acids) to those organs essential for survival (heart, brain and muscle). Sodium and water are retained and potassium is lost. There is also a reduction in the blood supply to 'non-essential' organs, especially skin and fat. The anabolic or flow phase follows the catabolic phase. During this time there is a positive nitrogen balance as muscle which has been lost is replaced. Fat stores are also replenished and there may be weight gain. This process may take several months to complete.

The endocrine changes

1. *Catabolic phase.* During this early phase there is a rise in the blood levels of cortisol, growth hormone, glucagon, ADH, prolactin and the catecholamines. The actions of insulin are suppressed. The initial response to emotion, pain and surgery is an increase in adrenergic activity with a resultant increase in circulating levels of catecholamines. Both epinephrine (adrenaline) and norepinephrine (noradrenaline) are released but the effects of epinephrine (adrenaline) predominate. Heart rate, cardiac contractility, and peripheral vascular resistance all rise resulting in an increase in BP and myocardial O_2 consumption. Stimulation of muscle β-adrenergic receptors results in glycogenolysis whilst α-adrenergic stimulation suppresses the release of insulin by the pancreas. The activity of the enzyme triglyceride lipase is increased, resulting in the release of free fatty acids.

Cortisol levels rise to up to five times normal during surgery and may remain elevated for several days. The magnitude and duration of the rise vary with the extent of the surgery. Cortisol causes a decrease in peripheral vascular resistance, an increase in cardiac output and an improvement in tissue blood flow. It promotes salt and water retention at the kidney and inhibits the actions of insulin. This, in combination with gluconeogenesis at the liver, results in hyperglycaemia. High circulating levels of cortisol are immunosuppressant and may increase susceptibility to infection and reduce wound healing. Growth hormone is released from the pituitary gland and results in hyperglycaemia and lipolysis. Its effects are anti-insulin.

The acute phase inflammatory response is characterized by a rise in several cytokines. Interleukin 6 (IL-6) is the major circulating pro-inflammatory cytokine.

It is predominantly produced by monocytes and its levels in the circulation correlate to the extent of tissue damage. This causes lymphocyte stimulation, hepatic production of acute phase proteins, haematopoiesis, fever and modulation of ACTH/cortisol production. There is, however, a complex system of pro- and anti-inflammatory cytokines at both tissue and circulating levels with the response to trauma varying between individuals. An exaggerated cytokine response to traumatic stimuli in some individuals may be implicated in the development of systemic inflammatory response syndrome.

2. Anabolic phase. Insulin is the main anabolic hormone involved in the stress response. Its actions are many and widespread. Its main effects are to increase the membrane transportation and hence utilization of glucose. It also stimulates amino acid synthesis and inhibits lipolysis.

The effect of anaesthesia on the stress response

Laryngoscopy, intubation and extubation cause a marked increase in adrenergic activity, but the effect of anaesthesia on the overall stress response is trivial by comparison with that of surgery. Anaesthetic agents or techniques may, however, modify the neuroendocrine response to the trauma of surgery.

1. Opioid analgesics. Certain of the metabolic responses to trauma may be regarded as undesirable, e.g. increased myocardial work and O_2 consumption. Attempts have been made to produce stress-free anaesthesia using high doses of potent opioid analgesics. Whilst high-dose fentanyl and morphine have been shown to obtund the peroperative haemodynamic and endocrine responses to intubation and surgery, neither agent has a lasting effect into the immediate postoperative period.

2. Efferent neuronal blockade. Much of the initiation of the stress response relies on the outflow of the sympathetic nervous system. Some success has been achieved in suppressing this response with the use of α- and β-receptor blockade. Cortisol release and hepatic glycogenolysis have both been reduced by the use of such agents.

3. Afferent neuronal blockade. Afferent nociceptive stimuli modulate the degree of response to trauma. Abolition of the neuroendocrine response depends upon the complete blockade of afferent somatic and autonomic nerves and is therefore probably only viable in the pelvis, eye and limbs. There is no evidence that abolition of neural input will alter the inflammatory response to surgery. Epidural analgesia has been shown to reduce the rise in glucose, epinephrine (adrenaline) and cortisol during surgery. However, the effects only lasted until the epidural wore off. Intrathecal local anaesthetics have similarly been shown to suppress the endocrine response but are also only effective for the duration of the blockade.

4. Etomidate. In sleep doses etomidate is a potent antiadrenal agent and modifies the cortisol response to surgery. Midazolam also contains an imidazole ring and may reduce the cortisol rise seen in abdominal and peripheral surgery. The volatile agents have no effect at clinical concentrations.

It remains unclear whether the abolition of the stress response to surgery is a desirable objective. There is as yet no reliable way of achieving such an aim beyond the operative period. Future developments in this field may lie with manipulation of both the hormonal and cytokine response to trauma.

Further reading

Desborough JP. The stress response to trauma and surgery. *British Journal of Anaesthesia*, 2000; **85:** 109–17.
Epstein J, Breslow MJ. The stress response of critical illness. *Critical Care Clinics*, 1999; **15:** 17–33.

Related topics of interest

Adrenocortical disease (p. 1); ARDS and ALI (p. 24); Diabetes (p. 89); Sepsis and SIRS (p. 229); Spinal and epidural anaesthesia (p. 241)

TEMPERATURE – HYPERTHERMIA

Hyperthermia is a core temperature > 37.5°C. Severe hyperthermia is defined as a core temperature > 40°C or an increase in body temperature at a rate greater than 2°C per hour. The aetiology of hyperthermia falls into two categories: increased heat production or decreased heat loss.

Increased heat production

1. ***Pyrogens/toxins.*** e.g. in sepsis, following burns, or blood transfusion reactions.

2. ***Drug reactions.*** As a consequence of excessive dosage of the drug or as an abnormal reaction to normal doses. Potential triggers include methylene-dioxymethamfetamine (MDMA, 'ecstasy'), thyroxine, monoamine oxidase inhibitors, tricyclic antidepressants, amfetamines and cocaine. Hyperthermia following a drug reaction may manifest as the neuroleptic malignant syndrome (NMS) or serotonin syndrome.

3. ***Endocrine.*** Associated with hyperthyroidism or phaeochromocytoma.

4. ***Hypothalamic injury*** following cerebral hypoxia, oedema, or head injury/trauma.

5. ***Malignant hyperthermia (MH).***

Decreased heat loss

- Excessive conservation especially in neonates and children.
- Heat stroke.
- Drug effects (e.g. as a predicted effect of anticholinergic administration).

Pathophysiology

Hyperthermia leads to an increased metabolic rate and oxygen consumption which in turn requires an increase in cardiac output and minute ventilation to meet demand. With increased carbon dioxide production the patient starts to develop an acidosis, initially compensated for by tachypnoea. As the oxygen debt worsens a metabolic acidosis develops secondary to lactic acid production. Subsequent sweating and vasodilatation result in a relative hypovolaemic state and worsening of the metabolic derangement if left untreated. Neurological damage, seizures, rhabdomyolysis, acute renal failure, myocardial ischaemia and infarction may all follow.

Management

1. ***General cooling measures:*** decrease ambient temperature, exposure of the patient, cold air fans, application of ice packs to extremities. Cold fluid given intravenously or intraperitoneally, cardiac bypass and cooling of blood volume.

2. _Definitive treatment_ of underlying condition using dantrolene (e.g. in MH, NMS, MDMA poisoning) mannitol (rhabdomyolysis, acute renal failure).

3. _General intensive care:_ invasive monitoring to optimize fluid balance, sedation and ventilation if required.

Neuroleptic malignant syndrome

This is an idiosyncratic complication of treatment with neuroleptic drugs such as the butyrophenones and phenothiazines. Patients are usually catatonic with extrapyramidal and autonomic effects including hyperthermia. The aetiology is unknown but appears to be related to antidopinergic activity of the precipitating drug on dopamine receptors in the striatum and the hypothalamus suggesting a possible imbalance between norepinephrine (noradrenaline) and dopamine. There is no evidence of an association with malignant hyperthermia.

Clinical features include hyperthermia, muscle rigidity and sympathetic overactivity, whilst treatment involves withdrawal of the agent and general supportive and cooling measures.

Malignant hyperthermia

This is a rare pharmacogenetic syndrome with an incidence between 1:10000 and 1:200000. It shows autosomal dominant inheritance with variable penetrance. The associated gene is on the long arm of chromosome 19. Other gene sites have been proposed and there may be considerable genetic heterogenicity. Malignant hyperthermia (MH) presents either during or immediately following general anaesthesia with a syndrome indicative of greatly increased muscle metabolism due to abnormal calcium ion flux, although it may occasionally be induced by severe exercise. The cardinal signs are hyperthermia, a combined respiratory and metabolic acidosis often with associated muscle rigidity. This is the end point of a dysfunction of the sarcoplasmic reticulum and abnormalities of intracellular ionic calcium. It results from enhanced calcium-induced release of more ionized calcium from the cytoplasmic reticulum into the cytoplasm causing myofibrillar contraction, depletion of high energy muscle phosphate stores, increased metabolic rate, hypercapnia and heat production, increased oxygen consumption and a metabolic acidosis. This entire sequence of events is caused by exposure of susceptible patients to a trigger agent.

The following drugs are all considered safe for use in MH patients: thiopental, propofol, non-depolarizing muscle relaxants, nitrous oxide, opiates, local anaesthetics, benzodiazepines, and droperidol.

The following drugs should not be used in MH patients: all volatile anaesthetic agents, suxamethonium, verapamil, nifedipine and diltiazem.

1. _Associated conditions._ There are two associated conditions, central core disease and the King-Denborough syndrome. Central core disease is an autosomal dominant, non-progressive congenital myopathy with abnormalities of the sarcoplasmic reticulum and t-tubules and a chromosome 19 defect. King-Denborough syndrome is a clinical diagnosis made over time based on the patient's appearance and physical characteristics, including short stature, slowly progressive myopathy, thoracic kyphosis, lumbar lordosis, undescended testes, pectus carinatum and an unusual facial appearance characterized by small low set ears and antimongoloid obliquity of the palpebral fissure.

Certain other neuromuscular conditions are associated with mild pyrexia, acidosis, hyperkalaemia, raised creatinine kinase and acute rhabdomyolysis. Although these signs and findings are all similar to the presentation of malignant hyperthermia, these patients are not found to be MH susceptible on formal testing. These include: muscular dystrophy (Becker's and Duchenne's), spinal muscular atrophy, myotonias, periodic paralysis, neuroleptic malignant syndrome, McArdle's syndrome, and carnitine palmitoyl transferase deficiency.

2. *Presentation.* Malignant hyperthermia may present with either or both of the following clinical pictures:

- Metabolic stimulation; hypercarbia, tachypnoea, metabolic acidosis, arrhythmias, hyperthermia, hypoxaemia.
- Abnormal muscle activity; failure of jaw to relax (masseter muscle rigidity), generalized rigidity, hyperkalaemia, myoglobinuria and acute renal failure, raised creatine kinase, DIC, cerebral and pulmonary oedema.

3. *Management.* Having made a diagnosis of possible MH, all trigger agents must be immediately stopped and the soda lime changed if being used. An alternative means of anaesthesia must be substituted e.g. propofol/midazolam infusion, and surgery postponed or expedited. The temperature, ECG, BP and CO_2 levels should all be monitored and arterial blood gas analysis performed. Venous blood should be sampled intermittently for potassium, creatinine kinase and myoglobin as well as FBC and a clotting screen. The urine output should be monitored and urine tested for myoglobin.

Dantrolene should be given in bolus doses of 1 mg/kg at 10 minute intervals until the patient responds to a maximum dose of 10 mg/kg. Dantrolene is a muscle relaxant acting by uncoupling the mechanism of excitation-contraction. It is a yellow/orange powder stored in a vial of 20 mg with 3 g of mannitol and sodium hydroxide. It is stored below 30°C and protected from light. Reconstitution is with 60 ml of sterile water (it takes some time to dissolve) and forms an alkaline solution of pH 9.5.

General cooling measures should be undertaken and any hyperkalaemia treated with insulin and dextrose, calcium chloride and hyperventilation. Intravenous fluids should be given and a diuresis promoted with furosemide (frusemide) or mannitol in order to prevent myoglobin-induced renal damage. DIC may develop.

4. *Investigation.* Investigation is undertaken after the immediate crisis has resolved. It involves a quadriceps muscle biopsy from the vastas medialis, which includes the muscle point. Histologically this is normal but the specimen is connected to a force transducer and exposed to caffeine (2 mmol/l) or halothane (2%). If a contracture occurs, generating a force in excess of 0.2 g, the test is positive. If both tests are positive the patient is deemed susceptible (MHS), if only one test is positive the patient is equivocal (MHE) and if both are negative the patient is non-susceptible (MHN). In view of the genetic disposition the immediate relatives of the susceptible patient should also be tested. Non-invasive testing using phosphorus magnetic resonance spectroscopy may be possible in the future.

Further reading

Hopkins PM. Malignant hyperthermia: advances in clinical management and diagnosis. *British Journal of Anaesthesia*, 2000; **85:** 118–129.

Adnet PJ, Gronert GA. Malignant hyperthermia: advances in diagnostics and management. *Current Opinion in Anaesthesiology*, 1999; **12:** 353–358.

Related topics of interest

Drugs of abuse (p. 97); Inherited conditions (p. 136); Sequelae of anaesthesia (p. 232); Temperature – hypothermia (p. 255)

TEMPERATURE – HYPOTHERMIA

Vital cellular processes require the temperature of the body to be controlled within 0.5°C of its normal (the 'set point'). Normal body temperature is thus 37°C +/– 0.5°C and it exhibits a circadian rhythm (lowest at 0400 hours and highest at 1700 hours). Thermoregulation depends on the balance between heat gain and heat loss. Heat is gained from metabolism, exercise and from hot foods. It is lost by radiation (40%), convection (30%), evaporation (20%), respiration (10%) and small amounts through conduction (unless the patient is wet = evaporation). Cutaneous and deep temperature sensors relay via the spinal cord to the anterior thalamus. Cold information is transmitted via A-delta fibres and warm information via unmyelinated C-fibres (also responsible for pain sensation). This explains why intense heat sensation cannot be distinguished from pain. Stimulation of the anterior thalamus causes cutaneous vasodilatation and heat loss while stimulation of the posterior thalamus causes shivering and vasoconstriction. The most effective responses to hypothermia are behavioural (moving to a warmer area, adding clothes).

The consequences of hypothermia (< 35°C) include a reduced cardiac output, hypovolaemia ('cold' polyuria from reduced ADH secretion), reduced tissue oxygen delivery, coagulopathy and abnormal platelet function (patients undergoing hip replacement have increased blood transfusion requirements when hypothermic), prolonged drug action (e.g. muscle relaxants), slow awakening due to reduced cerebral function, and shivering (increases oxygen demand, causes pain).

The consequences of severe hypothermia include coma, cardiac arrhythmias (atrial fibrillation < 35°C, ventricular fibrillation < 28°C), further hypovolaemia (loss of renal tubular function), and with prolonged hypothermia, gastric erosions and pancreatitis.

Problems

1. Identifying individuals at risk from hypothermia (those at the extremes of age and the sick).
2. Minimizing heat loss.

At risk individuals

Mild hypothermia in the anaesthetized patient is almost inevitable unless measures are taken to prevent it. The main reasons for this are: internal redistribution of heat, reduction in heat production, exposure of the body to a cool environment, and the effects of anaesthetic agents on thermoregulation. Children, especially neonates, are more at risk than adults because of their increased surface area to volume ratio.

The induction of anaesthesia rapidly results in peripheral vasodilatation and the internal redistribution of heat. Anaesthesia causes a decrease in the metabolic production of heat (no muscle activity, no shivering, decreased cellular metabolism) as well as preventing the behavioural control mechanisms. The overall amount of thermal energy available to compensate for the internal redistribution is thus less.

The body loses heat by conduction to air close to the skin. Clothing allows a layer of air warmed by the skin to remain in contact with the body and reduce further heat loss. Surgical patients are usually naked or near naked so air warmed by the skin is replaced by new, cold air and heat is lost by convection. Surgeons like operating in ambient temperatures of 20°C or less and the frequent air changes of modern operating theatres enhance loss of heat by conduction. Water conducts heat several thousand times more efficiently than air. No protective warm layer can exist around the skin in water.

Regional anaesthesia produces further heat loss. As well as the obvious internal redistribution of heat resulting from vasodilatation, epidural anaesthesia appears to lower the threshold temperature at which an efferent thermoregulatory response is initiated. Upper body shivering fails to compensate for the loss of lower body muscle activity. In addition local anaesthesia blocks the perception of skin temperature. Fentanyl added to an epidural decreases the shivering threshold further still and adds to the risk of hypothermia.

Intraoperative body temperature may be monitored at a number of sites.

- Rectal – affected by faeces, risk of viscus perforation.
- Nasopharyngeal. This reflects brain temperature and is affected by respiratory gases (unless the patient is intubated). A risk of bleeding and dislodging exists.
- Oesophageal. This reflects cardiac temperature.
- The tympanic membrane reflects brain temperature when approximated to the membrane. Infrared measurement avoids the risk of perforation and bleeding.
- Skin. This is dependent on cutaneous blood flow. The core/peripheral temperature gradient reflects perfusion and volume status particularly in infants.
- Blood, e.g. a pulmonary artery catheter reflects core temperature.
- Urinary catheter. A thermistor may be incorporated to measure core temperature.

Strategies for minimizing heat loss
- Increase the room temperature.
- Use radiant heaters, especially for neonates.
- Cover the patient, use forced-air warming blankets.
- Warm all fluids used on and in the patient.
- Warm and humidify gases.
- Provide extra inspired oxygen for the shivering patient.

Further reading

Davis AJM, Bissonnette B. Thermal regulation and mild intraoperative hypothermia. *Current Opinion in Anesthesiology*, 1999; **12**: 303–309.

Sessler DI. Central thermoregulatory inhibition by general anesthesia. *Anesthesiology*, 1991; **75**: 557–559.

Related topics of interest

THORACIC ANAESTHESIA

Thoracic surgery predominantly involves bronchoscopy (see Airway surgery), mediastinoscopy, and thoracotomy. This discussion is limited to thoracotomy.

Indications for one lung ventilation

1. Absolute (anaesthetic).
- Airway soiling from bronchiectasis, bleeding, a lung abscess or an empyema with a bronchopleural fistula.
- Gas leak. This may occur with a giant lung cyst (may form a flap valve), a bronchopleural fistula, tracheobronchial rupture, or bronchial surgery.

2. Relative (surgical). Improved access in pulmonary, oesophageal, anterior spinal or great vessel surgery.

Double-lumen tubes

Double-lumen tubes allow an independent channel for ventilation and suction of each lung. The endobronchial portion of the tube is cuffed, and extended at an angle which corresponds to the bronchial anatomy. The tracheal lumen ends distal to the tracheal cuff to allow ventilation of the other lung. The bronchial cuff of a right-sided tube usually includes an eye or slot, in order that the right upper lobe bronchus can be ventilated. This bronchus usually arises from the right main bronchus ~2.5 cm from the carina. However, considerable anatomical variation exists in the position of the right upper lobe bronchus (it may even arise from the middle lobe bronchus or directly off the trachea). For this reason a left-sided tube is usually chosen for all operations other than those involving surgery to the left main bronchus. Examples of double-lumen tubes with a carinal hook are a Carlen (left-sided) tube, a White (a right-sided version of a Carlen), and a Gordon-Green (a single lumen right-sided endobronchial tube). Examples of double-lumen tubes with no carinal hook are a Robertshaw (right or left), a Bryce-Smith (left-sided), a Bryce-Smith-Salt (right-sided) and a Bronchocath (left- or right-sided PVC tube). A recent development is the use of a single-lumen tracheal tube with an attached movable bronchial blocker (Univent tube). A double-lumen tube is inserted blindly and then its position checked using clinical signs. It is strongly recommended that the position is checked with a fibreoptic bronchoscope, and this is repeated after the patient is moved into the operative position.

Physiology of one lung ventilation

During two lung ventilation in a lateral thoracotomy position the upper lung is ventilated preferentially (the lower hemi-diaphragm encroaches further into the chest and the mediastinum compresses the lower lung). The lower lung, however, is better perfused. This V:Q mismatch is partially reversed when only the dependent lung is ventilated as there is increased pulmonary vascular resistance in the deflated lung. However, some blood still perfuses the deflated lung but this intrapulmonary shunt is limited by hypoxic pulmonary vasoconstriction (HPV). Any cause of a reduction in cardiac output causes a reduction in HPV. HPV is also inhibited by catecholamines, vasodilators, and inhalational anaesthetic agents. The degree to which gas exchange worsens during one lung ventilation (OLV) also depends on whether the deflated lung is diseased. The shunt will be worse if the lungs are healthy as a diseased lung results in preferential ventilation and perfusion in its healthy partner.

Minimizing hypoxia

1. Maintain the tidal volume that was used during two lung ventilation as much as airway pressures allow. If the peak airway pressure is too high, the tidal volume is reduced and the ventilatory rate increased.

2. Use an inspired oxygen concentration of at least 50%.

3. Insufflate the unventilated lung with O_2 at 4 l/min via a catheter. This reduces venous admixture but partially inhibits HPV. CPAP (5 cm H_2O pressure) may also be applied to this lung but this may impair surgical access. A compromise is to occasionally inflate the unventilated lung with 100% O_2, hold it open for a few seconds and then let it down again. This may help prevent a gradual deterioration in oxygenation during OLV.

4. Monitor O_2 saturation and arterial gases and encourage the surgeon not to compress the dependent lung or its blood vessels during traction.

PEEP is generally not of benefit in minimizing hypoxaemia during OLV as it increases pulmonary vascular resistance in the dependent lung and may increase the shunt fraction.

Oxygen delivery may be further compromised during OLV by a fall in cardiac output. The high intrapulmonary pressures of OLV add to the causes of hypotension during thoracotomy by lowering cardiac output.

Anaesthetic management

1. Assessment and premedication. History and examination determine the nature and extent of pulmonary disease. Chronic bronchitics complain of dyspnoea, cough and sputum production. They have airway obstruction, low V:Q ratios, hypoxaemia, and may have loss of CO_2 respiratory drive. The ECG may show cor pulmonale secondary to chronic hypoxic pulmonary vasoconstriction.

Patients with emphysema complain of cough and dyspnoea but little sputum production. They have a reduced compliance, increased V:Q ratio and no hypoxia. It is important to establish their normal minute ventilation as this will be increased to maintain a normal $PaCO_2$.

Investigation should include a CXR, ECG, respiratory function tests and arterial blood gases. Clinical evaluation such as the ability to blow out a match held 15 cm from the mouth lacks objectivity. Spirometry is performed to establish the FVC (normal = 60 ml/kg; <15 ml/kg = unable to cough). The maximum breathing capacity (MBC) is measured by multiplying the maximum respiratory rate by the tidal volume. Measurement periods of 15 seconds are used and the result multiplied by four to obtain the result for 1 minute. MBC is approximated by $FEV_1 \times 35$ or the PEFR $\times$ 0.25. Normal MBC = >60 l/min. MBC of 25–50 l/min is associated with severe respiratory impairment, whilst a patient with an MBC <25 l/min is a respiratory cripple. Flow volume loops may also be performed. The response to bronchodilators is also assessed. Lung resection reduces respiratory function values by 20% per lobe. A right pneumonectomy results in a reduction of 60% whilst a left produces a loss of 40%.

Lung resection is contraindicated if the FEV_1 is <0.8 litres. Sputum retention is a major problem if the FEV_1 is <1.0 litre. Measurement of pulmonary artery pressure has also been used to predict resection possibilities on an individual basis. CT scanning is frequently used to assess anatomical resection problems (distance of tumour from carina, etc.).

Opioid premedicants are generally avoided. Antisialogogues may increase sputum retention. Anxiolysis is provided by benzodiazepines unless sedation would compromise respiratory function. Bronchodilator therapy should be continued up to the time of surgery.

2. Conduct of anaesthesia. An intra-arterial catheter allows direct blood pressure measurement and sequential blood gas analysis. A pulmonary artery catheter is useful if cor pulmonale exists.

An inhalational induction may be used if there is a high risk of bronchospasm. Hypotension may occur peroperatively and result from blood loss, mediastinal movement, surgical retraction, myocardial ischaemia or the anaesthetic technique (e.g. sympathetic blockade from epidural analgesia or TIVA).

Hypoxaemia during surgery may result from pulmonary oedema, loss of lung volume, reduction in hypoxic pulmonary vasoconstriction, or an increased V:Q mismatch. Misplacement or displacement of the double lumen tube or a reduction in cardiac output, may also result in hypoxaemia.

Intravenous crystalloid infusions during thoracotomy may increase extracellular lung water and thus increase V:Q mismatch. Whole blood may increase the incidence of tumour recurrence (immunological effect), so packed cells should be given if transfusion is required.

3. Postoperatively. Before re-inflation the deflated lung is suctioned. Manual ventilation is then performed to re-inflate the lung, with direct observation while the chest is still open. Short-acting opioids may be used to provide analgesia during surgery but respiratory depressant agents should be avoided in the postoperative period. Local anaesthetic thoracic epidural blockade with 0.25% bupivacaine (1 ml per segment to be blocked) followed by a continuous infusion of 0.125–0.25% bupivacaine (4–5 ml/hour) can be used to provide analgesia for several days. A number of opioid analgesics have been added to bupivacaine to improve the quality of analgesia and to reduce the dose of local anaesthetic administered. Postoperative supervision in a high care area with oxygen therapy, physiotherapy, and monitoring of respiratory rate is required. Postoperative ventilation should be used only in those patients who have failed to maintain adequate gas exchange despite aggressive respiratory physiotherapy and good quality analgesia.

The perioperative mortality of lobectomy is 2–3%, pneumonectomy 5–8%, and oesophagectomy ~10%.

4. Bronchopleural fistula. The incidence of a fistula following surgical resection is ~1.5% after lobectomy and ~4.5% after pneumonectomy. It may also occur following trauma or oesophageal rupture. The typical history is of an infection in the pleural space causing an empyema. This erodes the bronchial stump which breaks down and the patient complains of the sudden onset of a productive cough. CXR signs of a fistula include a fluid level created as fluid leaks out of the space, failure of a hemithorax to opacify, and consolidation in the other lung from contralateral spill.

The anaesthetic requirements are that there must be no fluid contamination of the contralateral lung, further hypoxaemia must be prevented, and that positive pressure ventilation should be withheld until the fistula is isolated. The pleural space should be drained prior to surgery and an unclamped chest drain be *in situ* before induction. An endobronchial tube is essential. Classically intubation was performed under deep inhalational anaesthesia in an upright position but nowadays it is more usually performed after a rapid sequence induction.

5. Lung reduction surgery. This is performed for emphysema and provides a mechanical rather than physiological improvement. There is improved airflow with more efficient chest wall and diaphragm mechanics. As the mean intrathoracic pressure is reduced, venous return and right ventricular function are increased. Previously compressed alveoli are re-expanded improving gas exchange.

A thoracotomy is used for single lung surgery, or a sternotomy if bilateral procedures are performed. Dynamic hyperinflation with barotrauma must be avoided. Good postoperative analgesia is imperative.

Further reading

Conacher ID. Anaesthesia for the surgery of emphysema. *British Journal of Anaesthesia*, 1997; **79:** 530–538.
Pennefather SH, Russell GN. Placement of double lumen tubes – time to shed light on an old problem. *British Journal of Anaesthesia*, 2000; **84:** 308–310.
Plummer S, Hartley M, Vaughan RS. Anaesthesia for telescopic procedures in the thorax. *British Journal of Anaesthesia*, 1998; **80:** 223–234.

Related topics of interest

Asthma (p. 27); Myasthenia gravis (p. 158); Pain relief – acute (p. 199); Sequelae of anaesthesia (p. 232)

THYROID SURGERY

Patients may present for thyroid surgery with an enlarged thyroid gland or in a state of abnormal thyroid function. Enlargement of the thyroid gland may be due to a multinodular goitre, Graves disease (autoimmune), autoimmune thyroiditis (Hashimoto's disease), a solitary nodule (benign or malignant), iodine deficiency (pregnancy or diet) or may follow a viral infection (de Quervans thyroiditis).

Problems
- Airway obstruction from a thyroid swelling.
- Superior vena caval obstruction may be the result of a retrosternal goitre.
- Thyroid function. The patient may not be euthyroid.
- Autoimmune disease of other organ systems may be associated with thyroid disease.
- Malignant tissue infiltration may occur in the major structures of the neck causing, for example, vocal cord dysfunction.

Thyrotoxicosis
Thyrotoxicosis (hyperthyroidism) results from excessive production of the two thyroid hormones thyroxine (T4) and tri-iodothyronine (T3). It is most commonly caused by an autoimmune disease associated with human specific thyroid stimulator, an IgG immunoglobulin (Graves disease). Other causes are a multinodular goitre, or a solitary secreting nodule. The clinical features of special concern to the anaesthetist include the following.

- Enlargement of the gland may involve the upper trachea, cricoid and thyroid cartilages. The gland may extend retrosternally and cause lower tracheal compression or SVC obstruction. Collapse of the trachea (tracheochondromalacia) may occur following removal of the gland.
- The patient may have a resting tachycardia, increased cardiac output, and increased susceptibility to the development of arrhythmias. Atrial fibrillation is especially common.
- There may be abnormal glucose tolerance and the patient is likely to feel anxious.
- Exophthalmos may be present and cause difficulty in protecting the eyes during surgery.
- Thyrotoxic myopathy manifests as a proximal muscle weakness.

Thyrotoxic crisis
An acute manifestation of all the features of thyrotoxicosis may occur soon after a partial thyroidectomy. It is more common in patients who are still hyperthyroid at the time of surgery. Untreated it results in coma and is frequently fatal. Signs include:

- Pyrexia.
- Confusion, restlessness and delirium.

- Tachycardia, atrial fibrillation and high-output cardiac failure. Flushing, sweating and abdominal pain.
- Dehydration and ketosis. Treatment should be started urgently with β-blockers, sedation, cooling, rehydration, and antithyroid drugs. Esmolol and dantrolene have both been reported as specific treatments. Supplementary O_2 should be given. The patient may require mechanical ventilation and admission to an ITU should be considered as soon as the crisis manifests.

Hypothyroidism

This may be primary (typically occurring in middle-aged females) and be due to either atrophy or Hashimoto's disease, or be secondary to failure of thyroid-stimulating hormone production. The features of hypothyroidism of special anaesthetic interest include:

- Decreased metabolic rate and reduced mental and physical activity leading to obesity.
- CVS. Resting bradycardia with a predisposition towards myocardial ischaemia. Arteriosclerosis and hypertension are common. A pericardial effusion may occur.
- Hypothermia is common.
- The tongue may be enlarged and there may be a polyneuropathy.
- Addison's disease and pernicious anaemia are common.

Anaesthetic management

1. Assessment and premedication. Patients undergoing thyroid surgery should be in as normal a state of thyroid function as possible (euthyroid). The preoperative use of carbimazole to achieve this may result in depression of the white cell count and a recent history of sore throat or other infection should be sought. Propylthiouracil is an alternative. A careful assessment of the upper airway and tracheal deviation should be made. Thoracic inlet radiographs may be indicated. β-blockers, if used, should be continued up to the time of surgery. Benzodiazepine premedication is useful for anxiolysis.

2. Conduct of anaesthesia. A reinforced or armoured tracheal tube is usually passed in patients who are to undergo thyroid surgery. Some authors have advocated a laryngeal mask airway as this avoids non-depolarizing relaxants and allows assessment of vocal cord movement (recurrent laryngeal nerve integrity). The nerve is electrically stimulated, and the movement observed with a fibreoptic bronchoscope. Whichever airway is used it must be secured in a fashion to ensure tapes or ties do not encroach on the surgical field. Care should be taken to protect the eyes, especially in the presence of exophthalmos, prior to the placement of head towels. The anaesthetic breathing system should be securely attached to the tracheal tube connector as this will be inaccessible during the operation. A reverse Trendelenburg (head-up tilt) position may be requested by the surgeon to aid venous drainage and reduce blood loss in the field. This will predispose to the development of an air embolus.

3. *Postoperatively* Thyroid surgery may result in damage to one or both of the recurrent laryngeal nerves. The patient will have postoperative hoarseness, or, in the case of bilateral nerve damage, inspiratory stridor and acute respiratory obstruction. The patient should be extubated 'light' after direct inspection of vocal cord movement. Wound haematoma may also present as an acute upper respiratory emergency and the skin closure material should be readily removable e.g. clips. Tracheal oedema may occur and require treatment with dexamethasone. Pneumothorax is a potential complication especially if there has been dissection at the root of the neck or behind the sternum. Acute hypocalcaemia may occur, especially if the parathyroid glands have also been removed.

Further reading

Farling PA. Thyroid disease. *British Journal of Anaesthesia*, 2000; **85:** 15–28.
Griffen M, Russell J, Chambers F. General anaesthesia for thyroplasty. *Anaesthesia*, 1998; **53:** 1202–1204.

Related topics of interest

Air embolism (p. 9); Intubation – difficult (p. 141); Positioning (p. 207)

TIVA

Intravenous anaesthesia became popular with the use of althesin and etomidate. Neither is currently available for this use, and propofol is the universal drug of choice. It provides hypnosis with good recovery and little nausea and vomiting. Opioids by bolus or infusion can be given to provide analgesia. Spontaneous or intermittent positive pressure ventilation with oxygen-enriched air is given via a suitably secured airway. Nitrous oxide may be used as a supplement, utilizing its amnesic and analgesic effects.

Propofol may be given by an initial bolus followed by an infusion, or by a computer-controlled pump programmed to achieve a steady state blood concentration TCI (Target Controlled Infusion). This program uses observed blood propofol concentrations in a population to set its infusion characteristics. A three-compartment pharmacokinetic model is used to describe the distribution, redistribution and elimination of propofol and to predict population pharmacokinetics. Context-sensitive half time is used to predict time to awakening after the infusion is discontinued.

TIVA may be used as an alternative to volatile based anaesthesia in virtually all situations. It is however specifically suited for cardiac surgery during bypass, bronchoscopy using a venturi system for ventilation, when volatile anaesthetics are contraindicated and is commonly used for short procedures. It is becoming more popular for maintenance of anaesthesia for longer cases e.g. neurosurgical procedures.

Patient controlled sedation can be achieved using propofol in a standard PCA system.

TIVA – Pros

- Clinical indications as discussed above.
- Convenience of using TCI to administer TIVA.
- No atmospheric pollution in theatre.
- Less PONV than with volatile anaesthesia.

TIVA – Cons

1. Failure of intravenous access, connection of infusion lines, or infusion pump failure will result in inadequate anaesthesia. With volatile anaesthesia, ventilation monitoring and expired gas analysis assess drug delivery. No equivalent monitoring exists for TIVA.

2. Co-administration of drugs through the same venous access will alter delivery rates. Siphoning from TIVA syringes can occur if they are placed high above the patient and the plunger is not adequately secured.

3. Propofol causes a fall in blood pressure and SVR, and resets the baroreflex so that there is a lower heart rate than expected with hypotension. Ventilatory depression with initial apnoea is common.

4. Inter-individual variation of pharmacokinetics and pharmacodynamics is large (60–80%). 'One shoe does not fit all', resulting in frequent manual adjustment of the target concentration.

5. With TCI the target concentration is quoted as a blood concentration, although the site of action is the brain.

6. Depth of anaesthesia is clinically assessed. The intensity of surgical stimulation differs during an operation, and particularly between different operations.

7. Propofol at high plasma concentrations causes a fall in cardiac output which reduces hepatic clearance and peripheral distribution. Elimination and redistribution are therefore altered affecting TCI accuracy.

8. Opioids show pharmacodynamic synergism with propofol therefore affecting TCI efficacy. Nomograms for various opioid infusions have been developed to guide adjustments of propofol infusion rates.

9. TCI gives slower induction times with less propofol given than with a manual bolus. Maintenance doses are greater using TCI rather than a simple infusion. Induction dose added to maintenance doses results in total drug usage being similar. There is no faster emergence from anaesthesia with TCI than with a manual infusion system.

10. Time to emergence is similar with sevoflurane maintenance and propofol TIVA, although sevoflurane gives a significantly greater incidence of PONV.

11. Disease increases pharmacokinetic variability making TCI inaccurate, risking administering more TIVA than is required.

As with anaesthesia maintained with volatile agents, drug dosage and depth of anaesthesia must be titrated for each patient. For the future, the discovery of accurate depth of anaesthesia monitors would allow closed-loop systems for the administration of TIVA to be developed.

Further reading

Target Controlled Intravenous Anaesthesia using 'Diprifusor'. *Anaesthesia*, 1998; **53:** Supplement 1, 1–86.
Morton NS. Total intravenous anaesthesia (TIVA) in paediatrics: advantages and disadvantages. *Paediatric Anaesthesia*, 1998; **8:** 189–194.

Related topics of interest

Airway surgery (p. 12); Day surgery (p. 80)

TRACHEOSTOMY

A tracheostomy may be performed as an elective procedure. It should never be performed as a life-saving emergency. When immediate percutaneous airway access is required a cricothyroidotomy remains the procedure of choice. The vast majority of tracheostomies performed are percutaneous dilational tracheostomies (PDT). The opportunity for surgical trainees to gain experience of open tracheostomies has been virtually lost.

Positioning the patient with the neck straight and extended ensures a midline approach.

Indications

- Upper airway obstruction, when airway control has been assured.
- Prolonged ventilatory support, when modern ventilators with sensitive patient flow triggers permit assisted ventilation with minimal or no sedation.
- Difficulty in weaning from ventilation, again allowing less sedation and reducing respiratory work.
- Tracheobronchial toilet.
- Protection of lungs from soiling when the laryngopharyngeal reflexes are depressed.
- As part of a surgical or anaesthetic technique, e.g. laryngectomy.

Contraindications

1. **Absolute.** The need for immediate airway access.

2. **Relative**
- Ill defined anatomy.
- Coagulopathy.
- Haemodynamic instability.
- Neck extension contraindicated.
- High oxygen, PEEP and ventilatory requirement.

Complications

Comparative studies have shown that the incidence of early complications with PDT is lower than those associated with surgical tracheostomy. The minimal tissue damage makes infection (0–4% vs. 10–30%) and secondary haemorrhage less likely. The limited data available on long-term complications also suggest that PDT is less likely to cause tracheal stenosis than conventional, surgical tracheostomy.

1. **Immediate complications**
- Hypoxia due to failure of ventilation during procedure (accidental extubation or puncture of the tracheal tube cuff).
- Misplacement of tracheostomy tube; too high, paratracheal, through the posterior wall of the trachea, or into the oesophagus.
- Bleeding; minor – common, major – rare.

2. Intermediate complications

- Early displacement of the tracheostomy tube – an immature and/or very small tracheal stoma makes replacement difficult.
- Obstruction from blood or secretions.
- Infection.
- Secondary haemorrhage.
- Erosion through the tracheal wall.

3. Late complications

- Tracheal stenosis (26% when defined by a tracheal stenosis of >10%).
- Subglottic stenosis – rare.

The technique of PDT

Different techniques require specific approaches. All patients for PDT should be given 100% O_2. The tracheal tube should be withdrawn until the top of the cuff is across the cords. Alternatively, the tracheal tube can be replaced with a laryngeal mask airway (LMA) or intubating laryngeal mask airway (ILMA). A cannula is inserted between the 1st and 2nd or 2nd and 3rd tracheal rings and a guidewire passed through it. The use of a bronchoscope to observe and confirm entry of the needle and guidewire into the trachea is highly recommended. After the guidewire has been inserted the stoma is enlarged with a series of dilators (Ciaglia) or with forceps (Griggs). A size 8.0 mm tracheostomy tube will be adequate in most patients.

Post-tracheostomy care

Regular physiotherapy, tracheobronchial toilet with 'pre-oxygenation' prior to suctioning and checks on the cuff pressure (< 20 mmHg) should be performed. A CXR will confirm the correct positioning of the tracheostomy tube. The patient is nursed semi-recumbent. The wound is dressed daily and the tube changed after 1 week. Communication aids should be available to the awake patient with a tracheostomy.

Further reading

Holdgaard HO, Pederson J, Jensen RH *et al.* Percutaneous dilatational tracheostomy versus conventional surgical tracheostomy. *Acta Anaesthesiologica Scandanavica*, 1998; **42:** 545–550.
Soni N. Percutaneous tracheostomy: how to do it. *British Journal of Hospital Medicine*, 1997; **57:** 339–345.

Related topics of interest

TRANSFER OF THE CRITICALLY ILL

As specialists in the care of the critically ill and especially of ventilated patients, anaesthetists are frequently involved in the transfer of such patients. Transfers may be primary (to hospital from the site of the incident/accident) or secondary (between hospitals). Patients are also frequently transferred within a hospital. Transfer can be hazardous for the patient and rarely for accompanying personnel. Attention is increasingly being given to designated transfer teams and the development of transfer guidelines. Key points to consider when transferring the critically ill include:

- Communication between hospitals.
- Detailed patient assessment.
- Pre-transfer physiological stabilization.
- Anticipation of likely problems during transfer.
- Pre-transfer interventions.
- Equipment checks.
- Comprehensive handover.

General principles

Prior to transferring any critically ill patient the risks should be weighed against the potential benefits of treatment at the receiving unit. Transfer should be arranged if the appropriate level of care is not available at the original location. Early communication between senior clinical staff at the referring and the receiving hospital is essential. Ideally, the receiving hospital should take responsibility for the transfer and provide a team to perform it. Patients should be resuscitated and physiologically stable (unless the patient has a condition which can only be stabilized at the receiving hospital).

Potential hazards of transfer

- Removal of patient from secure hospital environment.
- Reduced number of carers who may themselves lack experience.
- Reduced or less effective monitoring.
- Reduced access to patient.
- No access to additional equipment.
- Difficulty in performing resuscitation or other practical procedures.
- Hostile environment: limited space, noise, motion sickness, fatigue.

When it is decided to sedate a patient with a head injury the neurological status before sedation should be carefully recorded. The neurological status of patients with suspected spinal injuries should be recorded before and after the transfer.

Unconscious patients should always be intubated before transfer. Virtually all head-injured patients with an altered level of consciousness will require intubation. The inspired oxygen concentration is noted and a current arterial blood gas analysis obtained. If a transfer ventilator is to be used, check an arterial blood gas 10 minutes after the patient is connected to it. Haemodynamic normality and stability should be achieved pre-transfer. Adequate intravenous lines should be inserted and fixed securely. Intravenous fluids should be warmed if necessary. Blood and blood products should be available if required. If infusions of inotropes are required spare infusions should be drawn up and labelled. Fractures should be splinted to prevent neurovascular damage.

A comprehensive written referral should accompany the patient. On departure, the receiving hospital should be contacted with an estimated time of arrival.

Personnel

Personnel accompanying a critically ill patient should be able to cope with all common problems. Ideally a transfer team should retrieve the patient from the referring hospital. Such teams are well established in paediatric practice but are not always available for adult patients. An appropriately trained doctor skilled in resuscitation and support of organ systems should always accompany the patient along with at least one appropriately trained assistant. The doctor supervising the transfer will often be an anaesthetist or intensive care doctor. Adequate death and injury insurance should be provided for the transfer team.

Equipment

All equipment should be checked before collecting the patient. Ideally it should be reliable, simple, and durable. The following basic equipment should accompany all critically ill patients:

- Mechanical ventilator (with facility for airway pressure monitoring, minute volume measurement and disconnect alarm).
- Oxygen – enough for the transfer plus enough for unforeseen delays; preferably with an independent alternative supply.
- Airway equipment – intubation and surgical airway equipment.
- Self inflating bag-valve-mask device.
- Effective suction apparatus.
- Intravenous access and infusion equipment and a stock of intravenous fluids.
- Syringe pumps (with fully charged batteries).
- Volumatic intravenous fluid pumps (infusion by gravity is unreliable during transfer).
- Defibrillator.
- Spare batteries.

Drugs

The following should always be carried:

- Resuscitation drugs (epinephrine (adrenaline) and atropine).
- Cardiovascular drugs e.g. nitrates, antiarrhythmics, inotropes.
- Anticonvulsants e.g. diazepam, thiopental.
- Analgesics.
- Hypnotic agents e.g. midazolam, propofol.
- Muscle relaxants.
- Respiratory drugs e.g. salbutamol.
- Other drugs such as naloxone, mannitol and glucose.

Monitoring

The ideal monitoring for critically ill patients during transfer is the same as would be used in theatre or on the intensive care unit. This may not always be possible but modern multifunction monitors allow several pressure waves to be displayed in addition to standard functions.

Non-invasive blood pressure monitoring is susceptible to vibration artifact as well as inaccuracy due to arrhythmias (e.g. atrial fibrillation). Where haemodynamic instability is a possibility intra-arterial pressure monitoring is the only reliable method of measurement. Pulse oximetry is mandatory, as is capnography in ventilated patients. Temperature should be measured, particularly in children. All critically ill patients should be catheterized and hourly urine output should be recorded. Central venous pressure should be monitored if necessary.

Modes of transport

The majority of interhospital transfers are carried out by road ambulance. The problems of road ambulance transfers are excessive movement, noise, lack of space, motion sickness and occasionally extended transfer times (either due to long distances or traffic congestion). If the patient deteriorates en route the ambulance should be stopped to allow effective resuscitation, intervention or examination of the patient.

Air transfers may be appropriate in certain circumstances. The usual indications are that the patient needs to be transferred a long distance or in a short period of time. Transfer may be by fixed-wing aircraft or by helicopter. Fixed-wing aircraft are used for long distances. Helicopters can travel moderate distances quickly and often land at, or very close to, the receiving hospital. Air transfers are expensive. Problems en route include poor patient access, limited space, motion sickness, high noise levels and vibration. Cabins are pressurized only to the equivalent of approximately 2000 m above sea level so supplementary oxygen should always be administered. The expansion of gases at altitude can be a problem where a patient has a pneumothorax or excessive gas in the bowel (e.g. in bowel obstruction) and where a tracheal tube is filled with air (saline should be substituted).

Transfers within hospitals

The general principles of transfers between hospitals are equally applicable to transfers within hospitals. The patient should not be moved until the receiving department is ready to commence the investigation or procedure. At least two people should accompany the patient on the transfer, a doctor and a nurse.

Further reading

Oakley PA. Interhospital transfer of the trauma patient. *Trauma*, 1999; **1**: 61–70.
Runci CJ, Reeve WG, Reidy J, Dougall JR. A comparison of measurements of blood pressure, heart rate and oxygenation during interhospital transfer of the critically ill. *Intensive Care Medicine*, 1990; **16**: 317–322.

Related topics of interest

CPR (p. 75); Head injury (p. 124); Sedation (p. 226)

UROLOGY

Patients requiring urological procedures tend to be paediatric or geriatric. Prostatectomy presents specific problems to the anaesthetist. There are four approaches to prostatectomy. They are transurethral resection (TURP), retropubic, transperineal and suprapubic (transvesical) resection. Absorption of irrigating fluid occurs during TURP. Warm glycine solution (1.5% isoosmotic) is used as it is a poor electrical conductor but has good optical properties giving the surgeon a clear view. Irrigation fluid is absorbed at about 20 ml/min, depending on the height of the fluid above the patient (hydrostatic pressure) and the number and size of open venous sinuses. Irrigation time should be limited to 1 hour and the height of the irrigation fluid restricted to less than 60 cm. If volume overload occurs then bradycardia, initial hypertension, raised CVP, pulmonary oedema and later CVS collapse may be seen. Hyponatraemia may occur with cerebral oedema causing confusion, headache, convulsions, coma and CVS collapse. The treatment is fluid restriction but if severe, hypertonic saline, loop diuretics and CVP monitoring may be required. Raising serum sodium by more than 2 mmol/l/h may cause demyelination, particularly in the central pontine region. If the sodium falls below 120 mmol/l a mortality rate of 50% is quoted. Glycine absorption may also cause CNS problems possibly by acting as an inhibitory transmitter. It is metabolized to ammonia and this may contribute to the symptoms.

Retropubic prostatectomy requires a laparotomy and large blood loss should be expected. General anaesthesia with epidural analgesia and invasive CVS monitoring is usually performed.

Problems

- Elderly males with concurrent diseases.
- The TURP syndrome of fluid overload and hyponatraemia.
- Risk of bladder perforation.
- Position – TURP is performed in lithotomy.
- Blood loss.
- Risk of burns and hypothermia with TURP.
- Fibrinolysis from urokinase release.

Anaesthetic management

1. Assessment and premedication. Particular attention should be paid to the CVS of patients presenting for prostatectomy. Prostatic hypertrophy may cause obstructive renal failure and surgery is delayed until catheterization has allowed renal function to normalize. Minimum investigations are a FBC, X-match, U+E, ECG and CXR. The serum sodium should be >130 mmol/l preoperatively. Other investigations may be required depending on the patient's health.

2. Conduct of anaesthesia. Each patient should be anaesthetized with consideration of their other pathologies. Regional anaesthesia with a sensory block higher than T10 is frequently used. Supplementary O_2 is given. Blood loss should be monitored, the haemoglobin concentration in irrigation fluid can be measured in theatre.

3. Advantages of regional anaesthesia
- Blood loss is reduced.
- Cerebral function is better assessed.
- Bladder perforation is more easily recognized with nausea, pain and abdominal wall rigidity and distension.
- Postoperative analgesia.
- Vasodilation increases the intravascular space.
- Incidence of DVT is reduced.

4. Disadvantages of regional anaesthesia
- Psychological and patient dignity.
- Potential technical failure.
- Cough is unsuppressed (may interfere with surgery, and increase bleeding from venous distension).
- Hypotension or excessively high block.
- Post-spinal headache.
- Hypoventilation.

Alternatively, general anaesthesia with or without a caudal block may be used. Antibiotics may be required if a urinary tract infection exists. If the TURP syndrome is suspected surgery should be terminated and the plasma electrolytes measured.

5. Postoperatively. To prevent clot retention following TURP, continuous bladder irrigation is usually performed until the bleeding has stopped. Careful CVS and neurological observation must be continued as the problems of hypo-osmolar volume overload may still occur. Resolution of the sympathetic blockade may decrease the intravascular space contributing to volume overload. TURP blood loss is difficult to assess and transfusion is often required. Intravenous crystalloid fluids should be given sparingly and dextrose solutions avoided.

Further reading

Gravenstein D. Transurethral resection of the prostate (TURP) syndrome: a review of the pathophysiology and management. *Anesthesia and Analgesia*, 1997; **84:** 438–446.
Jenson V. The TURP syndrome. *Canadian Journal of Anaesthesia*, 1991; **38:** 90–97.

Related topics of interest

Elderly patients (p. 107); Renal disease (p. 217); Spinal and epidural anaesthesia (p. 241)

VASCULAR SURGERY

The three major areas are carotid, aortic and peripheral vascular surgery. A number of general considerations of anaesthesia for vascular surgery can be applied before considering the specific problems relating to these areas of surgery.

1. **Age.** Patients are generally elderly.

2. **CVS pathology.** Hypertension, ischaemic heart disease, cerebrovascular disease, cardiac failure and hyperlipidaemia are common amongst patients for vascular surgery.

3. **Associated disease.** Diabetes mellitus, respiratory and renal disease.

4. **Smoking.**

5. **Polypharmacy.** These patients are often taking a large number of drugs.

Perioperative management

The history, examination and investigations determine the degree of CVS impairment together with the extent of associated pathologies. Sophisticated tests may be needed to optimize the preoperative condition and to evaluate risk. All patients should have an FBC, cross-match, clotting studies, U+E, liver function tests, ECG and a CXR. Further investigations are performed as indicated. An anxiolytic premedication minimizes psychological and CVS stress. Benzodiazepines, opioids or phenothiazines may be used. A single dose of β-blocker helps attenuate peroperative myocardial ischaemia. Any cardiovascular drug therapy should be maintained preoperatively although warfarin should be discontinued or converted to heparin.

Monitoring should include an ECG placed in the CM5 position to detect myocardial ischaemic change, a CVP if large blood volume changes are anticipated (PAOP may be better), an arterial line (direct pressure and gases), capnography, urine output and temperature.

1. **Regional anaesthesia.** This is frequently used for aortic and peripheral vascular surgery. Advantages include peripheral vasodilatation, postoperative analgesia and in aortic surgery a decrease in the effects of cross-clamping. An epidural catheter should be sited after checking clotting function and before heparin is given. There is increasing evidence that peripheral vascular surgery followed by a postoperative epidural infusion results in a better outcome. The reasons for this may be the attenuation of hypercoagulability or reduced vasoconstriction and improved blood flow in the affected limb. Epidural analgesia may also reduce the incidence of postoperative tachycardia, myocardial ischaemia and infarction in an at-risk patient group.

2. **General anaesthesia.** Haemodynamic stability is required during induction, intubation, surgery and postoperatively. Opioids form the common basis of a smooth anaesthetic with or without small doses of volatile agents. Intra-arterial

monitoring prior to induction is used to observe the effect of laryngoscopy on the blood pressure with further treatment given, if required, prior to intubation. Muscle relaxation with cardiovascularly stable agents such as vecuronium, or pancuronium if hypotension or bradycardia are present. Isoflurane may cause coronary steal (at > 2%) whilst enflurane depresses myocardial function.

Neuromuscular blockade is reversed with neostigmine and glycopyrrolate to minimize tachycardia.

Close attention to gas exchange, haemodynamics, analgesia and urine output may necessitate ITU/HDU care. Silent myocardial ischaemia is common postoperatively, and oxygen should be given for at least 48 hours.

Carotid surgery

Carotid endarterectomy reduces TIAs and prevents CVAs due to emboli from ulcerated atheromatous plaques if a stenosis of >70% exists. It is performed 20 times more often in the USA than the UK. Myocardial infarction is the commonest cause of perioperative mortality. Cross-clamping of the internal carotid artery leaves the ipsilateral hemisphere dependent upon perfusion from the Circle of Willis. Regional anaesthesia with a cervical plexus block or a cervical epidural allows neurological assessment of the awake patient. Under GA, stump pressures (distal to the clamp the pressure should be > 50 mmHg), or an EEG/CFAM or somatosensory evoked potentials may be used. The use of distal stump pressures is controversial. A temporary shunt during cross-clamping is often used. The effects on cerebral perfusion of changes in ICP, arterial pressure, venous pressure, PaO_2 and $PaCO_2$ should be considered. Brain protection with thiopental (reduces cerebral O_2 demands, decreases oxygen-free radical formation and blocks sodium channels) has been recommended. Nimodipine decreases vascular spasm. Heparin 5000 units is given before cross-clamping. Isoflurane is the best volatile as it maintains cerebral perfusion/ requirement coupling and a normal EEG at lower mean arterial pressures than halothane or enflurane. Nitrous oxide may be best avoided. Normocapnia, normotension and normovolaemia should be maintained. Mild hypothermia (34°C) and the prevention of hyperglycaemia are beneficial. Esmolol, nitroprusside or alfentanil are used to control the hypertension associated with intubation and extubation. Local anaesthetic infiltration around the sinus prevents perioperative autonomic stimulation.

Aortic surgery

Elective or emergency reconstruction (usually abdominal, but may be thoracic). Antibiotic prophylaxis and a nasogastric tube are required. An epidural is commonly used in elective cases. Special features include:

1. Renal preservation. Cross-clamping is rarely performed above the renal arteries but renal perfusion is nevertheless markedly impaired. Renal dopamine, mannitol and furosemide (frusemide) (once normovolaemia and an adequate perfusion pressure are restored) may stimulate urine output.

2. Cross-clamp. This raises the SVR by 40% with the potential for hypertension and myocardial strain (vasodilators/nitrates should be available). Release of the clamp must be preceded by adequate filling as the fall in the SVR and reperfusion of the ischaemic pelvis and legs (producing a systemic acid load) can cause severe hypotension. Bicarbonate, vasopressors, inotropes and calcium should be available.

3. Heparin (1 mg/kg) may be given via a central line prior to cross-clamping. It may need reversal at the end of the procedure (check the APPT or ACT).

4. Acute rupture. Resuscitation is likely to be inadequate until cross-clamping of the aorta gains control of the haemorrhage. A rapid sequence induction is performed once the surgeon is scrubbed. Two anaesthetists are needed. Massive blood transfusions, FFP and platelets are frequently required. The mortality rate is > 50%. Paraplegia may occur due to thrombosis of the anterior spinal artery.

Peripheral vascular surgery

Surgery may be elective or may be urgent for attempted limb salvage (thrombolysis/embolectomy/bypass grafting). Epidural/spinal anaesthesia provides increased graft flow, less blood loss, good postoperative analgesia and avoids the hazards of intubation. The risks are of prolonged surgery, inadequate block and the use of heparin (epidural haematoma). Regional anaesthesia prevents a perioperative rise in plasminogen activator inhibitor-1 and, as already noted, may decrease graft thrombosis. The epidural should be continued for at least 24 hours postoperatively. Epidural blockade established 3 days prior to amputation decreases the incidence of phantom limb pain.

Further reading

Colombo JA, Tuman KJ. Peripheral vascular surgery: does anaesthetic management affect outcome? *Current Opinion in Anaesthesiology*, 1998; **11:** 23–27.
Garrioch MA, Fitch W. Anaesthesia for carotid artery surgery. *British Journal of Anaesthesia*, 1993; **71:** 569–579.

Related topics of interest

Cardiac assessment (p. 55); Depth of anaesthesia (p. 86); Elderly patients (p. 107); Hypertension (p. 131); Neuroanaesthesia (p. 167); Preoperative preparation (p. 209); Spinal and epidural anaesthesia (p. 241); Stress response to surgery (p. 248)

VENTILATION
Kay Chidley

Mechanical ventilation has been the backbone of anaesthesia and intensive care medicine since its introduction in the 1950s during the polio epidemic. There has been a growing increase in the use and sophistication of ventilatory support, primarily in the intensive care unit but also in operating theatres.

Modes of ventilation

A mode of mechanical ventilation describes whether a breath is volume or pressure controlled. It also informs whether breaths are mandatory (delivered by the ventilator regardless of the patient's own respiratory effort) or spontaneously triggered. Despite the complexity of modern ventilators, Chatburn's original classification of ventilators based on the power source, drive and control mechanisms, and output remains applicable. Other variables such as the type of control, trigger, limits and cycling may be added for a more complete description of individual ventilators.

Modes of ventilation are usually volume controlled (volume constant, pressure variable) or pressure controlled (pressure constant, volume variable). A trigger initiates each breath. The duration of the breath is held constant by a limit variable (e.g. time) or non-constant when a cycle variable (e.g. volume) determines the end of inspiration.

PEEP may be added to a given mode of ventilation in an attempt to increase alveolar recruitment and thus oxygenation. Intrapulmonary shunting may also be reduced following the redistribution of lung water from the alveoli to the perivascular interstitial space. Providing there is no reduction in cardiac output, the use of PEEP may permit a reduction in the FiO_2 to achieve the same PaO_2.

1. Volume controlled ventilation. Assisted ventilation during anaesthesia is invariably volume controlled. Each breath is delivered at a pre-set volume over a fixed inspiratory time at the expense of variable airway pressures. Lung compliance determines the airway pressures generated. There is no compensatory ventilator response to alter frequency of breaths delivered if the patient makes any respiratory effort. Tidal volumes of 7 to 10 ml per kg are suitable for the majority of surgical patients.

2. Pressure control ventilation. This is less frequently used than volume control. It is only available as a mode of ventilation in the operating theatre with more modern anaesthetic machines. Pressure controlled ventilation (PCV) delivers a pre-set pressure to the patient. The resulting tidal volume depends on lung compliance, airway resistance and intrinsic PEEP. There is no direct control of delivered tidal volumes which depend on inspiratory flow rate and time. In a pressure control mode there are pre-set time factors starting and finishing the respiratory cycle.

Although it has no proven improvement in outcome PCV offers lung protection, by limiting plateau and peak alveolar pressures. It may also improve alveolar recruitment and oxygenation especially when delivered by inverse ratio ventilation (I:E ratios > 1:1).

Assisted ventilation

Assisted modes of ventilation, where each inspiration is triggered by the patient and is then boosted by the ventilator reduce atrophy of respiratory muscles which rapidly occurs with the abolition of spontaneous respiration.

These methods all rely on sensitive flow triggers allowing inspiration without too big a negative pressure deflection.

1. Assist control. The ventilator delivers a breath when triggered by the patient's inspiratory effort or independently if the patient does not trigger within a certain time. A background rate of 4–6 breaths/min less than the patient's own respiratory rate will cover any fall in patient self-ventilation.

2. Intermittent mandatory ventilation. The patient receives positive pressure breaths from the ventilator at a pre-set tidal volume and rate. This is in addition to the patient's own efforts. This mode ensures there will be a minimum minute volume. When weaning from ventilation the rate is initially high then decreased as the patient becomes decreasingly ventilator-dependent.

3. Pressure support ventilation. A pre-set pressure augments every spontaneous breath. Airway pressure is sustained until inspiratory flow drops to about 25% below the peak flow level. Patients find PSV a comfortable mode of ventilation to help wean from a ventilator. It has also been successfully used in non-invasive (mask CPAP or BIPAP) ventilation. The rate of respiration is not set as this is totally dependent on the patient's own intrinsic ventilatory rate.

Properties of an ideal ventilator

An ideal ventilator would:

- Be universal for all ages and sizes.
- Be easy to use.
- Have an accurate oxygen delivery system.
- Offer a range of ventilatory modes including CPAP, BIPAP, CMV, IMV, PSV and PEEP, as well as the ability to deliver extremes of tidal volume, rate and inspiratory flow rates.
- Utilize a breathing system of low resistance with the ability to nebulize and humidify gases.
- Have comprehensive monitoring and function alarms.
- Be reliable, as patient safety is essential.
- Be robust, easy to clean and maintain, and have cheap disposables.

Comparing ITU and theatre ventilators for surgical patients

Ventilators used in theatre tend to be sufficient to ventilate normal lungs for a period of time rarely exceeding several hours. Ventilation is usually controlled, continuous mechanical ventilation delivered via a volume or time cycled mode. Pressure limitation may also be a feature. Attempts to compensate for desaturation by increasing inspiratory time may lead to gas trapping and barotrauma.

Intensive care ventilators are more patient-responsive with multiple ventilatory modes available. Many ITU ventilators have their own self-checking and diagnostic functions, performing automatic corrections to maintain a stable tidal volume, inspiratory flow rate and waveform. These ventilators accommodate patient effort and triggering and ultimately the process of weaning from ventilation.

Ventilating the lungs of ITU patients who require surgery can be especially challenging. Patients with acute respiratory failure ventilated with an intensive care type of ventilator have been found to maintain better intraoperative oxygen exchange than those patients ventilated with a theatre type of ventilator. Patients at high risk (minute ventilation >15 l/min and peak inflation pressures >50 cmH$_2$O) had an improved outcome if ventilated with an ITU type of ventilator for their operation. Patients in acute respiratory failure requiring mechanical ventilation for surgery benefit from a ventilator with pressure/flow characteristics (i.e. high inspiratory flow) similar to that used in the intensive therapy unit. This minimizes intraoperative deterioration in pulmonary gas exchange.

Further reading

Bramson RD. New modes of mechanical ventilation. *Current Opinion in Critical Care*, 1999; **5**: 33–42.
Schapera A, Marks JD, Minaghi H *et al.* Perioperative pulmonary function in acute respiratory failure: effect of ventilator type and gas mixture. *Anesthesiology*, 1989; **71**(3): 396–402.

Related topics of interest

Asthma (p. 27); Breathing systems (p. 42); Thoracic anaesthesia (p. 257); TIVA (p. 264)

VOMITING

Postoperative nausea and vomiting (PONV) are the most common side-effects of anaesthesia and surgery, causing considerable patient morbidity. The overall incidence is approximately 30% and thus prevention is a vital part of every anaesthetic procedure. Vomiting causes misery, pain, electrolyte imbalance (hypokalaemic alkalosis), raised IOP and ICP, and places the patient at risk of aspiration, the Mallory-Weiss syndrome or oesophageal rupture. It may also complicate a surgical procedure e.g. by causing wound dehiscence.

Physiology

1. Central control. The vomiting reflex is controlled by the vomiting centre (VC) which is within the reticular formation in the medulla at the level of the olivary nuclei. The VC is within the blood–brain barrier and receives afferent nerve fibres from the cerebrum, the chemoreceptor trigger zone (CTZ), the vagus, the sympathetic nervous system and the oculo-vestibular apparatus. Neural transmission within the VC is predominantly mediated by acetylcholine.

The CTZ lies in the area postrema, outside the blood–brain barrier in the lateral wall of the fourth ventricle. Transmission here is via doperminergic and $5HT_3$ and opioid receptors. Once activated the CTZ then stimulates the VC. It mainly produces vomiting in conditions such as uraemia and pregnancy, and following certain drugs and radiotherapy.

2. Vomiting reflex. Efferent output from the vomit centre travels in somatic and autonomic nerves, mainly in the 5th, 7th, 9th, 11th and 12th cranial nerves as well as the spinal nerves. Immediately prior to vomiting a large breath is taken, the diaphragm is fixed and the glottis closed. The abdominal muscles then contract. This increases intragastric pressure and when the cardiac sphincter relaxes gastric contents are expelled. Pyloric sphincter tone increases to prevent forward flow.

Causes

1. Sensory.
- Somatic, e.g. gag reflex, airway manipulation.
- Visceral, e.g. distension, inflammation or traction of bowel, cervix, kidney, bladder or gonads. Chemo- or mechanoreceptors with vagal afferents.

2. Labyrinthine stimulation e.g. motion pressure (N_2O), or ear disease.

3. Hypotension e.g. with spinal anaesthesia or shock.

4. Drugs.
- Induction agents, in descending order of emetic properties; etomidate, ketamine, methohexitone, thiopental (propofol appears to be antiemetic).
- Inhalational agents, including N_2O.
- Opioid analgesics.
- Cytotoxic agents particularly cisplatinum.

5. **Metabolic** e.g. uraemia, radiotherapy, diabetes and Addison's disease.

6. **CNS** causes include raised ICP, infection and migraine.

7. **Pain** e.g. following MI or postoperatively.

8. **Higher centres input** e.g. fear, smell, sight, anticipation and anorexia nervosa.

9. **Systemic infections** e.g. viral hepatitis.

10. **Hypoxia.**

11. **Pregnancy** particularly the first trimester.

12. **Surgery** particularly ocular, ENT, gynaecological and gut.

13. **Patient factors** e.g. age, gender or a history of PONV or motion sickness. Being a child or female increases the incidence.

14. **Miscellaneous** factors such as mask ventilation, prolonged surgery and early oral postoperative fluids which increase PONV.

Treatment

The potential causes of PONV, including their mediation, should be considered thus allowing appropriate techniques or drugs to be used. If the causes are likely to be VC-mediated then an anticholinergic that crosses the blood–brain barrier is logical e.g. hyoscine or cyclizine (also has antihistamine actions). If stimulation of the CTZ is likely then an antidopaminergic agent should be chosen, e.g. phenothiazines or butyrophenones. Metoclopramide has predominantly antidopaminergic actions and is prokinetic. $5HT_3$ antagonists such as ondansetron, granisetron and tropisetron act at the CTZ and in the gut. Acupuncture between the tendons of flexor carpi radialis and palmaris longus decreases the incidence of PONV. Propofol as an antiemetic for chemotherapy has been advocated.

Pulmonary aspiration

The estimated incidence of pulmonary aspiration following general anaesthesia from a number of large studies ranges from approximately 1:2000 to 1:14 000 anaesthetics. The estimated mortality ranges from 1:50 000 to 1: 240 000 anaesthetics. It is particularly likely to occur in emergency procedures and in pregnancy. The clinical consequences of pulmonary aspiration of gastric contents depends upon the particulate content, bacteriological content and pH of the aspirate. From animal work, a critical pH of less than 2.5 and volume of aspirate of more than 0.5 ml/kg has been described in order to produce a severe clinical problem. Prophylaxis with H_2 antagonists, antacids or prokinetic drugs has been advocated for at-risk patients, though there is no evidence to support such action and it may even be harmful.

Patients who aspirate gastric content and develop clinical signs such as dyspnoea, wheezing, cyanosis, haemodynamic instability, hypoxia, hypercarbia and acidosis should be given supportive treatment (ventilatory support, airway suction, physiotherapy and haemodynamic support as appropriate). The CXR may show unilateral diffuse infiltration or an ARDS picture. There is no evidence to support the use of steroids, and antibiotics are given if infection is evident.

Further reading

Engelhardt T, Webster NR. Pulmonary aspiration of gastric contents in anaesthesia. *British Journal of Anaesthesia*, 1999; **83:** 453–460.

Postoperative nausea and vomiting. *British Journal of Anaesthesia*, 1992; **69:** Supplement 1.

Related topics of interest

Preoperative preparation (p. 209); Sequelae of anaesthesia (p. 232)

INDEX

TURP, 271

Urology, **271**

V/Q scan, 103
Vascular surgery, **273**
Ventilation, **276**

and ARDS, 25
jet, 14
Ventricular fibrillation, 75, 77
Ventricular septal defect, 72
Ventricular tachycardia, 75, 77
Vomiting center, 279
Vomiting, **279**